Policy and practice in promoting public health

Promoting public health: skills, perspectives and practice

This book forms part of an innovative series of structured teaching texts from The Open University, aiming to improve readers' understanding of modern multidisciplinary public health. The series consists of three books, *Theory and research in promoting public health* edited by Sarah Earle, Cathy E. Lloyd, Moyra Sidell and Sue Spurr, *Policy and practice in promoting public health*, edited by Cathy E. Lloyd, Stephen Handsley, Jenny Douglas, Sarah Earle and Sue Spurr, and *A Reader in promoting public health: challenge and controversy*, edited by Jenny Douglas, Sarah Earle, Stephen Handsley, Cathy E. Lloyd and Sue Spurr. These books form the core texts for The Open University's third-level undergraduate course, K311 *Promoting public health: skills, perspectives and practice*.

The books have four core themes:

- **power** and control and the ways these influence public health
- **change** in policy and practice and challenges to inequalities in health
- **diversity** of views, experiences and values about health and wellbeing
- **values and evidence** and how these inform public health theory and practice.

Policy and practice in promoting public health

Edited by Cathy E. Lloyd, Stephen Handsley, Jenny Douglas, Sarah Earle
and Sue Spurr

 The Open University

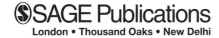 SAGE Publications
London • Thousand Oaks • New Delhi

Published by

Sage Publications
1 Oliver's Yard
55 City Road
London EC1Y 1SP

in association with

The Open University
Walton Hall
Milton Keynes MK7 6AA

First published 2007

Edited and designed by The Open University.

Typeset in India by Alden Prepress Services, Chennai.

Printed and bound in the United Kingdom by The Alden Group, Oxford.

This book forms part of an Open University course K311 *Promoting public health: skills, perspectives and practice*. Details of this and other Open University courses can be obtained from the Student Registration and Enquiry Service, The Open University, PO Box 197, Milton Keynes MK7 6BJ, United Kingdom: tel. +44 (0)870 333 4340, email general-enquiries@open.ac.uk

http://www.open.ac.uk

A catalogue record for this book is available from the British Library.

Library of Congress Control Number: 2006925334.

ISBN 978-1-4129-3072-7 (hardback)

ISBN 978-1-4129-3073-4 (paperback)

1.1

Contents

About the authors

Cathy E. Lloyd is a Senior Lecturer in Health and Social Care at the Open University. She has worked in public health and epidemiology for more than twenty years, both in the UK and USA. Her research interests include psycho-social aspects of longterm conditions, mental health, and minority ethnic health issues. She is Honorary Secretary of the Psychosocial Aspects of Diabetes Study Group, and has written a range of publications in national and international journals. She is currently principal investigator of a study examining alternative modes of data collection in South Asian communities in the UK. Before coming to the Open University nine years ago she was a Research Fellow at the University of Birmingham, Department of Epidemiology and Public Health.

Stephen Handsley is a Lecturer in Health and Social Care at the Open University. He is a medical sociologist whose research interests include public health, death, dying and bereavement, and mental health. Since returning to education in 1995, he has taught widely in a number of higher education institutions. Before coming to the Open University two years ago he was a Research Fellow at the University of Warwick, Department of Sociology. His published works include articles, book chapters and conference papers on the following: promoting public health; the impact of sudden death on family equilibrium; reproductive loss; cultural constructions of mourning in the Irish Catholic community in Britain; death and contagion; and personal and social transformation through training and education.

Jenny Douglas is a Senior Lecturer in Health Promotion at the Open University. She has worked in health promotion and public health for more than twenty years. Her current research interests include 'race', ethnicity, gender and health; the organisational positioning of health promotion specialists; and cigarette smoking in African-Caribbean young women. Jenny has undertaken research and written widely about the health experiences of minority groups. Jenny chairs the Public Health and Health Promotion Research Group at the Open University. She is co-editor of *Promoting Health: Knowledge and Practice* (Palgrave/ Open University, 2000), *The Challenge of Promoting Health: Exploration and Action* (Palgrave/ Open University, 2002) and *Debates and Dilemmas in Promoting Health* (Palgrave/ Open University 2003).

Sarah Earle is a Lecturer in Health and Social Care at the Open University and has been teaching in higher education for nearly fifteen years. She is a medical sociologist with an interest in reproductive health, sexuality, and healthcare education and practice. She convenes the British Sociological Association's Human Reproduction Study Group and chairs the Birth and Death Research Group at the Open University. She is the co-author of *Sex in Cyberspace: Men who Pay for Sex* (Ashgate, 2007) and co-editor of

The Sociology of Healthcare: A Reader for Health Professionals (Palgrave, 2007), *Sociology for Nurses* (Palgrave, 2005) and *Gender, Identity and Reproduction: Social Perspectives* (Palgrave, 2003) and has written many other book chapters, papers and articles.

Sue Spurr is a Course Manager in the Faculty of Health and Social Care. She has edited and contributed to a range of co-published Open University core texts, and has a particular interest in complementary and alternative medicine.

Moyra Sidell was a Senior Lecturer in the Faculty of Health and Social Care at The Open University until 2003. She has published in the fields of women's health and the health of older people, and has carried out research commissioned by the Department of Health on end of life care in care homes for older people.

Linda Jones is Professor of Health at the Open University, with research and teaching interests in health and social policy. She has published widely on environmental aspects of children's health, and in the 1990s led the development of the first OU course on public health: *K301 Promoting Health: Skills, Perspectives and Practice*. She is currently Pro-Vice Chancellor for Curriculum and Awards at the Open University.

David J. Hunter is Professor of Health Policy and Management at Durham University, where he is also the director of the Centre for Public Policy and Health in the School for Health and Wolfson Research Institute. With a background in political science and medical sociology, he has worked in the field of health policy for over thirty years. His research interests include public health policy and implementation, and the organisation of public health systems both in the UK and elsewhere. David has published widely on aspects of health policy, including the reform of the NHS and the evolution of public health policy in the UK. David chairs the UK Public Health Association. He is author of *Public Health Policy* (Polity, 2003), co-editor of *New Perspectives in Public Health*, now in its second edition (Radcliffe Publishing, 2006), and editor and main author of *Managing for Health* (Routledge, 2007).

Mark Dooris is Director of the Healthy Settings Development Unit and Principal Lecturer in Public Health Policy and Practice at the University of Central Lancashire, where he is also strategic lead for the Health-Promoting University initiative. Mark studied at Oxford University and Southbank Polytechnic, and has a background in health promotion, public health, community development, healthy cities, and environmental and transport policy. He has worked in a range of roles within local government, the health service and in voluntary sector settings, and has carried out consultancy work for the WHO and other agencies. He has researched and written on healthy settings, arts and health, nature and health, sustainable development, corporate citizenship and impact assessment. Mark was co-chair of the

UK Health for All Network from 1992 to 1994. He currently chairs the Joined-up Healthy Settings working group for the International Union of Health Promotion and Education. He is also on the editorial board of *Critical Public Health* and a member of the UK Sustainable Development Panel.

John Kenneth Davies is Principal Lecturer in Health Promotion and Director of the International Health Development Research Centre in the Faculty of Health and Social Science, University of Brighton. With over twenty-five years experience as an academic and practitioner in health promotion and public health in the UK and overseas, he has served as WHO Consultant in Health Promotion, as European Vice-President and as Global Vice-President for Scientific and Technical Development with the International Union for Health Promotion and Education. He has initiated and led a number of major EU-funded multinational projects on health promotion and public health.

Kythé Beaumont is a Senior Lecturer and Staff Tutor in the Faculty of Health and Social Care at the Open University. She has a background in community work and has taught in adult and higher education since 1980. She has a research interest in complementary and alternative medicine and a particular interest in public health.

Tom Heller is a General Practitioner working in a deprived area of north Sheffield. For the last twenty years he has also been a Senior Lecturer in Health Studies within the Faculty of Health and Social Care at the Open University and been involved in the production of a series of Open University courses on a wide variety of subjects.

Pam Foley is a Senior Lecturer in the Open University's Faculty of Health and Social Care. She researches, writes and publishes in the fields of children's health care policy and practices associated with children's emotional and social development, and is a co-editor of *Children in Society: Contemporary Theory Policy and Practice* (Palgrave Macmillan, 2001).

Angela Scriven is a Reader in Health Promotion at Brunel University, London. She has been teaching and researching in the field of health promotion for over twenty years and has published widely, including the following edited books: *Health Promotion Alliances: Theory and Practice* (1998), *Health Promotion: Professional Perspectives* (1996; 2001 second edition), *Promoting Health: Global Perspectives* (2005), *Health Promoting Practice: The Contribution of Nurses and Allied Health Professionals* (2005) and *Public Health: Social Context and Action* (2007). Her research is centred on the relationship between health promotion policy and practice within specific contexts.

Anita Noguera is a freelance consultant in health promotion and health impact assessment. She is also an Associate Lecturer in Health and Social Welfare with the Open University. Qualifying originally as a nurse, she obtained a first degree with the Open University, then studied for a MA in the philosophy and ethics of mental health, followed by a PhD in ethics and sociology at the University of Warwick. She became a Research Fellow there and also taught in the Faculty of Sociology and the post-graduate medical school. She has worked for the Health Development Agency and the World Health Organization's European Office for Health and Development, Venice. She has written extensively on social exclusion, the social determinants of health, health impact assessment, health issues in minority ethnic communities and ethics in mental health practice.

Other contributors

This book has grown out of debates and discussions in the K311 course team at The Open University. Besides the named authors, other team members who have contributed to the development of the book include Diane Charlesworth (Regional Academic, South West Region, in the Faculty of Health and Social Care), Philip Greaney (editor), Liz Rabone (editor), Gill Gowans (Copublishing), Cherryl Lewis (Course Team Assistant) and Liliana Torero de Clements (Course Team Assistant). The Open University course team would like to thank critical readers and developmental testers for their valuable comments on earlier draft chapters, and especially Professor Jackie Green, Leeds Metropolitan University, who, in her capacity as External Assessor, provided insightful and valuable comments.

Introduction

Cathy E. Lloyd

Promoting public health involves all of us in various ways, and is something that occurs at different levels and in a wide range of settings. Although health can be influenced by individual choice, it is also influenced by whole governments and government agencies, policy makers and other powerful groups in society. How policy is made and changed, and the effects of this on public health, are the key considerations of this book. Multidisciplinary public health in the twenty-first century is a global as well as a local issue. Individual and group action at the local and national level can have global health consequences, just as the global context impacts on the health and wellbeing of individuals and the communities in which they live. This book considers promoting public health at the level of community, and the relationship between the local and the global in terms of the policies designed to address inequalities in health and disease. The reader is encouraged to reflect on how those involved in multidisciplinary public health can use and influence policy in order to inform practice.

Key issues or themes woven into the book include a recognition of differences in power and opportunities for change, as well as the diversity of both health experiences and the myriad settings in which multidisciplinary public health practice takes place. A further theme – of values and evidence – encourages the reader to question just whose values, and what evidence, underpin policy and practice in public health. Thinking points – short pauses for consideration – have been included and are designed to encourage the reader to take a critical stance on the issues and debates contained within this book.

This book is in two parts. Part I, 'Promoting public health through public policy', considers the relationship between local, national, international and global policy and the promotion of public health. Part II, 'Promoting public health at a local level', focuses on local and community action for health. Each part contains six chapters. The final chapter in each part focuses on a substantive public health question in order to draw together the key issues discussed in that particular part.

Part I considers key issues in policy and practice, including the question of how policy decisions made at the global level impact on health at national and local levels. Making and changing policy, and the organisations and settings within which promoting public health takes place, are examined, before this part of the book concludes with a case-study of poverty in order to explore the ways in which healthy public policy seeks to address the effects of poverty on health.

Part II focuses on promoting public health at the local level and on the potential for public health action that engages with and empowers individuals and communities. The underlying principles of public health work at a local level are applied to a range of settings, and particular ways of assessing need and evaluating action are addressed. This second part of the book concludes with a case-study on mental health, drawing together the key themes and concepts by considering the ways in which mental health can be promoted through public health action.

This book is part of the third-level Open University course *Promoting public health: skills, perspectives and practice* (K311) and is published together with a companion volume *Theory and Research in Promoting Public Health*. Both books are designed to engage the reader in a systematic review and critical assessment of current ways of working to promote public health. They offer the skills, knowledge and understanding for the development, implementation and evaluation of multidisciplinary public health practice.

In writing this book, the authors made use of text and illustrations from *The Challenge of Promoting Health: Exploration and Action* (edited by Linda Jones, Moyra Sidell and Jenny Douglas), published by Palgrave Macmillan for the preceding Open University course *Promoting Health: Skills, Perspectives and Practice* (K301). Any substantial use of this has been indicated in the list of authors of a particular chapter, but special thanks go to Linda Jones and Pat Thornley.

Part I
Promoting public health through public policy

Public health promotion occurs in different settings and is carried out by a range of people, but wherever it takes place – and no matter who is involved – public policy is a key feature of public health promotion in the twenty-first century. Public policy provides the context within which individuals, organisations and agencies can promote public health. In turn, individuals, organisations and agencies can also influence public policy making to develop policies that support and enable health-promoting societies. In Part I of this book, the focus is on promoting public health through the development of healthy public policy.

Chapter 1, 'Promoting public health in a global context', begins by exploring the relationship between the global and the local, and introduces the reader to public policy making in a global context. The chapter examines the global politics of public health, focuses on globalisation, and explores global inequalities in health. It also introduces three key contemporary public health issues: global reproductive and sexual health, the policy and politics of global pharmaceuticals, and the global public health workforce.

In Chapter 2, 'The development of healthy public policy', the focus is on the development of healthy public policy in the UK. The chapter begins by exploring the development of national strategies to promote public health in England, Northern Ireland, Scotland and Wales. It then reflects on the potential of healthy public policy to transform society through the promotion of equity and social justice. Chapter 2 discusses the development of social welfare policy and the contribution of this to public health; it concludes by focusing on environmental politics and sustainability.

The next chapter – Chapter 3, 'Making and changing healthy public policy' – focuses on the policy-making process. Drawing on a range of theoretical concepts and models, it explores three key questions: Who is involved in policy making? How is policy made? And what influences policy? In this chapter these issues are explored by focusing on the case-study of smoking policy.

In Chapter 4, 'Organisations and settings for promoting public health', emphasis is given to the places in which people live, work and play, recognising that these settings have an enormous influence on health and wellbeing. The chapter starts by exploring the origins of a settings approach and considers the role of healthy public policy in developing and supporting health within different settings and contexts. Drawing on both theory and practice, this chapter explores the importance of culture and leadership within the context of organisational development and change management.

Chapter 5, 'Partnerships and alliances for health', explores the potential for promoting participation, collaboration and empowerment through partnerships and alliances for health. Using a range of national and international examples, the chapter examines definitions and explanations for partnership working, exploring the values that underpin this approach. This chapter also explores the policies that support partnerships for health, and discusses some of the challenges of working in partnership.

The final chapter in this part of the book – Chapter 6, 'Addressing poverty and health' – brings together the material introduced in previous chapters and focuses on the relationship between poverty, health and public policy. The chapter begins by defining poverty and exploring the groups in society most likely to experience it. It considers the health consequences of poverty and examines both national and international policies to address poverty and inequalities in health.

Chapter 1

Promoting public health in a global context

Sarah Earle

Introduction

Every day, individuals make choices that influence health, and public health promotion often focuses on the individual at a local level. However, when an individual buys a favourite chocolate bar, shops at a preferred supermarket, or decides how much they are prepared to pay for a bunch of bananas, these choices have far-reaching consequences for people and communities across the globe. Although such choices may have a global impact, in turn the global context also influences the lives and choices of people at local, regional and national levels. Terrorism, natural disasters, global warming, sex trafficking and infectious diseases, among many others, are some of the global issues that cross national borders to threaten health and wellbeing.

This chapter examines modern multidisciplinary public health in a global context and the role of public policy in providing a framework for change. Modern multidisciplinary public health is referred to as 'public health' in this book and consists of:

> a range of activities, performed by different people in a variety of settings and levels, and is thus both complex and diverse. It includes people working within different paradigms, or worldviews, and ... with different yet overlapping sets of values. It also embraces a range of multidisciplinary approaches to health research, planning, evaluation, policy making and action ...
>
> (Earle, 2007a, pp. 7–8)

The chapter begins by outlining, in Section 1.1, the relationship between global policy, politics and public health and introduces the concept of globalisation. Section 1.2 then begins to consider the policy process (which is examined in more detail in later chapters), and explores why understanding policy is important for promoting public health and discussing different types of policy. This is followed by a discussion of global policy and the impact of this on public health. Section 1.3 draws on specific case-studies to explore the relationship between globalisation and public health, focusing on reproductive and sexual health, global pharmaceuticals and the global public health workforce. Finally, Section 1.4 reflects on local action in a global context and some of the opportunities for promoting public health.

1.1 Global policy, politics and public health

Globally, health has been steadily improving. For example, since the 1950s life expectancy has increased by twenty years and child mortality (child death under the age of five) has decreased by approximately seven million since the 1970s (WHO, 2003). However, these improvements are not, by any means, equally distributed and there is enormous inequity between people living in different parts of the world (see Box 1.1).

Box 1.1 Global inequalities in health

- Global life expectancy has increased, but there is a very large gap in life expectancy between developed countries (such as Canada, Japan and the UK) and high-mortality developing countries (in Sub-Saharan Africa, parts of South America and Eastern Europe).

- Global levels of child death are in decline, but approximately 98 per cent of all child deaths occur in developing countries.

- In developing countries there are continuing high levels of maternal mortality due to conditions such as haemorrhage, sepsis and obstructed labour, and subsequent high levels of disability resulting from these conditions.

- In developed countries, communicable disease (e.g. HIV/AIDS and tuberculosis) accounts for only 5 per cent of the total disease burden; in developing countries it ranges from 40 to 60 per cent.

(Adapted from WHO, 2003)

Inequalities exist within countries as well as across them, an issue which has received particular attention in developed rather than developing countries, although significant inequalities also exist within the latter. For example, McDaid and Oliver (2005) note that, within many developed countries, there are considerable disparities in public health expenditure between the rich and poor. Thus, although global health has improved, there are clearly many continuing inequities. It is also worth noting here that there is no established definition for the difference between 'developed' and 'developing' countries – the terms that are used in this book – although the term 'developed' usually refers to those countries with high income per capita. Elsewhere, other authors refer to First and Third World countries, to North and South, or to high-, low- and middle-income countries (see, for example, Graham, 2007).

Since the beginning of the twentieth century, the world population has also increased exponentially; it now stands at approximately 6.5 billion and is expected to continue to rise to over 9 billion by 2050, with population growth at its highest in developing countries (UNDESA, 2005). Globally, the population is also ageing. In developed countries, 20 per cent of the population is currently aged 60 years or over, and in developing countries the figure is 8 per cent. However, by 2050, the projected figures are expected to rise to 32 per cent and 20 per cent respectively (UNDESA, 2005). These population changes and projections can determine patterns of health and disease and can, therefore, have enormous implications for global and local policy, particularly since health concerns vary across age groups (Davey, 2005).

Global policy and the global political landscape are increasingly important features of public health. Local action can have far-reaching global consequences and global change can, and does, influence action at local and national levels. The section below explores some of these global changes by focusing on the concept of globalisation.

1.1.1 Globalisation

Globalisation is a much discussed and debated concept which has significant implications for global, as well as local, health. Globalisation has been variously described as a concept, a process, a project and a revolution, and it is associated with some of the major worldwide changes that have occurred since the late twentieth century (Scriven, 2005). Globalisation refers to the transformation of human interaction across social, political, economic and technological spheres, in relation to spatial, temporal and cognitive change (Buse et al., 2002). Seeking to critically theorise the concept of globalisation, Kellner argues that:

> the key to understanding globalization is theorizing it as at once a product of technological revolution and the global restructuring of capitalism in which economic, technological, political, and cultural features are intertwined. From this perspective, one should avoid both technological and economic determinism and all one-sided optics of globalization in favor of a view that theorizes globalization as a highly complex, contradictory, and thus

> ambiguous set of institutions and social relations, as well as one
> involving flows of goods, services, ideas, technologies, cultural
> forms, and people.
>
> (Kellner, 2002, p. 285)

In essence, globalisation can be seen primarily as an economic phenomenon – the global, borderless expansion of capitalism (Geertz, 1998). However, changes in information and communication technologies (ICTs) are also part of globalisation. For example, mobile telephony and the increasing use and availability of the internet facilitate communication, commerce and exchange across borders, which transcend time and space, and in a way never seen before in history.

Some writers, however, question the very existence of globalisation, arguing that contemporary economic trends are not unique, and that they are international but not really global (Hirst and Thompson, 1996). Such writers prefer to use the term 'internationalisation' rather than globalisation. Although most would agree that globalisation exists, there is considerable disagreement about why and how this transformation is taking place and about what the implications of globalisation might be for the future (see, for example, Castells, 1996). There is considerable discord as to whether globalisation should be seen as a positive force for good or a negative force which creates and perpetuates poverty and inequalities.
Pro-globalisation groups (such as the International Policy Network, 2007, or World Growth, 2007) argue that free trade, in the form of goods, services, ideas and technologies, creates global wealth which, in turn, creates peaceful, prosperous and healthy societies. In contrast, anti-globalisation groups (such as Consumers International, 2007, or Friends of the Earth International, 2007a) argue that free trade is not fair trade, and that globalisation destroys traditional cultures, communities and local economies, leading to poverty and inequalities in health.

Thinking point: do you think that globalisation might have a negative or a positive effect on public health?

There is considerable debate as to whether globalisation should be viewed positively or negatively, although most writers agree that globalisation is 'Janus faced'; that is, that it can have both a positive and a negative effect on public health (Guillén, 2001). McMichael and Beaglehole (2003) argue that accelerated economic growth and technological advances have led to global increases in life expectancy and, for many people, have dramatically enhanced health and wellbeing. Of course, enhanced health is not enjoyed equally by all populations either within or across countries. Some of the health risks posed by the global flow of goods, services, ideas, technologies, cultural forms and people are outlined in Box 1.2.

Box 1.2 Some of the health risks posed by globalisation

- The continuation of poverty, and other factors, which create and maintain patterns of illness and disease between and within developed and developing countries.

- Global environmental degradation, such as the spread of invasive species, the dispersal of organic pollutants and atmospheric changes.

- Increased power of global capital, together with fragmentation of labour markets, leading to lower standards of occupational health and safety.

- The expansion of the international drug trade.

- The expansion of trafficking in people.

- Increased international travel leading to the spread of infectious diseases.

- Increasing prevalence of mental health problems in ageing, urban communities.

(Adapted from McMichael and Beaglehole, 2003, p. 12, Box 1.1)

This section has explored briefly the relationship between global policy, politics and public health. The next section examines policy in greater depth and discusses the role of the key global policy-making agencies and organisations and the part they play in promoting (or not promoting) public health.

1.2 Understanding policy

Policy making is complex; it is a political activity which crosses national borders. Policies can be made by individuals and organisations, as well as by governments and other agencies, and they can be made at a local level, as well as at regional, national and international levels. Policies at local and national levels often emerge from other policies that have been determined at a global level; however, local policy and practice can also influence global policy making.

Thinking point: in what ways do you imagine policy influences you?

Policy affects everyone: this is why it is so important to understand what policy is, how it is made and how it can be changed. For example, a healthy school might have a policy relating to the kind of food and drink children may bring in their packed lunches. A doctor's surgery or a hospital clinic may have policies that determine appointment bookings, consultation and waiting times. In a local authority, policies will determine when, where and how waste is collected and disposed of. All these policies have implications for public health at local and global levels.

1.2.1 What is policy?

The term 'policy' is hard to define because it is often used to mean different things within different contexts. Sometimes it is not defined at all, and interpretation of any implied definition can lead to confusion, and to very different policy outcomes. Guba (1984) suggests that there are eight different definitions of 'policy': these are outlined in Box 1.3.

Box 1.3 Eight definitions of the term 'policy'

1   Policy is an assertion of intents or goals.

2   Policy is the accumulated standing decisions of a governing body by which it regulates, controls, promotes, services, and otherwise influences matters within its sphere of authority.

3   Policy is a guide to discretionary action.

4   Policy is a strategy undertaken to solve or ameliorate a problem.

5   Policy is sanctioned behavior, formally through authoritative decisions, or informally though expectations and acceptance established over (sanctified by) time.

6   Policy is a norm of conduct characterized by consistency and regularity in some substantive action area.

7   Policy is the output of the policy-making system: the cumulative effect of all the actions, decisions, and behaviors of the millions of people who work in bureaucracies. It occurs, takes place, and is made at every point in the policy cycle from agenda setting to policy impact.

8   Policy is the effect of the policy-making and policy-implementing system ...

(Guba, 1984, pp. 64–5)

Drawing on the work of Easton (1953), Ham (2004) highlights the importance of values – defined as rewards and sanctions – and notes that, in any society, values are allocated by means of policies. More straightforwardly, however, Titmuss defines policy as 'the principles that govern action directed towards given ends. The concept denotes action about means as well as ends and it, therefore, implies change: changing situations, systems, practices, behaviour' (Titmuss, 1974, p. 23). Simply put, 'policy' can refer to a principle, or set of principles, and it can be written or unwritten. Most importantly, policy is about taking action and implementing change.

'Policy' is an umbrella term, but there are many different types of policy: for example, public policy, social policy, health policy and healthy public policy (see Box 1.4). Each of these types of policy focuses on particular principles and actions, and you will come across all these terms in this and subsequent chapters.

Box 1.4 Defining different types of policy

Public policy refers to the general actions (and inactions), regulations and laws developed by governments.

Social policy refers to the way in which 'governmental and other organizations throughout the world attend to, promote, neglect or undermine our wellbeing' (Dean, 2006, p. xii).

Health policy refers to the actions of governments that relate specifically to health and the healthcare services.

Healthy public policy refers to placing 'health on the agenda of policy makers in all sectors and at all levels, directing them to be aware of the health consequences of their decisions and to accept their responsibilities for health' (WHO, 1986, p. 2).

Local, regional, national and international policies can intersect in ways that do, or do not, promote public health. The section below considers some of the global policies that influence public health.

1.2.2 Global policies and governmental policy-making organisations

This section examines global policy and the role of international agencies and organisations in global governance (the systems and processes by which societies operate) and policy making. Principally, there are three different kinds of international governmental organisations: the international financial institutions (such as the World Bank), the United Nations (UN) (including the World Health Organization) and policy forums (such as the G8). These international organisations, and their functions, are outlined in more detail in Figure 1.1.

Figure 1.1   The principal international governmental organisations (Source: adapted from Dean, 2006, p. 37, Table 3.1)

Types	Names	Functions
International financial institutions	International Monetary Fund (IMF)	Ensuring monetary stability/providing credit facilities to nations in economic difficulty
	World Bank	Financing social and economic development programmes and projects
		Promoting and overseeing: human rights, world peace, social and economic development
United Nations (UN)	World Health Organization (WHO)	
	International Labour Organization (ILO)	
	UN Development Programme (UNDP)	
	UN High Commissioner for Human Rights (UNHCHR)	
	UN High Commissioner for Refugees (UNHCR)	
	UN Children's Fund (UNICEF)	
	UN Educational, Scientific and Cultural Organization (UNESCO)	
	World Trade Organization (WTO)	Regulation of world trade systems
Policy forums or 'clubs'	Organization for Economic Co-operation and Development (OECD)	Economic co-operation and development in thirty 'developed' nations
	G8	Co-ordination between the eight richest nations
	G77	Co-ordination between 133 (originally seventy-seven) 'developing nations'

The World Bank and the International Monetary Fund (IMF) are now two of the world's most influential policy-making organisations (McMichael and Beaglehole, 2003). Created after the Second World War, both organisations (together with the World Trade Organization which was created in 1995) provide the context for a globalised market through free trade policies, structural adjustment programmes, corporate taxation concessions and investment incentives, together with the relaxation of wage controls and standards of health and safety at work (McMichael and

Beaglehole, 2003). Both organisations also play a role in promoting global public health. For example, the World Bank sets out to provide technical and financial assistance to developing countries, one of its goals being the eradication of poverty and the improvement of living standards. However, free trade policies, such as the World Trade Organization's (WTO) multilateral trade agreements, often benefit developed rather than developing countries, and the structural adjustment programmes imposed by the IMF often reduce public expenditure on public health services. Arguably, although these financial institutions recognise their role in the global health agenda, they are often criticised for harming, rather than promoting, public health (McMichael and Beaglehole, 2003).

The governance of the World Health Organization (WHO) – which has played a central role in promoting public health worldwide and is discussed in detail below – has been overshadowed by the global economic governance and power enacted by the World Bank and IMF. Poku and Whiteside (2002) argue that this shift has led to two important changes in the global health context: first, a move away from the traditional concepts of social justice and equity, in favour of the laissez-faire principles and policies of free trade and the market; and, second, a shift away from seeing public health expenditure as a necessary and productive investment for wellbeing and economic growth, towards a view in which spending on healthcare, and public health more generally, is seen as a drain on national resources.

In spite of the enormous influence of the international financial institutions, the UN is still a hugely influential agency which, as shown in Figure 1.1, consists of a range of organisations and programmes, such as the WHO and the UN Development Programme (UNDP). Over the years, the WHO, in particular, has been especially influential in promoting public health and developing healthy public policy. Its definition of health as 'a state of complete physical, mental and social well-being and not merely the absence of disease or infirmity' (WHO, 1946), for example, is frequently quoted. The history and role of the WHO is discussed in detail elsewhere (see, for example, Earle, 2007a). However, one of its most significant landmarks included the launch of the Global Strategy for Health for All by the Year 2000 (WHO, 1977). This strategy stated that the role of governments and the WHO should be the attainment by all people of the world – by the year 2000 – of a level of health that would permit them to lead a socially and economically productive life. In 1978, the WHO adopted the Declaration of Alma Ata, reintroducing the concept of 'health for all', which emphasised the importance of primary care in achieving the highest levels of health, and recognising the problem of global inequalities in health: 'The existing gross inequality in the health status of the people particularly between developed and developing countries as well as within countries is politically, socially and economically unacceptable and is, therefore, of common concern to all countries' (WHO, 1978, paragraph II).

In 1980, the first European Health for All strategy was launched and this has been updated and evaluated periodically. In 1985, the first set of European policies and indicators was established to include sixty-five indicators linked to thirty-eight regional targets (WHO, 1985). In 1998, a revised European Health for All policy framework was adopted, which became known as Health 21 (WHO, 1998). The goal of Health 21 is to achieve the full health potential of all citizens by promoting and protecting people's health, reducing the incidence of injury and disease, and alleviating the suffering these cause. Health 21 is underpinned by the values of equity, solidarity, participation and accountability, and by the belief in health as a fundamental human right.

Since the 1980s, the WHO has also been the cornerstone of the health promotion and new public health movements, the principles of which have been elaborated in numerous health promotion conferences and charters, the most recent being the Bangkok Charter for Health Promotion in a Globalized World (WHO, 2005). Indeed, the first of these charters, the Ottawa Charter for Health Promotion (WHO, 1986), is the foundation for public health practice in the UK and elsewhere. The Ottawa Charter emphasised the importance of healthy public policy and endorsed a settings approach, which seeks to enable social environments to maximise their potential to promote public health. The influence of the settings approach, and of the values adopted by the Health for All movement, can be seen in the WHO Healthy Cities programme, which originally began in Europe. The Healthy Cities programme:

> engages local governments in health development through a process of political commitment, institutional change, capacity building, partnership-based planning and innovative projects. It promotes comprehensive and systematic policy and planning with a special emphasis on health inequalities and urban poverty, the needs of vulnerable groups, participatory governance and the social, economic and environmental determinants of health. It also strives to include health considerations in economic, regeneration and urban development efforts.
>
> (WHO, 2006b)

At the time of writing, there are 1,200 cities and towns from over thirty countries in the Healthy Cities movement in the WHO European Region.

In March 2005, the WHO also established a Commission on Social Determinants of Health. Operating for three years, the Commission is responsible for recommending policies to improve public health and reduce inequalities through action on the factors that influence health. In particular, the Commission will compile evidence to support policy change, especially for low-income developing countries.

Although the WHO has played a hugely influential role in global health policy and the development of healthy public policy, other UN organisations and programmes play an increasingly important role. In 2000, for example, the UN Millennium Declaration was adopted by the heads of state, who promised to 'uphold the principles of human dignity, equality and equity at the global level', particularly as they affect the most vulnerable in society (UN, 2000). The UN Millennium Development Goals (MDGs) were formulated from the Millennium Declaration (see Figure 1.2).

Figure 1.2	United Nations Millennium Development Goals (Source: adapted from UNDP, 2006)	
1	Eradicate extreme poverty and hunger	
	Target 1:	Reduce by half the proportion of people living on less than a dollar a day
	Target 2:	Reduce by half the proportion of people who suffer from hunger
2	Achieve universal primary education	
	Target 3:	Ensure that all boys and girls complete a full course of primary schooling
3	Promote gender equality and empower women	
	Target 4:	Eliminate gender disparity in primary and secondary education preferably by 2005, and at all levels by 2015
4	Reduce child mortality	
	Target 5:	Reduce by two-thirds the mortality rate among children under five
5	Improve maternal health	
	Target 6:	Reduce by three-quarters the maternal mortality ratio
6	Combat HIV/AIDS, malaria and other diseases	
	Target 7:	Halt and begin to reverse the spread of HIV/AIDS
	Target 8:	Halt and begin to reverse the incidence of malaria and other major diseases
7	Ensure environmental sustainability	
	Target 9:	Integrate the principles of sustainable development into country policies and programmes; reverse loss of environmental resources
	Target 10:	Reduce by half the proportion of people without sustainable access to safe drinking water
	Target 11:	Achieve significant improvement in lives of at least 100 million slum dwellers, by 2020

8	Develop a global partnership for development	
	Target 12:	Develop further an open trading and financial system that is rule based, predictable and non-discriminatory, and includes a commitment to good governance, development and poverty reduction – nationally and internationally
	Target 13:	Address the least developed countries' special needs. This includes tariff- and quota-free access for their exports; enhanced debt relief for heavily indebted poor countries; cancellation of official bilateral debt; and more generous official development assistance for countries committed to poverty reduction
	Target 14:	Address the special needs of landlocked and small island developing states
	Target 15:	Deal comprehensively with developing countries' debt problems through national and international measures to make debt sustainable in the long term
	Target 16:	In co-operation with developing countries, develop decent and productive work for youth
	Target 17:	In co-operation with pharmaceutical companies, provide access to affordable essential drugs in developing countries
	Target 18:	In co-operation with the private sector, make available the benefits of new technologies – especially information and communications technologies

The MDGs recognise the impact of globalisation and the global context of development. They also recognise the broad determinants of health and wellbeing. Three of the eight MDGs relate specifically to health, although it could be argued that all relate generally to health.

In an increasingly globalised world, the policy forums also provide an arena within which countries can share the principles, values and policies which are vital to international economic development and prosperity. For example, the Organization for Economic Co-operation and Development (OECD), which shares a commitment to democratic governance, produces decisions and recommendations across a range of social and economic issues including trade, education and development. The OECD works with other countries, non-governmental organisations (NGOs) and civil society organisations (e.g. trade unions and faith organisations). The G8, which held its first annual summit in 1975, comprises Canada, France, Germany, Italy, Japan, Russia, the UK and the USA, and seeks to work co-operatively to manage the effects of globalisation by securing informal political agreement on major global issues. For example, it lobbied for the Heavily Indebted Poor Countries (HIPC) Initiative – a programme initiated by the IMF and World Bank – to agree a process to cancel the debt of the world's poorest countries. It also set up the Global Health Fund to Fight AIDS, Tuberculosis and Malaria in countries such as India and Sierra Leone.

However, critics of the G8 argue that this, and other similar policy forums, serves the needs of the richest developed countries rather than the needs of others. In a critique of the G8 Gleneagles summit in 2006, Oxfam International have described the approach of the G8 leaders to cancelling debt and tackling poverty as 'late and light', arguing that they 'must do far more, far faster' (Oxfam International, 2006).

1.2.3 Non-governmental organisations in the global policy context

Although governmental organisations and agencies such as the World Bank, the WHO and the G8 have a major role to play in policy making, NGOs also play a vital part in influencing policy at a global level. There are tens of thousands of NGOs, both big and small; some of these operate locally, regionally or nationally, whereas others work at a global level. The Global Policy Forum (2000) estimates that there are over 25,000 NGOs operating at international level. NGOs act as critics of other global policy-making organisations and some, such as Oxfam International, can be involved in service delivery, particularly within developing countries and in areas where centralised services do not reach the most disadvantaged communities.

Some NGOs work towards global justice. For example, the Peoples' Health Movement calls for a greater emphasis on the principles of the Declaration of Alma Ata (WHO, 1978) and a revision of all policies which impact negatively on public health. Others use a 'name and shame' approach to expose corporate violations and environmental crimes. One such NGO is CorpWatch, which describes itself as 'part of a diverse global movement for human rights, social justice, environmental sustainability, peace, corporate transparency and accountability' (CorpWatch, 2006). In 1997, CorpWatch was responsible for exposing poor working conditions in Nike factories in Vietnam, forcing them to change some of their corporate policies (O'Rourke, 1997). In 2004, through their website http://www.warprofiteers.com, CorpWatch exposed the companies (e.g. Boeing, BP and Shell Oil, USA) said to profit from the war in Iraq (CorpWatch, 2004) (see Figure 1.3).

NGOs, such as Friends of the Earth International, the International Rivers Network and Greenpeace, also campaign on global environmental policy, particularly on issues relating to deforestation, GM crops, climate justice, fair trade and the privatisation of essential services such as water supplies. In a press release following the publication of the World Bank report, *Clean Energy and Development Towards an Investment Framework* (World Bank, 2006), Friends of the Earth International criticise the World Bank, arguing not only that their plans do not address climate change, but that the poorest and most disadvantaged countries and communities will fare the worst (Friends of the Earth International, 2006).

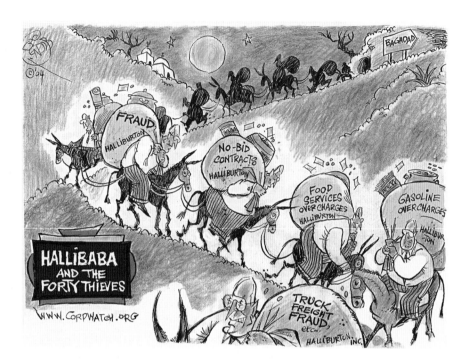

Figure 1.3   'Hallibaba and the forty thieves': the NGO CorpWatch exposes war profiteers

Thinking point: how do NGOs influence global policy making?

Whereas some NGOs focus on the pursuit of social action and social justice, and others on development and sustainability issues, yet others, such as Christian Aid or Médecins Sans Frontières, focus on giving immediate relief to victims of war, accidents and natural disasters. Many NGOs work across all of these areas, sometimes in coalitions. However, whatever the type of work they do, the actions of NGOs can be analysed on three levels: micro-policy, macro-policy and norm setting (Global Policy Forum, 2000). Micro-policy refers to actions taken to change or challenge legislation or policy, macro-policy refers to the ways in which NGOs can influence or challenge strategic approaches to policy, and norm setting refers to the influence of NGOs on public opinion. Although there is no doubt that many NGOs have enormous influence on global policy making – and, indeed, many have a consultative status with the UN – there are some who question their independence from governmental organisations and agencies. For example, Mudingu writes:

> The term Non-Governmental Organisations is actually a misnomer. The NGOs are financed and directed by the various imperialist agencies, the imperialist governments and the comprador regimes. They act as the liaison between the people and the governments. They are the vehicles through which the exploiters seek to influence the opinions of 'civil society'.

> They are the servants of imperialist capital. Almost all the NGOs are directed by the invisible hand of the imperialists who set them up or fund them in accordance with their strategic goals.
>
> (Mudingu, 2006)

NGOs play a role in shaping, changing and challenging global policy, as well as innovating in areas such as service delivery and relief aid. However, the private commercial interests of the multinational corporations can often have the greatest influence on global policy and these are discussed below.

1.2.4 Private commercial interests and global public health policy

Anti-globalisation organisations are highly critical of the international financial institutions and other governmental organisations such as the WTO, but lay the blame for the 'evils' of the global capitalist expansion at the feet of the large multinational corporations. In many countries around the world, essential services, ranging from laundry and cleaning in hospitals to refuse collection, have been contracted out and are now delivered by private commercial interests. At a global level, public–private partnerships are recognised as a powerful new force of global governance. Indeed, the Bangkok Charter for Health Promotion in a Globalized World (WHO, 2005) highlights the importance of partnerships with private-sector organisations to ensure that corporate practice promotes public health. These partnerships include donation programmes where pharmaceutical companies donate a drug to eliminate a particular disease (e.g. in Africa, Merck have donated ivermectin to cure river blindness), as well as the involvement of the 'new philanthropists' who donate money for specific health initiatives (e.g. the Melinda and Bill Gates Foundation which donated $6 billion for vaccines) (Poku and Whiteside, 2002).
Public–private partnerships are often successful; however, private donors can sometimes stipulate conditions and policies which harm, rather than promote, public health.

Outside the public health sector, multinational corporations have been blamed for many public health problems and health-related issues. Restaurants and food and beverage companies, for example, have been criticised for promoting unhealthy food and drink (Earle, 2007b); the travel and hospitality industry is blamed for social, environmental and cultural degradation (UNDESA, 2006); and, as you read in Section 1.2.3 above, some companies have been exposed for their exploitation of workers and poor health and safety records.

Although multinational corporations are criticised for their contribution to poverty and inequalities in health, they also have opportunities to promote social justice, health and wellbeing. Corporate Social

Responsibility Europe – a European business network – seeks to ensure that sustainable development can co-exist within an entrepreneurial and competitive business environment. To this aim, it outlines ten key goals for corporate social responsibility (CSR): these are given in Box 1.5.

Box 1.5 Ten goals for corporate social responsibility?

1   **Innovation and entrepreneurship** to meet the constant demand for affordable and sustainable products and services, particularly in developing countries.

2   **Skills and competence building** for life-long learning, ensuring a balance between home and work.

3   **Equal opportunities and diversity** in the workplace to help bring businesses closer to their markets.

4   **Health and safety** within businesses and the communities within which they are located, as well as within those along the supply chain.

5   **Environmental protection** through innovative research and development to reduce emissions and energy consumption.

6   **Corporate responsibility in the mainstream of business** to ensure that business objectives, values and strategies are aligned with corporate responsibility policies.

7   **Stakeholder engagement** that is proactive and helps anticipate and resolve social and environmental concerns.

8   **Leadership and governance** for corporate responsibility as a prerequisite.

9   **Communication and transparency** in order to build trust and, therefore, competitiveness.

10 **Businesss-to-business co-operation and alliances** to help innovate for responsible solutions to business challenges.

(Adapted from Corporate Social Responsibility Europe, 2006, pp. 7–8)

Thinking point: do you think that corporate social responsibility can help promote public health?

There are many who are sceptical of the concept of corporate social responsibility. Henderson (2001), for example, argues that it is far from harmless and, indeed, that it is likely to threaten the development of the poorest, as well as the richest, countries. Others, however (e.g. Christian

Aid, 2004), argue that most companies – and the global multinationals in particular – do very little except pay lip-service to CSR. In a report which exposes the 'real face' of CSR, Christian Aid (2004) argues that CSR simply cannot live up to its promises. The two case-studies given in Box 1.6 detail some of the corporate violations perpetrated by companies which claim to act according to their CSR policies.

Box 1.6 The real face of corporate social responsibility?

Shell claims that it has turned over a new leaf in Nigeria and strives to be a 'good neighbour'. Yet it still fails to quickly clean up oil spills that ruin villages and runs 'community development' projects that are frequently ineffective and which sometimes divide communities living around oilfields.

British American Tobacco stresses the importance of upholding high standards of health and safety among those working for it, and claims to provide local farmers with the necessary training and protective clothing. But contract farmers in Kenya and Brazil say this does not happen and report chronic ill-heath related to tobacco cultivation.

(Christian Aid, 2004, p. 2)

The next section explores the relationship between globalisation and public health, focusing on three specific public health issues.

1.3 Promoting public health in a globalised world

Terrorism, climate change, sex trafficking, non-communicable chronic disease pandemics, drug trafficking, the globalisation of tobacco and natural disasters are only some of the many public health issues that cross national frontiers, posing some of the greatest challenges for global governance ever seen (see, for example, Porter et al., 2002; Scriven and Garman, 2005). Of course, it is not possible to explore all these issues in depth, so this section explores some of the ways in which globalisation impacts on public health by focusing on three specific health issues: global reproductive and sexual health, the policy and politics of global pharmaceuticals, and the global public health workforce.

1.3.1 Global politics and reproductive and sexual health

Reproductive and sexual health is a global issue which cuts across cultural, socio-economic and national boundaries (Mayhew and Watts, 2002). It is a key component of gender equality, and gender equality plays a major role in eradicating poverty and inequalities in health. As such, improving global reproductive and sexual health is necessary if the MDGs are to be achieved by 2015 (UNFPA, 2003). Indeed, three of the eight MDGs relate specifically to reproductive and sexual health – the goals to reduce child mortality; improve maternal health; and combat HIV/AIDS, malaria and other diseases – and the other five relate generally to health, and to reproductive health. A rights-based approach to public health adopts the view that good health is a fundamental human right (Earle, 2007a). It follows, therefore, that good reproductive and sexual health permits all people, and women in particular, to lead a socially and economically productive life.

Thinking point: why do you think that reproductive and sexual health entered the global public health agenda?

Since the 1950s, grassroots women's organisations across the world have been campaigning for improved reproductive healthcare and reproductive and sexual rights, and it is this that has helped place reproductive and sexual health on the global (and subsequently national) public health agenda. In the 1970s and 1980s, feminist writers and activists were also extremely vocal, especially in their critique of population control policies. Hartmann (1987), for example, argued that population control programmes were motivated by the needs of the rich, rather than the poor and disadvantaged. She also argued that abortion and sterilisation were used coercively, that medical care was inadequate and that women lacked safe contraceptive methods. This campaigning prompted some re-evaluation of these policies and a greater concern for ensuring that women's voices was heard. However, it was only in 1994 that the concept of population control was replaced with that of reproductive rights, at the International Conference on Population and Development held in Cairo. Drawing on the WHO's (1946) definition of health, the UN Programme of Action of the International Conference on Population and Development defines reproductive health as:

> a state of complete physical, mental and social well-being and not merely the absence of disease or infirmity, in all matters relating to the reproductive system and to its functions and processes. Reproductive health therefore implies that people are able to have a satisfying and safe sex life and that they have the capability to reproduce and the freedom to decide if, when and how often to do so.
>
> (UNFPA, 1994, paragraph 7.2)

It was at this point that values and beliefs began to change at a time when some governments still believed that draconian population control policies were legitimate and acceptable. As Eager (2004) notes, the concept of reproductive rights, women's engagement and voluntary participation emerged as the new norm. Since then many policy changes have taken place. For example, in 1998 the WHO (2006a) developed a 'gender tool' (a method of conducting gender evaluations) to ensure that reproductive health research promotes, rather than hinders, gender equality and hence can contribute effectively to promoting reproductive and sexual health within developing countries, in particular.

However, in the developing world, pregnancy and childbirth can still be life-threatening (WHO, 2004a). Of the estimated 210 million pregnancies worldwide, eight million women suffer life-threatening conditions and, of these, an estimated 529,000 die during pregnancy and childbirth from preventable causes. Ninety-nine per cent of these deaths occur in developed countries. Between 50 and 80 per cent of women in the poorest developing countries also give birth without the assistance of a midwife or other skilled birth attendant, and between 50 and 80 per cent of women receive no antenatal care during pregnancy. Millions of people also lack access to contraception and to sexual health services, meaning that sexually transmitted infections, including HIV, and reproductive tract infections remain undiagnosed and untreated. Of the 45 million unwanted pregnancies that are terminated each year, approximately 19 million are unsafe, and unsafe abortions account for 13 per cent of all pregnancy-related deaths worldwide (WHO, 2004b). Poor reproductive health is not 'just' a matter of life and death or of sickness and health: in some countries it can mean that women are shunned by their husbands, families and communities, leaving them with nowhere to live and no means of earning a living (UNFPA, 2005).

Even in developed countries, reproductive and sexual rights are by no means secure. For example, women cannot obtain abortion 'on demand', and in some countries, such as Ireland, abortion remains illegal. Even in countries where abortion is legal, there are frequent legal and legislative challenges which aim to restrict abortion laws. There are also considerable disparities in reproductive and sexual health within and between developed countries. For example, in the UK, breastfeeding rates are the lowest in Europe, and initiation rates for breastfeeding vary considerably according to factors such as socio-economic status and educational attainment (TIC, 2006). In England, and in other developed countries, the burden of sexual illness is borne, in particular, by the most vulnerable in society (DoH, 2001).

The WHO has developed its first strategies for reproductive and sexual health with the aim of ensuring that global development goals and targets are met. The reproductive health strategy (WHO, 2004a) identifies five key action areas to help improve reproductive health (see Box 1.7).

Box 1.7 Improving global reproductive health

Five key action areas are:

1   strengthening health systems capacity

2   improving information for priority setting

3   mobilising political will

4   creating supportive legislative and regulatory frameworks

5   strengthening monitoring, evaluation and accountability.

(Adapted from WHO, 2004a, p. 23)

The sexual health strategy (WHO, 2006a) focuses on the prevention and control of sexually transmitted infections. In the short term it highlights the importance of targeted interventions and, in the longer term, the importance of 'user-friendly' services. It also recognises that reproductive and sexual health is not just women's business and that, to be successful, policy making and implementation must ensure men's, as well as women's, involvement and motivation.

1.3.2 The policy and politics of the global pharmaceutical industry

Petryna and Kleinman (2006) argue that global health pandemics are influenced by the policy and choices made at international level. For example, they argue that the failure to respond adequately at a global level to the AIDS pandemic contributed to the alarming growth of infection in South Africa and other regions. The governance of the global pharmaceuticals industry is achieved within a 'field of consent' (Fox et al., 2006) in which several stakeholders represent their own interests and commitments. Government and other regulatory bodies are responsible for protecting and maximising public health, as well as for economic development and policy. Professional groups, such as medicine and pharmacy, are responsible for knowledge and expertise in pharmaceutical prescribing. The global pharmaceutical industry, on the other hand, has commercial responsibilities as well as a public responsibility for improving public health and eradicating disease. Patients and consumers have interests in their own health and wellbeing as well as expectations regarding freedom from exploitation; many patient and consumer groups support these interests.

The global pharmaceuticals industry – although highly regulated – has come under increasing scrutiny and attention is being paid, in particular, to three interrelated issues: research and development activities; marketing strategies and policies; and the inequities in access between developed and developing countries. These three issues are discussed below.

Why are the research and development activities of the global pharmaceuticals under scrutiny? Quite simply, the pharmaceutical industry (together with other stakeholders) can create a demand for a new treatment. In other words, pharmaceuticals play a part in the social construction of health, illness and disease. Palmlund (2006), for example, argues that the menopause – the cessation of women's menstrual bleeding – has been transformed from a normal physiological process into a time of illness and disease. She argues that the pharmaceutical industry (together with doctors and women themselves) forms 'a triangle, where ideas about menopause as a health risk and an illness have been constructed and reinforced' (Palmlund, 2006, p. 542). The research and development activities of pharmaceutical companies are under scrutiny, not because their activities revolve around improving public health and eradicating disease, but because – some would argue – their activities revolve around the increase of profits.

To this end, the pharmaceutical industry spends an enormous proportion of its resources on marketing and advertising activities. These activities include re-branding, magazine advertorials, sponsoring and funding, as well as gifts, payments and hospitality (Petryna et al., 2006). A study conducted by Consumers International (2006) – a federation of consumer organisations – reveals that, although approximately US $60 billion is spent on marketing by the top twenty global pharmaceuticals each year, very little is known about what, exactly, the money is spent on. At first glance, the report argues, it would seem that marketing and advertising practices appear tightly regulated, particularly in European countries. However, promotion activities can be characterised as 'nice and friendly marketing', which refers to the way in which the industry has created a false sense of trust among consumers. In Europe (unlike the USA, for example), pharmaceuticals are not allowed to market prescription drugs directly to patients. Instead, Consumers International (2006) argues, they adopt subtle tactics to promote prescription drugs to pharmacists and medical students, and via patient groups, internet chat groups and product information websites. The same report reveals that, between 2002 and 2005, 972 serious and repeated breaches of marketing policy were reported. Consumers International argues: 'Such breaches further support our claim that drug promotion does not operate with consumer interests in mind, but rather is more focussed on generating profits by maximising sales revenue' (Consumers International, 2006, p. 16).

It would not be unreasonable to expect that, in a globalised world, access to medicines would be easier and cheaper, but this is not the case. Heywood argues:

> while there has been a globalisation of medical research, and a globalisation of knowledge about medicine, there has been only a partial globalisation in the availability of medicines. A doctor working in impoverished areas of Botswana or Malaysia can read about effective medicines on the internet, but has no hope of obtaining these medicines for her patients or getting to a health centre that can obtain them.
>
> (Heywood, 2002, pp. 222–3)

Thinking point: why might there be inequity in access to medicines?

There is enormous inequity in access to medicines between developed countries, where there is an increasing state of over-consumption, and developing countries, where there is often scarcity. This is the problem, Heywood (2002) argues, when something that is as essential to survival as water is commodified and privatised. Global pharmaceuticals make more money developing and selling medicines that can be used by a large number of people over long periods of time, rather than those used to treat the infectious diseases in developing countries. Busfield (2006) is critical of sociologists, social scientists and others, suggesting that more attention should be paid to the global pharmaceuticals industry because:

1   they are a major power within global – and national – economies
2   they are a major force in shaping healthcare, in developing societies in particular
3   they contribute to the cultural shift in seeing medicines as a way of solving socially constructed illnesses.

She argues that scepticism towards global pharmaceuticals should not be grounded in the claims that modern therapeutic drugs have little value – since many are invaluable – but because the pharmaceutical industry is unwilling to focus on the health problems of developing countries and unwilling to sell them life-saving drugs at prices that they can afford.

1.3.3 Health and the global public health workforce

The global public health workforce is complex and diverse. It consists of a range of individuals employed in a variety of occupations who work to protect and promote public health in populations, as well as working with individuals, groups and communities. In all countries, the public health workforce is essential to the delivery of healthcare services as well as to the performance of health systems more generally. However, most governments have neglected public health workforce development (Beaglehole and Bonita, 2001) and in some developing countries, the situation is particularly acute.

The *World Health Report 2006* (WHO, 2006c) states that there are fifty-seven countries – mostly in Sub-Saharan Africa and South-East Asia – with critical shortages of doctors, nurses and midwives; this is equivalent to 2.4 billion workers worldwide. The skill mix balance is also problematic with a shortage of workers in public health, and in health policy and management, in particular. In addition, there is inequity between urban populations, where there can be high concentrations of health workers, and rural populations, where there is scarcity at unsafe levels. The WHO suggests a strategy framework to tackle world health problems and help meet the MDGs by the year 2015, which focuses on the three key decision-making junctures in the global health workforce: entry, workforce and exit (see Figure 1.4).

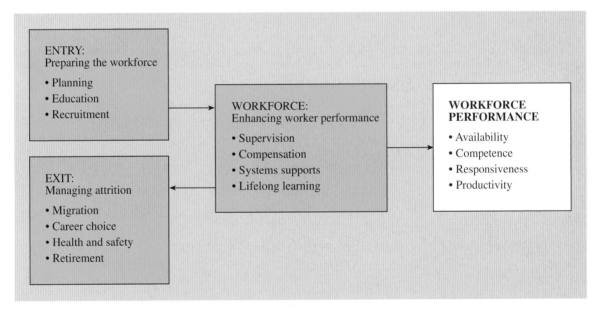

Figure 1.4   A strategy framework for the working lifespan (Source: WHO, 2006c, p. xxi, Figure 4)

In an increasingly globalised world, the migration of people across borders is ever more common. Whereas poorer countries often rely on NGOs for health service delivery, richer countries such as the UK are able to recruit health workers from other countries. In developing countries in particular, instability and economic deterioration can often have a very negative impact on the healthcare workforce, which, in turn, has negative consequences for public health. Writing specifically about African countries, Sanders et al. (2003) argue that the 'brain drain' of health professionals from Africa to the developed world and to other developing countries (such as South Africa) is one of the most serious problems facing

African countries today. This expatriation means that those healthcare workers remaining have increased workloads, thus leading to low productivity and poor service delivery which, in turn, leads to further migration out of the system.

Thinking point: in what ways might the migration of health workers improve public health?

The movement of health workers can have advantages. For the recipient country, the advantages are obvious since migrant workers help to resolve shortages or skill mix gaps. When migrants return home they bring back with them a wealth of experience, skills and expertise, and while they are working away, remittances (money sent back home by migrants) we thought to reduce poverty in their country of origin. However, some countries are trying to encourage migrants to return home. For example, the Philippine Overseas Employment Administration has developed an incentive programme, including tax-free shopping, subsidised business loans and scholarships, to encourage migrants to return to the Philippines (WHO, 2006c).

Although national policies and incentive programmes are helpful, given the global context of world health problems such as HIV/AIDS and the humanitarian crises posed by war, terrorism and natural disasters, a global response to the health workforce crisis is needed. The WHO suggests that a global solidarity is needed on three specific fronts:

1 **catalysing knowledge and learning** to include the pooling of experience and expertise to help countries tap into the best talent and practices, including identification and support for priority research issues

2 **striking co-operative agreements** to protect the health and safety of global migrants, relief workers and volunteers, the adoption of ethical recruitment practices and a willingness to commit human resources to assist in humanitarian emergencies

3 **responding to workforce crises** in the poorest developing countries to include both the immediate and long-term financing of the healthcare workforce.

(Adapted from WHO, 2006c, p. xxiv)

All these public health issues, and others, place a considerable burden on the organisations and agencies charged with global governance. However, globalisation and public health can be changed at local and global levels. The next section considers local action in a global context.

1.4 Local action in a global context

International organisations, whether governmental or non-governmental, play a major role in making and influencing global policy and in controlling, or affecting, the global context for public health. Public health practitioners, for example, are influenced (in what they can and cannot do) by the global political and economic context which determines all manner of health-related issues, such as housing, transport and climate, as well as healthcare issues, such as the availability of primary care, hospital services and pharmaceutical drugs (Prowse, 2003). The global and political economic context might, therefore, seem to be quite disempowering (Raeburn and Macfarlane, 2003). However, global change can be effected by lay people and by local public health practitioners.

1.4.1 The global challenge for public health practitioners

Beaglehole and Bonita (2001) argue that public health has yet to fulfil its promise and potential to improve the health of the poorest and most disempowered people in society. They suggest that globalisation is one of the key challenges of the twenty-first century and argue that 'The challenges facing public health practitioners have always been great. Today, they are even more daunting' (Beaglehole and Bonita, 2001, p. 81). Agreeing with this, Prowse (2003) argues that, although public health practitioners are constrained by the global context, the ability to lobby others in relation to globalisation and public health is one of the most important skills that a public health practitioner can possess. Writing specifically about the role of health promotion in meeting the challenges and opportunities of the global world, Mittelmark (2005) argues that practitioners must either forge new alliances, or risk complacency and stagnation. He emphasises, in particular, the need to build alliances between public health and the corporate social responsibility movement.

Thinking point: how else might public health practitioners meet the challenges and opportunities of the global world?

Changes in ICTs have developed alongside, and are part of, the globalisation process. They, too, can offer considerable opportunities for public health practitioners to meet the challenges and opportunities of globalisation. ICTs can facilitate local action within a global context; for example, mobile telephony can be used to co-ordinate activities, whereas email and the internet can facilitate communications exchange; and both can play an important role in non-violent (and violent) direct action. For example, the NGO Friends of the Earth International (2007b) has developed a cyberactivist network to provide information and to canvass support for their email actions and campaigns. ICTs can also play a part in promoting public health within communities across the world. For instance, ICTs can be used to educate and promote good health to particular groups or on particular topics – a good example of this is the website of the organisation Sexwise (http://www.ruthinking.co.uk), which provides information for young people on sex, pregnancy and relationships. The use of ICTs can also empower individuals and communities by encouraging networking and participation. In the late 1990s/early 2000s, for example, a community development network project was established to extend broadband access to economically disadvantaged neighbourhoods in New York (Venkatesh et al., 2004). ICTs can also be used in therapeutic contexts and, even outside of these, can serve a therapeutic role in the guise of online discussion forums and support groups: examples of these include Fertility Friends (http://www.fertilityfriends.co.uk) which supports people with experiences of infertility.

Thinking point: what are some of the potential problems of using ICTs in public health promotion?

Of course, ICTs cannot provide all the solutions and they do not solve public health problems overnight! There are many who are sceptical about the role of ICTs in public health. Drawing on a small, interview-based study of members of a health promotion team, Marshall (2004) notes that practitioners can be sceptical and cautious of ICTs. They are also well aware of the inequalities in access among some groups, such as older people. However, Marshall argues that these views can often be used to defend traditional means of communication (such as providing leaflets), wrongly positioning new technologies as dehumanising. In contrast, Marshall argues that ICTs can be a powerful tool in promoting public health, particularly when individuals and communities are involved in the design and development of ICTs to best meet their needs.

1.4.2 Local action for global governance

In the preface to the UK *White Paper on International Development* (DfID, 2006), Hilary Benn, Secretary of State for International Development, argues that governance: 'from the global right down to the village level – is about people and their relationships, one with another, more than it is about formal institutions. What makes the biggest difference to the quality of governance is active involvement by citizens – the thing we know as politics' (DfID 2006, pp. ix–x). In effect, local action can make a difference to the global context.

Thinking point: how might you get involved in lobbying for global change to improve public health?

There are many ways in which individuals can get involved in effecting change for better global health. Box 1.8 lists some of these.

Box 1.8 Lobbying for global health at a local level

Self-help and self-advocacy

For example, people with learning disabilities being responsible for creating change rather than being on the receiving end.

Letter writing

For example, to government leaders and others.

Campaigning

Organising local activities or sponsored events, signing action cards or petitions, volunteering, fundraising, buying merchandise

Joining a movement

For example, the peace movement, or the women's movement.

Developing partnerships and collaboration

For example, collaboration between lay people and public health practitioners.

Direct action (non-violent and violent)

Examples of non-violent direct action include picketing, boycotting, negotiation and striking; violent direct action can include sabotage, the destruction of property, vandalism, physical attacks, bombings and arson.

Campaigns such as Make Poverty History (probably the largest ever anti-poverty campaign), War on Want (which campaigns for trade justice) and Stamp out Poverty (which aims to increase sufficient revenue to realise the UN's Millennium Development Goals) provide good examples of the way in which lay people can involve themselves in lobbying for global change. All these campaigns encourage citizens to lobby for change through letter writing, buying merchandise and petitioning, as well as by organising local activities to raise awareness and increase political pressure.

Conclusion

Globalisation is a highly complex process. It predominantly refers to the global restructuring of the capitalist economy, resulting in the flow, as Kellner (2002, p. 285) argues in the quotation given in Section 1.1.1, 'of goods, services, ideas, technologies, cultural forms, and people'. Globalisation is Janus-faced; that is, it offers opportunities for change, development and prosperity, but it also poses threats to the health and wellbeing of individuals and communities in both developed and developing countries. However, as this chapter has shown, the threats posed by globalisation are felt unequally, and globalisation poses the greatest threat to the poorest and least empowered individuals, communities and countries across the world.

Policies are increasingly developed, implemented and changed within a global political context since important public health issues, such as terrorism, climate change and poverty, cross national boundaries. This chapter has introduced you to some of the different types of policy that are explored in later chapters in this book, and has discussed and examined some of the global policies and global policy-making organisations and agencies. Building on this, the next chapter examines the development of healthy public policy within a (predominantly) UK context and explores the relationship between global and UK policies.

Globalisation offers both opportunities and challenges for local action in a global context. While governmental agencies, such as the IMF and WHO, and non-governmental organisations, such as Oxfam, CorpWatch and Médecins Sans Frontières, are key players in the global political and policy-making context, global change can be effected by local people and by public health practitioners working at a local level with individuals and within communities. Indeed, individual and community action, in both local and global settings, plays a vital role in global governance for a healthy society.

References

Beaglehole, R. (ed.) (2003) *Global Public Health: A New Era*, Oxford, Oxford University Press.

Beaglehole, R. and Bonita, R. (2001) 'Challenges for public health in the global context – prevention and surveillance', *Scandinavian Journal of Public Health*, vol. 29, pp. 81–3.

Buse, K., Drager, N., Fustukian, S. and Lee, K. (2002) 'Globalisation and health policy: trends and opportunities' in Lee et al. (eds) (2002).

Busfield, J. (2006) 'Pills, power, people: sociological understandings of the pharmaceutical industry', *Sociology*, vol. 40, no. 2, pp. 297–314.

Castells, M. (1996) *The Rise of the Network Society*, Cambridge, MA, Blackwell.

Christian Aid (2004) *Behind the Mask: The Real Face of Corporate Social Responsibility*, London, Christian Aid.

Consumers International (2006) *Branding the Cure: A Consumer Perspective on Corporate Social Responsibility, Drug Promotion and the Pharmaceutical Industry in Europe*, London, Consumers International.

Consumers International (2007) [online], http://www.consumersinternational.org/ (Accessed 16 February 2007).

Corporate Social Responsibility Europe (2006) *European Roadmap for Business: Towards a Sustainable and Competitive Enterprise*, Brussels, Corporate Social Responsibility Europe.

CorpWatch (2004) [online], http://www.warprofiteers.com (Accessed 16 February 2007).

CorpWatch (2006) *Vision and Guiding Principles* [online], http://www.corpwatch.org/article.php?id=13399 (Accessed 9 August 2006).

Davey, B. (2005) 'Key global health concerns for the twenty-first century' in Scriven and Garman (eds) (2005).

Day, P. and Schuler, D. (eds) (2004) *Community Practice in the Network Society: Local Action/Global Interaction*, London, Routledge.

Dean, H. (2006) *Social Policy*, Cambridge, Polity Press.

Department for International Development (DfID) (2006) *Eliminating World Poverty: Making Government Work for the Poor. A White Paper on International Development*, London, The Stationery Office.

Department of Health (DoH) (2001) *Better Prevention. Better Services. Better Sexual Health. The National Strategy for Sexual Health and HIV*, London, The Stationery Office.

Eager, P.W. (2004) 'From population control to reproductive rights: understanding normative change in global population policy (1965–1994)', *Global Society*, vol. 18, no. 2, pp. 145–73.

Earle, S. (2007a) 'Promoting public health: exploring the issues' in Earle et al. (eds) (2007).

Earle, S. (2007b) 'Understanding obesity' in Earle et al. (eds) (2007).

Earle, S., Lloyd, C.E., Sidell, M. and Spurr, S. (eds) (2007) *Theory and Research in Promoting Public Health*, London, Sage/Milton Keynes, The Open University.

Easton, D. (1953) *The Political System*, New York, Knopf.

Fox, N., Ward, K. and O'Rourke, A. (2006) 'A sociology of technology governance for the information age: the case of pharmaceuticals, consumer advertising and the internet, *Sociology*, vol. 40, no. 2, pp. 315–34.

Friends of the Earth International (2006) Press Release: *World Bank Misses Double Dividend on Poverty and Climate Change* [online], http://www.foei.org/media/2006/0423.html (Accessed 9 August 2006).

Friends of the Earth International (2007a) [online], http://www.foei.org/ (Accessed 16 February 2007).

Friends of the Earth International (2007b) *Get Involved – Support Our E-mail Actions and Campaigns* [online], http://www.foei.org/cyberaction/index.html (Accessed 16 February 2007).

Geertz, C. (1998) 'The world in pieces: culture and politics at the end of the century', *Focaal: Tijdschrift voor Antropologie*, vol. 32, pp. 91–117.

Global Policy Forum (2000) *NGOs and Global Policy Making* [online], http://www.globalpolicy.org/ngos/analysis/anal00.htm (Accessed 11 August 2006).

Graham, H. (2007) 'Poverty and health: global and national patterns' in Douglas, J., Earle, S., Handsley, S., Lloyd, C.E., and Spurr, S. (eds) *A Reader in Promoting Public Health: Challenge and Controversy*, London, Sage/Milton Keynes, The Open University.

Guba, E.G. (1984) 'The effect of definitions of policy on the nature and outcomes of policy analysis', *Educational Leadership*, vol. 42, no. 2, pp. 63–70.

Guillén, M. (2001) 'Is globalisation civilising, destructive or feeble? A critique of five key debates in the social science literature', *Annual Review of Sociology*, vol. 27, no. 1, pp. 235–60.

Ham, C. (2004) *Health Policy in Britain: The Politics and Organisation of the National Health Service* (5th edn), London, Palgrave Macmillan.

Hartmann, B. (1987) *Reproductive Rights and Wrongs: The Global Politics of Population Control and Contraceptive Choice*, New York, Harper & Row.

Henderson, D. (2001) *Misguided Virtue: False Notions of Corporate Social Responsibility*, London, Institute of Economic Affairs.

Heywood, M. (2002) 'Drug access, patents and global health: "chaffed and waxed sufficient"', *Third World Quarterly*, vol. 23, no. 2, pp. 217–31.

Hirst, P. and Thompson, G. (1996) *Globalisation in Question*, London, Polity.

International Policy Network (2007) [online], http://www.policynetwork.net/main/index.php (Accessed 16 February 2007).

Kellner, D. (2002) 'Theorizing globalization', *Sociological Theory*, vol. 20, no. 3, pp. 285–305.

Lee, K., Buse, K. and Fustukian, S. (eds) (2002) *Health Policy in a Globalising World*, Cambridge, Cambridge University Press.

Marshall, A. (2004) 'ICTs for health promotion in the community: a participatory approach' in Day and Schuler (eds) (2004).

Mayhew, S.H. and Watts, C. (2002) 'Global rhetoric and individualistic realities: linking violence against women and reproductive health' in Lee et al. (eds) (2002).

McDaid, D. and Oliver, A. (2005) 'Inequalities in health: international patterns and trends' in Scriven and Garman (eds) (2005).

McMichael, T. and Beaglehole, R. (2003) 'The global context for public health' in Beaglehole (ed.) (2003).

Mittelmark, M. (2005) 'Global health promotion: challenges and opportunities' in Scriven and Garman (eds) (2005).

Mudingu, J. (2006) 'How genuine are NGOs?', *The New Times*, 7 August [online], http://www.newtimes.co.rw/index.php?option=com_content&task=view&id=6636&Itemid=1 (Accessed 11 August 2006).

O'Rourke, D. (1997) *Vietnam: Smoke from a Hired Gun, A Critique of Nike's Labor and Environmental Auditing in Vietnam as Performed by Ernst and Young* [online], http://www.corpwatch.org/article.php?id=966 (Accessed 8 November 2006).

Oxfam International (2006) Press Release: *G8 'Late and Lite' on Africa, Says Oxfam*, 16 July [online], http://www.oxfam.org/en/news/pressreleases2006/pr060716_g8_africa (Accessed 10 September 2006).

Palmlund, I. (2006) 'Loyalties in clinical research on drugs: the case of hormone replacement therapy', *Social Science and Medicine*, vol. 6, no. 2, pp. 540–51.

Petryna, A. and Kleinman, A. (2006) 'The pharmaceutical nexus' in Petryna, Lakoff and Kleinman (eds) (2006).

Petryna, A., Lakoff, A. and Kleinman, A. (eds) (2006) *Global Pharmaceuticals: Ethics, Markets, Practices*, Durham and London, Duke University Press.

Poku, N.K. and Whiteside, A. (2002) 'Global health and the politics of governance: an introduction', *Third World Quarterly*, vol. 32, no. 2, pp. 191–5.

Porter, J., Lee, K. and Ogden, J. (2002) 'The globalization of DOTS: tuberculosis as a global emergency' in Lee et al. (eds) (2002).

Prowse, J. (2003) 'International influences on public health' in Watterson, A. (ed.) *Public Health in Practice*, Basingstoke, Palgrave Macmillan.

Raeburn, J. and Macfarlane, S. (2003) 'Putting the public into public health: towards a more people-centred approach' in Beaglehole (ed.) (2003).

Sanders, D., Dovlo, D., Wilma, M. and Lehmann, U. (2003) 'Public health in Africa' in Beaglehole (ed.) (2003).

Scriven, A. (2005) 'Promoting health: a global context and rationale' in Scriven and Garman (eds) (2005).

Scriven, A. and Garman, S. (eds) (2005) *Promoting Health: Global Perspectives*, Basingstoke, Palgrave Macmillan.

The Information Centre (TIC) (2006) *The Infant Feeding Survey 2005: Early Results*, London, The Stationery Office.

Titmuss, R.M. (1974) *Social Policy: An Introduction* (eds B. Abel-Smith and K. Titmuss), London, Allen & Unwin.

United Nations (UN) (2000) *United Nations Millennium Declaration* [online], http://www.un.org/millennium/declaration/ares552e.htm (Accessed 13 August 2006).

United Nations Department of Economic and Social Affairs (UNDESA) (2006) *Sustainable Tourism* [online], http://www.un.org/esa/sustdev/sdissues/tourism/tourism.htm (Accessed 13 August 2006).

United Nations Department of Economic and Social Affairs (UNDESA) (2005) *World Population Prospects: The 2004 Revision Highlights*, New York, United Nations.

United Nations Development Programme (UNDP) (2006) *Millennium Development Goals* [online], http://www.undp.org/mdg/goallist.shtml (Accessed 29 August 2006).

United Nations Population Fund (UNFPA) (1994) *Programme of Action of the International Conference on Population and Development*, New York, United Nations Population Fund.

United Nations Population Fund (UNFPA) (2003) *Achieving the Millennium Development Goals: Population and Reproductive Health are Critical Determinants*, New York, United Nations Population Fund.

United Nations Population Fund (UNFPA) (2005) *Ending the Silent Suffering: Campaign to End Fistula*, New York, United Nations Population Fund.

Venkatesh, M., Nosovitch, J. and Miner, W. (2004) 'Community network development and user participation' in Day and Schuler (eds) (2004).

World Bank (2006) *Clean Energy and Development: Towards an Investment Framework*, Washington, DC, World Bank.

World Growth (2007) [online], http://www.worldgrowth.org/ (Accessed 16 February 2007).

World Health Organization (WHO) (1946) *Preamble to the Constitution of the World Health Organization as Adopted by the International Health Conference*, New York, 19 June–22 July 1946; signed on 22 July 1946 by the representatives of 61 States (Official Records of the World Health Organization, no. 2, p. 100) and entered into force on 7 April 1948.

World Health Organization (WHO) (1977) *Global Strategy for Health for All by the Year 2000*, Geneva, World Health Organization.

World Health Organization (WHO) (1978) *Declaration of Alma Ata*, International Conference on Primary Health Care Alma Ata, USSR, 6–12 September.

World Health Organization (WHO) (1985) *Health for All in Europe by the Year 2000, Regional Targets*, Copenhagen, World Health Organization Regional Office for Europe.

World Health Organization (WHO) (1986) *Ottawa Charter for Health Promotion*, Geneva, World Health Organization; also available online at http://www.euro.who.int/ AboutWHO/Policy/20010827_2 (Accessed 31 July 2006).

World Health Organization (WHO) (1998) *Health 21 – the Health for All Policy Framework for the WHO European Region*, Copenhagen, World Health Organization Regional Office for Europe.

World Health Organization (WHO) (2003) *The World Health Report: Shaping the Future*, Geneva, World Health Organization.

World Health Organization (WHO) (2004a) *Reproductive Health Strategy: To Accelerate Progress Towards the Attainment of International Development Goals and Targets*, Geneva, World Health Organization.

World Health Organization (WHO) (2004b) *Unsafe Abortion: Global and Regional Estimates of Unsafe Abortion and Associated Mortality in 2000* (4th edn), Geneva, World Health Organization.

World Health Organization (WHO) (2005) *The Bangkok Charter for Health Promotion in a Globalized World*, Bangkok, World Health Organization.

World Health Organization (WHO) (2006a) *Global Strategy for the Prevention and Control of Sexually Transmitted Infections: 2006–2015*, Geneva, World Health Organization.

World Health Organization (WHO) (2006b) *Healthy Cities and Urban Governance* [online], http://www.euro.who.int/healthy-cities?PrinterFriendly=1& (Accessed 13 August 2006).

World Health Organization (WHO) (2006c) *Working Together for Health: World Health Report 2006*, Geneva, World Health Organization.

Chapter 2

The development of healthy public policy

Jenny Douglas and Linda Jones

Introduction

Public policy in the UK does not develop in isolation. Rather, it is informed and influenced by a range of local, national, international and global imperatives and priorities. Having considered the relationship between public health and public policy at a global level in Chapter 1, this chapter focuses more closely on the development of healthy public policy in the UK. It starts by briefly putting the current public health policies of the four nations of the UK in context, keeping in mind their very transitory nature and the relationship between global and national policies. The contribution of modern multidisciplinary public health to debates in healthy public policy are then considered in Section 2.2, before subsequent sections move on to consider who and what, in the UK, influence the development of healthy public policy. These influences include social welfare policies, and Section 2.3 focuses on the relationship between social policy and public health promotion, illustrated by two particular case-studies, in housing and child health. A further key influence on healthy public policy is environmentalism, and this is the focus of the final section of this chapter.

2.1 Developing healthy public policy: the four nations of the UK

There has been international recognition of the need for governments to 'ensure that health is explicitly considered in the development of public policy' (WHO, 1998, p. 42). However, at the heart of healthy public policy is the question about the extent to which the state should intervene in promoting public health (Jochelson, 2005). While proponents of healthy public policy might argue that the state has a vital role to play in ensuring that all citizens have the right to good health, promoting public health may also be seen as a matter of individual choice. Notwithstanding these concerns, UK government policy has demonstrated a growing commitment to tackling health inequalities through the development of healthy public policy and partnership working.

The Wanless Review, *Securing Our Future Health: Taking A Long-Term View* (Wanless, 2002), focused attention on the function of public health throughout the UK, and called for a change in the way in which public health was invested in and delivered. It set out the full economic cost of predicted National Health Service (NHS) spending in a number of scenarios, from 'fully engaged' to 'slow progress' – the least optimistic. The review argued for the importance of taking account of the evidence available to inform effective public health interventions. One of the major themes of the report was the improvement of people's 'health literacy' so that they may become fully engaged with the public health agenda and the choices they need to make in order to lead healthier lives. The report further recommended the sharing of knowledge and information between the newly devolved health departments, as well as the gathering and comparison of health information on an international basis. This would lead to a better understanding of 'the role of income and other socio-economic inequalities in explaining differences in health outcomes' (Wanless, 2002, Annex A, p. 124).

In his final report two years later, Wanless (2004) concluded that, despite all the public health policy statements that had appeared over the previous thirty years or so, the results remained disappointing. There was a serious gap between the rhetoric and the implementation of policy, and the NHS remained a sickness rather than a health service. Wanless saw addressing this imbalance as the main challenge to government. There was no need for new policy. Rather, effort should be devoted to achieving change and implementing effective interventions to improve health.

Thinking point: are the four nations of the UK likely to diverge or converge in terms of healthy public policy?

In terms of healthy public policy, devolution in 2000 gave rise to a potentially and increasingly dis-United Kingdom. The four countries making up the UK – England, Wales, Scotland and Northern Ireland – have begun to diverge in respect of devolved policy sectors, including health (Hazell and Jervis, 1998; Greer, 2001, 2006). At the time of writing, Northern Ireland remains without an assembly, which was suspended as a result of the continuing troubles there, with the result that policy development has, for the most part, been in a state of limbo. In Wales and Scotland, a series of policy statements in recent years has stressed the importance of an 'upstream' public health agenda and sought to place the improvement of health as a priority on a par with improvements in the healthcare system. (An 'upstream' health agenda is an agenda that focuses on national or international policies which act on the main determinants of health, such as poverty, housing, etc., whereas 'downstream' policies tend to focus on individual behaviour change.) Much prominence has been given to the English strategies for health so that it has seemed that they are overall UK policy. However, the other countries of the UK have fiercely guarded their right to set their own policy agendas, and it is to these developments that you now turn.

2.1.1 England

In recent years in England, public health policy and practice have been placed high on the agenda of health and social care agencies concerned with improving health. After a long period of consultation and many changes to the publication date, the White Paper *Saving Lives: Our Healthier Nation* was published in 1999 (DoH, 1999). Four target areas were identified – cancer, coronary heart disease and stroke, accidents and mental health – which still related to a 'medical model' of health and disease prevention (Naidoo and Wills, 2000). However, in 2001 the government announced two targets: to reduce inequalities in infant mortality rates and to reduce the gap in adult life expectancy between the poorest and the more affluent geographical areas (Milburn, 2001).

Saving Lives: Our Healthier Nation aimed to avoid nanny state social engineering and individual victim blaming by proposing a contract for health in which the government promised to provide national co-ordination and leadership, ensuring that policy making across government took full account of health. This strategy recognised the need to work across sectors, involving the statutory, voluntary and private sectors in initiatives, and addressing politically sensitive issues such as working with the food industry and tobacco advertising.

The later White Paper, *Choosing Health: Making Healthy Choices Easier* (DoH, 2004), was very much a response to the issues thrown up by the Wanless review (Wanless, 2002, 2004). It set out proposals for action on a range of public health issues, including sexual health, obesity, smoking and alcohol abuse, and for significant changes to smoking in public places and to advertising aimed at children. *Choosing Health* was underpinned by three principles: informed choice, personalisation and working together. Focusing on the health of children and families, it committed further support for Sure Start, modernisation of the school nursing services and the development of healthy schools. The NHS as an employer, as well as provider of health services and healthcare, was highlighted as an important setting for public health. *Choosing Health* outlined ways in which the government would work with the food industry and the food standards agency to implement appropriate food labelling. In spite of all these recommendations, however, critics argued that the White Paper still failed to offer a workable strategy to reduce inequalities in health: 'Indeed, the concentration on choice and the focus on individuals as consumers rather than citizens, is a significant and beguiling distraction from the urgent need to address the social, economic and environmental issues which lie at the root of health inequalities' (UKPHA, 2005, p. 1).

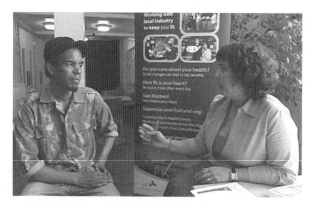

Figure 2.1   There is a range of public health initiatives in England, including this health promotion intervention in the West Midlands

In many ways, *Choosing Health*, and the strategies for health improvement that it put forward, was not dissimilar to the Green Paper *Prevention and Health: Everybody's Business* which was published much earlier, in 1976 (DHSS, 1976). *Choosing Health* re-emphasised health education, social marketing and theories of behaviour change, which had become somewhat obscured in the focus on structural factors to promote health and upstream policies to reduce inequalities in health. However, it also acknowledged the concerns laid out in the Wanless report (Wanless, 2004) with regard to the need for a stronger evidence base for public health, with the proposal (now implemented) to bring together the Health Development Agency and the National Institute for Clinical Excellence to form one body called the National Institute for Health and Clinical Excellence (NICE). The benefits of this were seen to be the development of a stronger evidence base and the building of an 'internationally recognised organisation promoting excellence in public health' (DoH, 2004, Annex B, p. 190). Although international influences on the development of the *Choosing Health* strategy were not explicitly indicated in the document itself, the importance of working nationally, regionally and across government departments, as well as with the voluntary sector, were seen as vital components to promoting public health.

2.1.2 Scotland

In Scotland's White Paper, *Towards a Healthier Scotland* (Scottish Office, 1999), the burden of promoting public health lay with the health boards. With devolution and the greater self-governing powers vested in the Scottish Parliament, the potential for divergence from England, in Scotland's strategy for promoting health, became greater. The Green Paper *Working Together for a Healthier Scotland* (Scottish Office, 1998) set targets proposing that Scotland's main 'illness' priorities were coronary heart disease and stroke, sexual health (including teenage pregnancies and HIV/AIDS), dental and oral health, and accidents. Thus, it also had a medical approach on disease prevention similar to that of England. However, this document also stated that tackling inequalities should be the first challenge for each of the priorities. When *Towards a Healthier Scotland* was published, mental health was included as a priority, although no target was set for this.

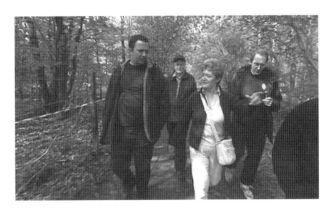

Figure 2.2   Towards a Healthier Scotland included mental health as a priority: the Be Active Stay Active (BASA) group is one such public health intervention

Towards a Healthier Scotland expressed a clearer commitment to tackling inequalities in health by monitoring inequality within each target area, and endorsed the use of Health Impact Assessment to monitor health inequality. A Public Health Strategy Group, chaired by Scotland's Minister for Health and Community Care and drawing representatives from the public, private, community and voluntary sectors, was established to monitor the implementation of the strategy.

Following a review of the public health function in Scotland, undertaken in 1999 (Scottish Executive, 1999), a Public Health Institute of Scotland was established in January 2001, with the threefold remit of improving the public health evidence base, information base and skills base. This was later combined with the Health Education Board for Scotland, becoming Health Scotland.

Improving Health in Scotland: The Challenge, was published in 2003 (Scottish Office, 2003a) to accompany the White Paper on health in Scotland, *Partnership for Care* (Scottish Office, 2003b). Rather than stating new strategies, *Improving Health in Scotland* aimed to pull together many existing strategies and targets. The overarching aim of this new strategy was to tackle health inequalities. As part of the rationale for its strategy, The Scottish Office cited the success of other countries' attempts to increase life expectancy rates (seen as a key indicator of health improvement), and used data from the World Health Organization (WHO) to support its focus on promoting good mental health: 'Other countries have already succeeded ... there is every reason to believe that Scotland can achieve similar success' (Scottish Office, 2003a, p. 3).

The document stressed the importance of leadership, both national and local, and involvement from the 'NHS, local government, voluntary and private sectors' (Scottish Office, 2003, p. 5), in a way similar to the English strategy. The Scottish strategy incorporated a strong 'top-down' approach to public health, with the reorganisation of departments and the development of new processes and ways of working. At the same time, there was an acknowledgement of the importance of individual choice, with one of the 'tools' available to help improve health being: 'Strengthening individuals – developing the confidence, resilience and capacity of individuals and families to make choices that support health while also making healthier choices the easier choices' (Scottish Office, 2003a, p. 11).

2.1.3 Wales

In 1998, *Better Health, Better Wales: A Consultation Document* was produced by the Welsh Office (Welsh Office, 1998), drawing on advice from the Welsh Office and a wide range of key organisations in the public and voluntary sectors. The Welsh strategy was more far reaching than the English strategy; it had a stronger commitment to reducing health inequalities and focused more sharply on the economic and social context of health. By the time the White Paper *Better Health: Better Wales* was published in March 2000 (Welsh Assembly Government, 2000), the fifteen health gain targets which had been set out previously, in 1997 (Welsh Office, 1997), and which provided a framework for measuring progress, were extended to include separate targets for improving children's health and wellbeing.In *Better Health, Better Wales*, local authorities and health bodies had a duty to collaborate in promoting public health.

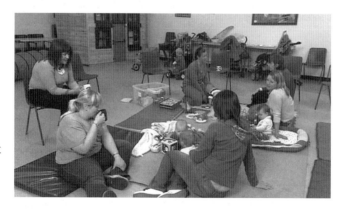

Figure 2.3   A key aspect of Welsh public health policy is the Sure Start initiative

In September 2003, the *Wales: A Better Country* strategy was published (Welsh Assembly Government, 2003). As in earlier strategies, improving health was given a high priority in this 2003 document, but the scope was widened. This strategy outlined a new vision for Wales in the twenty-first century, and indicated the importance of working within a European context and with international partners to promote health. It was followed in February 2004 by the launch of *Health Challenge Wales* (Welsh Assembly Government, 2004), the aim of which was to provide a new and inclusive national focus to secure greater ownership, commitment and action for better health, as part of a co-ordinated and sustained effort to promote public health (see Box 2.1).

Box 2.1 Health Challenge Wales

Health Challenge Wales is a call to everyone – all people and organisations – to do as much as they can to improve health.

It is a challenge to:

- You as an individual to do what you can to improve your own health and the health of your family.

- Government, national and local, to help create the conditions that are needed to help you and your family to lead a healthy life.

- Organisations to do as much as they can to help their employees, their customers and the people who use their services to improve their health.

Creating better health in Wales is not something the Welsh Assembly or the NHS can do on their own. It is a job for all of us.

(Welsh Assembly Government, 2006)

Health Challenge Wales represented a shift from an emphasis on socio-economic causes of illhealth in earlier Welsh strategies, to a focus on lifestyle factors which is similar to that of England (Greer, 2006).

2.1.4 Northern Ireland

The Northern Ireland health strategy *Well into 2000* was published in 1997 (DHSSPS, 1997) and, like the Welsh and Scottish strategies, it continued to emphasise the principles of tackling social exclusion and health inequalities, presenting a vision for improving health and wellbeing in Northern Ireland. It further endorsed the regional targets that had been outlined in the earlier *Health and Well-Being* strategy (DHSSPS, 1996) and proposed the comprehensive use of Health Impact Assessment similar to Scotland. A Minister for Public Health was appointed, and an interdepartmental Ministerial Group for Public Health was established to co-ordinate public health policy.

In March 2002, the White Paper *Investing for Health* was published, which set out explicitly the Northern Ireland strategy for health improvement within an international context. It started from the premise of health as defined by the World Health Organization (WHO, 1946), and as determined by the social, economic, physical and cultural environment, and stated that the health strategy of Northern Ireland was built on the WHO Health 21 policy framework for Europe (DHSSPS, 2002; WHO, 1999). It also put forward a partnership approach (in line with the Health 21 agenda) as the way to improve health and prevent illhealth; and promoted partnership between departments, public sector bodies, voluntary bodies, local communities and district councils.

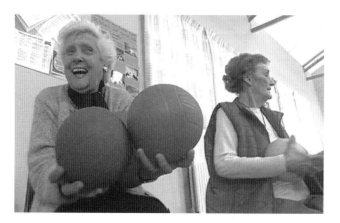

Figure 2.4 Public health promotion in Northern Ireland takes place in diverse ways and in a range of settings

Central to the Northern Ireland strategy was a commitment to ensuring equality of opportunity and tackling social disadvantage, and an endorsement of the settings approach, focusing on four settings – homes, communities, schools and colleges, and workplaces. The strategy outlined the role of all government departments and public sector bodies in improving health, and set out plans to assess the health impact of public sector policies and programmes. In 2006, the outcome of the Review of Public Administration in Northern Ireland was published, which heralded further changes in the public sector, including the amalgamation of the existing district councils into seven local authorities, in line with the seven local commisioning bodies of the strategic health authority (Review of Public Administration, 2006). Although the latest structure provides opportunities for greater development of healthy public policy across the statutory sector, health is being separated from social care services, with the creation of five new health trusts.

Thinking point: do the strategies for public health in each of the UK countries have a different focus?

2.1.5 Summary of the public health strategies of the four nations

In assessing the differences in public health policy between the four countries of the UK, the English, Welsh and Scottish strategies have focused much more on lifestyle issues, health education and behaviour change, and on targeted measures to address social exclusion (Greer, 2006). The Northern Ireland strategy is firmly committed to addressing inequalities. With the exception of the strategy for Northern Ireland, however, current policies have been more inward-looking, and have been concerned with developments only within their own country. The Northern Ireland strategy acknowledges the influence of international and global policy, and outlines the importance of sharing ideas, learning from the experience of other countries, and international co-operation 'in the search of new measures to prevent disease' ((DHSSPS, 2002). International influences are certainly present in the strategies of all four UK countries, albeit in varying degrees and different ways. Chapter 1 outlined the relationship between global public policy and health and considered the influence of globalisation on health and healthy public policy. Of course, the development of policy is influenced by other factors too, and the following sections of this chapter focus on some of these, beginning in Section 2.2 with the contribution of multidisciplinary public health to healthy public policy.

2.2 Healthy public policy and multidisciplinary public health

As already discussed, healthy public policy is concerned with creating a healthy society and acknowledges that, in order to do so, not only the physical but also the social, cultural and economic aspects of health and wellbeing must be addressed. Healthy public policy is nothing less than the transformation of society through giving priority to a health agenda so that public policy changes also deliver greater equity and democracy. In the UK, one way in which this has been expressed is through modern multidisciplinary public health, which has evolved from the sometimes separate, often overlapping disciplines of public health and health education, which have been considered elsewhere (Earle et al., 2007).

2.2.1 The contribution of public health

Kickbusch (1989) claimed that 'public health is ecological in perspective, multisectoral in scope and collaborative in strategy', a comment that echoes Milio's claim (1987) about healthy public policy. Public health traditions have undoubtedly provided an inspiration for healthy public policy (Milio, 1987). Public health has made a major intellectual contribution to the healthy public policy approach. It embraces a tradition of collective action at local and national levels to protect health and deal with health problems, even if, in the early twentieth century, this approach was neglected as attention focused on biomedical advances. Public health has recently sought to free itself from a medical model and to recreate a broader role. Health improvement and the strengthening of the public health function became a statutory requirement under the Health Act of 1999. Health authorities, in partnership with other statutory and voluntary organisations, were required to develop health improvement programmes annually, which were local strategies for improving health and healthcare. This focus has continued with the development of local strategic partnerships. In reviewing the progress of public health, Wanless (2004) noted that the major drivers for public health were identified in the 1970s, but although there had been some successes in relation to healthy public policy, implementation of this was very weak and a comprehensive evidence base was lacking.

Tensions arise in developing healthy public policy when the focus of attention is a 'whole-population' approach, but some practitioners argue that attention should be focused instead on high-risk groups. Debates such as this bring to the centre of discourse on healthy public policy the issue of whose values take precedent in the setting of policy. Libertarian reactions to calls for healthy public policy in the UK on issues such as rising obesity and cigarette smoking, have argued that this is the 'nanny state' interfering with personal freedom by telling people what to do (Joffe and Mindell, 200; Jochelson, 2005).

2.2.2 Health education and healthy public policy

Health education, it has been claimed, is an essential building block of healthy public policy (Tones and Green, 2004). Health education can create knowledge, critical consciousness and the pressure to change to healthier policies. In turn, this process creates the institutional frameworks and supportive environments within which people are enabled to change to healthier lifestyles, and institutions can become more health supporting. In this view, health education is essential for healthier public policy. Public policy acts on the socio-economic and physical environment to create the conditions in which people can be more healthy and choose more healthy ways of life, but it is public pressure, networking, lobbying, and so on – the products of raised consciousness and community action – that are seen as essential to forcing the legislators and regulators to act (Figure 2.5).

Thinking point: if you were trying to reduce child injuries, how would a health education approach be useful?

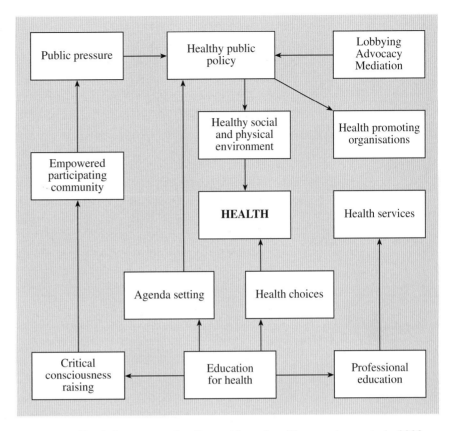

Figure 2.5   The influences on healthy public policy (Source: Jones et al., 2002, p. 109, Figure 6.1)

The example of working at a local level to reduce child injuries highlights many of the key influences illustrated in Figure 2.5. It would include a health education dimension: for instance, educating children about making safer choices when they cross roads and negotiate traffic. Another aspect of health education would be critical consciousness raising in the local area, not only about accidents as a health issue, but about the infrastructural changes that might be developed at a political level to reduce accidents. This could result in public pressure (by the 'empowered participating community') and active agenda setting for change. Another way of working for change could be evidence gathering, lobbying and mediation by professionals who work on child safety issues. For example, there may be opportunities to write targets for change into health contracts. The outcome of the whole process, if successful, could be the introduction of healthier public policies, such as traffic calming or new speed restrictions by the local highway authority.

In the 'real world' of transport policy, making such policies might be (and has been) resisted on the grounds that, although they might be safer for children, they would bring economic disbenefits by slowing up traffic and adding to congestion (Davis and Jones, 1996). So one important part of a health-educating role might be to demonstrate why, in this case, health considerations should outweigh economic considerations. This example illustrates the role that public health practitioners and other individuals can play in developing healthy public policy.

2.3 The contribution of social welfare policy to public health

The aim of healthy public policy is to steer through policies that offer maximum 'health gain,' and this begins with the recognition of how people operate within a complex environment which is social, cultural and economic as well as physical. Milio (1987) emphasised that healthy public policy must be ecological in perspective, multi-sectoral in scope and participatory in strategy (Milio, 1987). Healthy public policies 'improve the conditions under which people live: secure, safe, adequate, and sustainable livelihoods, lifestyles, and environments, including housing, education, nutrition, information exchange, child care, transportation, and necessary community and personal social and health services. Policy adequacy may be measured by its impact on population health' (Milio, 2001, p. 622). The relationship between healthy public policy and social welfare, public health and environmentalism is shown in Figure 2.6.

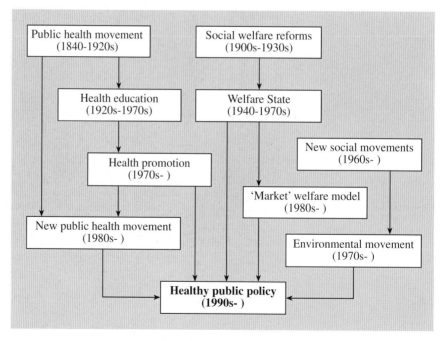

Figure 2.6   The emergence of healthy public policy (Source: Jones et al., 2002, p. 114, Figure 6.3)

2.3.1 The welfare state in the UK

The origins of the modern welfare state in the UK lie in Liberal government reforms before the First World War. During the 1940s, these modest initiatives translated into a more comprehensive welfare state, including a national health service and national insurance, needs-related and free at the point of use; a reformed national education system, which included state education for all to the age of fifteen; and a broader role for public sector council housing and social services. The welfare system in the twenty-first century has grown in complexity. Some policies and services, such as education and health, are now determined and provided at the level of the individual nations, while others, such as social security, are still decided at a UK level. Box 2.2 gives some major features of the UK benefits system today.

Box 2.2 Main benefits of the UK welfare system in the twenty-first century

National Insurance   This is still paid by almost every worker, but contributions are graduated according to earnings. National Health Service treatment does not depend on insurance contributions, but state old age pensions and unemployment benefit depend on a sufficient contribution record and provide a standard benefit. Incapacity benefit is paid to all those deemed incapable of all work.

Child Benefit   This was developed in the 1970s to give all families with children, in particular the prime carer (usually the mother), a small income that was independent of the breadwinner's wage, and thus combat child poverty.

Tax Credits   These replaced Family Credit and include working tax credit for low-paid workers, child tax credit and pension credit. Working tax credits are set against tax liability, administered by the Inland Revenue and paid through employers. A statutory minimum wage was introduced in 1999. These are all redistributive in their effects, adding resources to the poorest tenth of families and combating child poverty.

Income Support   This replaced National Assistance as a range of means-tested benefits to non-earners, not only the long-term unemployed but also pensioners (through the Minimum Income Guarantee). It has expanded massively, far outstripping the residual role envisaged for it in 1945.

Housing Benefit   This was developed as a separate means-tested system to provide support for council and private tenants, but it also indirectly supports many older people in private and local authority residential and nursing homes.

Disability Living Allowance   This is paid to disabled people to enable them to live independently. An Invalid Care Allowance gives low-level financial support to carers.

(Adapted from Jones et al., 2002, p. 174, Box 9.1)

In the first decades after the Second World War, there was a considerable degree of political agreement that the cost of the welfare state was compensated for by full employment, increased efficiency, political stability and economic growth. But this consensus was challenged by researchers and politicians on both the Right and the Left. 'New Left' critics highlighted the continued existence of poverty in the UK and the need for an expansion of welfare services (Townsend, 1979). 'New Right' economic liberals criticised the mounting bureaucracy, cost and ineffectiveness of the 'nanny' welfare state (Murray, 1994).

When 'New' Labour came to power in 1997, it offered a middle or 'Third Way' which continued some Conservative policies such as privatisation, but also introduced measures such as tax credits and the statutory minimum wage to help the poorest families. Sure Start was a Labour initiative created to enhance the functioning of young children and their families in the most deprived areas through the improvement and targeting of existing services (see Sure Start, 2007). New Labour sought to introduce choice, competition and differentiation into services such as education and health, while retaining and investing in them as public sector services. Its electoral success persuaded its opponents of the merits of occupying this middle ground and, by the mid-2000s, a significant degree of consensus on social policy had emerged once more.

2.3.2 Social policy theories and health

Social policy as a discipline offers theories and models of distinctive welfare approaches that can be valuable to those engaged in working for health. Public health work, of whatever type, does not happen in a vacuum, but within a dynamic and complex set of social structures and forces. It is important, therefore, to frame multidisciplinary public health within a critical analysis of wider economic, political and socio-cultural policy debates (Beattie, 1991; Caplan, 1993; Collins, 1997).

Some of the key theoretical debates in social policy in recent times have reflected ideological differences over equity and social justice, the responsibilities of the state and the individual, and the extent to which comprehensive social welfare is compatible with capitalism. For example, the New Right claimed not just that state welfare was ineffective and expensive, but also that the state had no business interfering in people's lives in this way. Rather, it should create conditions in which markets could flourish most effectively and in which citizens could take responsibility as sovereign consumers for determining and meeting their needs (Green, 1992). New Left analysis focused on harnessing the power of the state to improve welfare provision: to create greater equity, redistribute income through taxation, end poverty, reduce health inequalities, and counter race, class and gender discrimination.

Third Way ideology in the UK combined elements of New Right and New Left thinking and drew on the work of the sociologist Anthony Giddens (1998), who argued that a new way forward was needed to acknowledge shifts in society and the economy by the end of the twentieth century. Capitalism had not collapsed – indeed, the fall of communism in Eastern Europe left capitalism triumphant. Espousing economic growth within a market economy, therefore, was the only effective way to deliver the resources needed to pay for welfare and drive towards social justice (Borrie Commission, 1994). Social movements – the environmental, feminist and peace movements, for example – had highlighted individuals and groups as active agents, rather than passive consumers of welfare; hence greater choice and flexibility in service provision was deemed essential. Postmodernist thinking, although it has found few converts in social policy, has drawn attention to difference and identity (Lewis et al., 2000). The state could no longer be the sometimes oppressive, monopoly provider of welfare services; the Third Way offered a blend of public and private provision based on a pragmatic view of 'what worked best' (Blair, 1998). Third Way theorists therefore claimed a position between the state and the market (Powell, 2002), an approach that is attaining the status of political orthodoxy.

Thinking point: are there similarities between debates about social welfare policies and debates about promoting public health?

Debates about the relative responsibility of the state and the individual have characterised the whole history of public health and health promotion, as have debates about equality. In England in the 1980s, the New Right banned the phrase 'health inequalities' and instead used 'health differences', implying that these were natural and could not be remedied by state action. By the mid-2000s, the Third Way language of choice and partnership had become dominant in the health sector too.

Social policy has also influenced health workers by offering accounts and interpretations of key issues. Two examples – housing and childcare policies – highlight the significance of policy shifts for public health.

2.3.3 Housing and health

The link between health and housing was first made explicit in the nineteenth century and then again in the 1940s when the expansion of the public and private house-building programme was a main priority. By the end of the 1970s, however, with general housing and living standards much improved, it was argued that housing was no longer a social issue.

The demise of housing as an area of social policy is seen clearly in expenditure: between 1978–79 and 2002–03 combined spending on housing (rent subsidies, housing benefits and new construction) fell from 7 per cent to 4.2 per cent of total public expenditure, whereas spending on healthcare rose from 10 per cent to 15.7 per cent (Hills, 2004). In the 1980s, the government had required local authorities to increase rents substantially and to sell off much public sector housing (Malpass, 1985). Legislation allowed tenants to vote to opt out of local authority control to a private landlord or housing association. New Labour endorsed public/private partnerships in housing, seeing its focus as being on 'what works' and directing financial support to housing associations and other registered social landlords (Mullins and Murie, 2003).

Research highlighting the impact of poor housing on health (Strachan, 1988; Bines, 1994; Best, 1995) helped to move housing higher up the public policy agenda after 1997. An early Treasury-led initiative, the 'New Deal for Communities', focused on thirty-nine multiply-deprived neighbourhoods in order to improve housing and the physical environment, as well as increase job prospects (Hills, 2004). The Social Exclusion Unit, set up in 1997, had as a priority to focus on the 'worst estates' and consider housing, employment, health and community renewal together, as did equivalent initiatives in the rest of the UK; for example, the Social Exclusion Networks in Scotland. In 2005, *Making it Happen in Neighbourhoods: The National Strategy for Neighbourhood Renewal Four Years On* (ODPM, 2005a) and the five-year strategy for housing *Sustainable Communities: Homes for All* (ODPM, 2005b) both explicitly recognised the health implications of run-down neighbourhoods and poor housing.

The UK national strategies for health, in turn, highlight the importance of adequate housing in improving health. The Northern Ireland health strategy for 1997–2002 had commented that 'although major improvements have been made in tackling unfit and substandard housing ... problems remain in terms of high levels of unfitness in certain localities and in ensuring that the needs of special groups and those in acute need are met' (DHSSPS, 1996). The English public health strategy implementation document *Delivering Choosing Health* (DoH, 2005) identified how targets in the five-year strategy for housing, *Sustainable Communities: Homes for*

All (ODPM, 2005b) would help deliver reductions in health inequalities. The relevant service agreement targets pledge to:

> Tackle social exclusion and deliver neighbourhood renewal, ... narrowing the gap in health, education, crime, worklessness, housing and liveability outcomes between the most deprived areas and the rest of England, with measurable improvement by 2010. ODPM [2005b]
>
> [...]
>
> By 2010, bring all social housing into a decent condition with most of this improvement taking place in deprived areas, and for vulnerable households in the private sector, including families with children, increase the proportion who live in homes that are in decent condition. ODPM [2005b]
>
> (Reported in DoH, 2005, pp. 21–2)

Although in the UK housing and public health strategies there is clear recognition of links between housing, health and neighbourhood renewal, their ability to influence the quality of the existing housing stock is less certain since so much is now privately owned or rented. Some evidence from the twenty-six Health Action Zones in England indicates that integrated schemes to target specific groups can make a difference; for example, improvements to housing and transport services can assist older people (Baggott, 2000; Bauld et al., 2005). For those working for public health, such evidence is significant, encouraging the view that helping to reverse the downward spiral of illness due to poor housing might be achievable within the remit of everyday practice.

2.3.4 Policies for children

During the last few years, children have been key beneficiaries of a policy characterised as 'selective universalism' (Hills and Lelkes, 1999). While New Labour maintained the benefits system in general, it targeted extra help on those seen as having the greatest need (see again Box 2.2). Several Labour government initiatives were specifically aimed at children and their families in an effort to improve their health, income levels and functioning.

Strong evidence had accumulated by the late 1990s not only of high levels of poverty in one-parent families, large families and black and minority ethnic families (Glendinning and Millar, 1987; Nazroo, 1997; Gordon et al., 2000), but also of rising illness (Donkin et al., 2002). Three times as many people had incomes below half of mean income in the early 1990s as did in the late 1970s (Hills, 2004).

In this climate, Tony Blair pledged to halve child poverty by 2010 and eradicate it by 2020 (Blair, 1999). Child Benefit was increased, Child Tax

Credits introduced, direct support for childcare expanded substantially, and Child Trust Funds were established. The latter were £250 tax-free accounts (£500 for children in poverty) for all children born after September 2002, with a further government endowment at the age of seven. These financial benefits began to show results and relative child poverty fell by around 8 per cent between 1997 and 2004 (Hills, 2004; Millar and Gardiner, 2004). In Scotland, a separate national survey also concluded that 'the percentage of both children and pensioners in low-income households has been falling' (Palmer et al., 2004, p. 10).

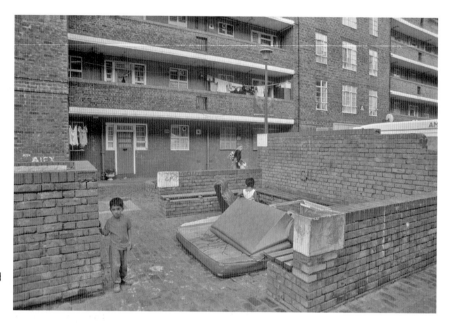

Figure 2.7   Blair pledged to eradicate child poverty by 2020

In addition to financial benefits, other policy initiatives were launched. The Social Exclusion Unit aimed to enhance services for a range of disadvantaged groups, including children excluded from school, and teenage parents. Sure Start was aimed at families with children under the age of four years in poor areas, using community-based interventions to provide more support to parents, enhance their parenting skills and provide more formal and informal childcare. Three thousand five hundred children's centres were planned by 2010 to provide a range of support services, and the 'extended school' concept added in breakfast clubs, after-school clubs and other services. Early years education was extended to include, in particular, at least part-time nursery places for all children aged three and above from 2004. *Every Child Matters: Next Steps* (DfES, 2004), and Children's Bills for the four UK countries, set out a radical agenda for restructuring, focused on integrating services and staff to meet common, agreed outcomes across all services that work with children. Children's Trusts are designed for joint planning, commissioning, financing and delivery of services by education, health, social services and other agencies.

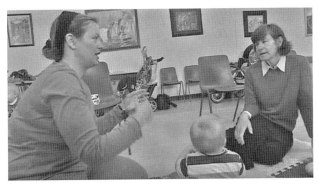

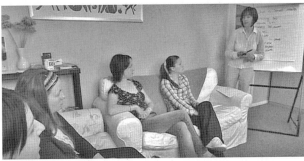

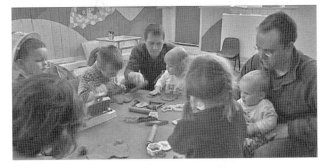

Figure 2.8 There is a range of interventions designed to promote public health within the Sure Start initiative in Powys, Wales

Thinking point: to what extent is this targeting of children and families also a feature of health policies?

There are strong links to health, where reducing health inequalities by 10 per cent by 2010, starting with children under the age of one year, became a key objective in *Delivering Choosing Health* (DoH, 2005). Improving physical activity levels, launching media campaigns aimed at children, extending the healthy schools initiative and developing the school nurse role were all seen as 'big wins' in the English public health strategy, as well as those of the other UK countries. Two priority themes in *Tackling Health Inequalities* (DoH, 2002) focused on providing a sure foundation for early childhood and improving opportunity for children. Health Action Zones were set up to tackle inequalities by improving and co-ordinating service delivery, and health improvement programmes (later local strategic partnerships) were designed to plan coherently across agencies to enhance health.

These policy changes also offer new opportunities for public health practitioners. Children's Trusts are likely to change quite significantly how health professionals working with children are trained and how health services for children are delivered. They offer the prospect of creating a broader understanding of health by other childcare professionals and for the upstream approaches of multidisciplinary public health to be integrated into the core of work with children.

2.4 Environmental politics and public health

This section explores UK and international debates about the environment, focusing in particular on 'sustainable development' and the convergence of the environmental and public health movements. As far back as 1977, the WHO Health For All strategy acknowledged the importance of a healthy environment, and more recent policy statements have clarified how people at all levels might take action to protect the environment. At the same time, sustainable development policies have increasingly acknowledged the centrality of health and, at the United Nations (UN) World Summit on Sustainable Development held in Johannesburg in 2002, health was one of five priority planning areas for delegates (UN, 2002).

So, how far should public health practitioners incorporate the messages of sustainability into everyday practice, and how might this be done? What is the relevance of 'green consumerism'? Can those working to promote health make new partnerships that will help deliver more sustainable development and improved environmental health outcomes?

2.4.1 The rise of the environmental movement

In the 1970s and 1980s, environmentalism, in the shape of the 'green' movement in particular, became more prominent (Dobson, 1991). Many would date the birth of green politics as coinciding with the publication in 1962 of Rachel Carson's campaigning book *Silent Spring*, which warned of the disastrous environmental consequences of indiscriminate use of pesticides, fungicides and herbicides on the land. As a powerful mix of prophecy and science, it both detailed the increasing use of chemicals in every aspect of daily life and characterised the future 'silent spring' in the following vision:

There was once a town in the heart of America where all life seemed to live in harmony with its surroundings ...

[...]

The countryside was famous ... for the abundance and variety of its bird life [and for] the streams, which flowed clear and cold out of the hills and contained shady pools where trout lay ...

Then a strange blight crept over the area and everything began to change. Some evil spell had settled on the community: mysterious maladies swept the flocks of chickens; the cattle and sheep sickened and died ... The farmers spoke of much illness among their families. In the town the doctors had become more and more puzzled by new kinds of sickness appearing among their patients ...

There was a strange stillness. The birds, for example – where had they gone? ... The few birds seen anywhere were moribund; they trembled violently and could not fly. It was a spring without voices ...

[...]

The roadsides, once so attractive, were now lined with browned and withered vegetation as though swept by fire ... Even the streams were now lifeless ...

[...]

No witchcraft, no enemy action had silenced the rebirth of new life in this stricken world. The people had done it themselves.

(Carson, 1965. pp. 21–2)

2.4.2 Sustainable development

The concept of 'sustainable development' came into prominence in the later 1980s with the publication of The Brundtland Report by the UN World Commission on Environment and Development (1987). Sustainable development was defined as: 'Development that meets the needs of current generations without compromising the ability of future generations to meet their needs' (UN World Commission on Environment and Development, 1987, p. 8).

Thinking point: consider what view of economic growth underpins the concept of sustainable development.

The concept of sustainable development carried with it the demand that economic growth should be balanced against resource depletion and the recognition of ultimate dependence on the natural environment. If growth outstripped resources then the ability of future generations to live in a similar way to the present generation would be compromised. Elsewhere in the Brundtland Report this was described as 'non-declining per capita utility (satisfaction or well-being)'. In other words, economic growth should be such that it could deliver to people similar levels of satisfaction or wellbeing in 2050 or 3000 as it delivered in the current year.

The Brundtland Report was radical in other ways. It emphasised that sustainable development was not just about policy making 'at the top', but about popular participation in decision making, and empowering groups and individuals to protect the environment. In this it reflected the increasing interest of ordinary people in the environment, the growth of green pressure groups – such as Friends of the Earth and Greenpeace – and greater responsiveness of politicians to the environmental issues. It also recognised that sustainable development would require social and economic change and argued that: 'overriding priority should be given to the essential needs of the world's poor ... Development involves a progressive transformation of economy and society ... Even the narrow notion of physical sustainability implies a concern for social equity between generations that must logically be extended to equity within each generation' (UN World Commission on Environment and Development, 1987, p. 165–6).

This positioned sustainable development as a radical approach concerned with achieving greater equity between countries or within societies. Some core ideas within sustainable development are set out in Box 2.3.

Box 2.3 Core ideas within sustainable development

1   Environment–economy integration: integrating economic development and environmental protection in planning and implementation.

2   Futurity: explicit concern with the impact of current activity on future generations.

3   Environmental protection: reducing pollution and environmental degradation and protection of the non-human world.

4   Equity: commitment to meeting the basic needs of the poor of the present generations and to equity between generations.

5   Quality of life: recognition that human well-being is constituted by more than economic growth and prosperity alone.

6   Participation: recognition that sustainable development requires institutions to be restructured to allow all voices in society to be heard in decision making.

(Connelly and Smith, 2003, p. 6)

Following the Brundtland Report, the principles of sustainable development have been fleshed out in various ways. One emphasis is on the 'precautionary principle', which means acting to prevent likely harm even without conclusive evidence. This was adopted as Principle 15 by the UN World Conference on Environment and Development – the so-called 'Earth Summit' – at Rio de Janiero in 1992 in the following terms: 'Where there are threats of serious or irreversible damage, lack of full scientific certainty shall not be used as a reason for postponing cost-effective measures to prevent environmental degradation' (UNCED, 1993, p. 9).

Another principle is that 'the polluter pays', which means that the costs of pollution are met by those who pollute rather than by the wider society. A chemical leak into a river from an industrial plant, for example, should be the responsibility of the polluter rather than the local government authority.

A more contentious principle is integrated pollution control (IPC), especially as it may involve international action. IPC requires anticipating and assessing the effects of all pollution on land and in the sea and air, and takes into account how pollution might spread from one medium to another. For example, an oil spillage could have repercussions not only for marine life, but also for coastal communities and for tourism. Atmospheric pollution might lead to physical effects on plant life.

2.4.3 Global policy-making for sustainable development

The Brundtland Report marked the beginning of a new era of global environmental policy making. In 1992, the Earth Summit developed a programme of action on sustainable development: Agenda 21. This endorsed principles central to sustainable development and proclaimed the right of all people to a 'healthy and productive life in harmony with nature' (UNCED, 1993, p. 9). Perhaps its greatest achievement was in gaining agreement on environmental impact assessment in each case where proposed actions 'are likely to have a significant adverse impact on the environment' (UNCED, 1993, p. 9), although the definition of 'significant' remained unclear.

In 2000, the UN adopted eight 'Millennium Development Goals', including a goal to 'ensure environmental sustainability' (UNDP, 2006, Goal 7) (see also Chapter 1, Section 1.2.2 in this volume, in particular Figure 1.2). This set targets, including a 50 per cent cut in the numbers of people without safe drinking water and a significant improvement in the lives of 100 million slum dwellers, both by 2010. Building on this, delegates to the 2002 UN World Summit on Sustainable Development in Johannesburg pledged to 'act together, united by a common determination to save our planet' (UN, 2002, p. 5). The Report was outspoken on issues of equity, commenting that: 'Eradicating poverty is the greatest global challenge facing the world today and an indispensable requirement for sustainable development, particularly for developing countries ... concerted and concrete measures are required at all levels to enable developing countries to achieve sustainable goals' (UN, 2002, paragraph 7).

The Report highlighted inequalities within and between societies, the 'deep fault line that divides human society between rich and poor' and the particular threats posed by the uneven distribution of the costs and benefits of globalisation (UN, 2002, paragraphs 11–12, 14). It noted the need to change unsuitable patterns of consumption and production and to 'de-link economic growth and environmental degradation' by finding more sustainable routes to economic development (paragraph 15). But as in previous reports, some of the hard questions about how to restrain demands for resources from developed countries, control the operations of multinationals, and limit economic growth remained unanswered. Friends of the Earth calculated that the average UK citizen creates a hundred times more carbon dioxide than the average citizen of Malawi (FoE, 2004).

Within Europe, a range of European Union (EU) regulations require member states to control hazardous activities, develop public participation in planning, and meet a whole range of objectives for specific protection of water and air quality, noise levels, radiation, soil pollution, and so on. The UK was slow to develop integrated pollution control until it was spurred into action in the 1990s by European regulation (Connelly and Smith, 2003). Since 2000, it has had to respond to further EU regulation, such as the Integrated Pollution Prevention and Control Act of 1999, which requires EU countries to prevent pollution problems rather than manage them. It now has a range of New Environmental Policy Instruments (NEPIs), including incentives for companies to invest in green technologies, an emissions trading scheme and a climate change levy.

2.4.4 Integrating health and sustainable development

By the early 1990s, sustainability had become incorporated into the health sector. In the UK, for example, many of the aims of the 'new' public health movement in the early 1990s focused on 'avoiding or countering hazards in the environment' (Draper, 1991, p. 7). Hazards included the thinning of the ozone layer, the greenhouse effect, deforestation and over-use of pesticides, as well as poverty, unemployment and inappropriate economic growth.

The Ottawa Charter for Health Promotion (WHO, 1986) had already identified 'building healthy public policies' and 'creating sustainable environments' as key elements of its health promotion strategy:

> Our societies are complex and interrelated. Health cannot be separated from other goals. The inextricable links between people and their environment constitutes the basis for a socio-ecological approach to health. The overall guiding principle for the world,

> nations, regions and communities alike, is the need to encourage reciprocal maintenance – to take care of each other, our communities and our natural environment. The conservation of natural resources throughout the world should be emphasized as a global responsibility.
>
> (WHO, 1986, p. 1)

Within health promotion, the Sundsvall Conference on Supportive Environments (WHO, 1991) and the Jakarta Conference (WHO, 1997) helped to clarify how sustainable development could be translated into everyday health-promoting action. WHO drew on the work of the Earth Summit to produce Health 21, which emphasised a healthy and safe physical environment (WHO, 1999). In target 10, Health 21 advocated environmental taxes to promote health and reduce pollution, signalling the significant convergence between health and environmental aims.

The current framework of UK action demonstrates this integration of health and environment. The Department of Trade and Industry's *Environment and Health Action Plan, 2004–2010* identifies four areas for action, including climate change, biodiversity, waste and 'environment, health and quality of life' (DTI, 2004). The Department of Health's *Choosing Health* strategy (DoH, 2005) has a whole action plan on diet, including action on sustainable farming and food, and its physical activity action plan focuses on a range of environmental improvements to deliver health targets for combating obesity.

2.4.5 Action on sustainable development

The plurality of actors, agencies, reports and regulations that have been noted here illustrates part of the challenge for environmentalists. How can collective action be successful when they are so many different groups to consult, co-ordinate and convince? Moreover, getting workable solutions may require persuading some groups or countries to restrain themselves for the common good. Take the example of over-fishing:

> although there is general recognition of the problem, it is still extremely difficult in practice to prevent it. It remains in the interest of individual countries to continue present practices even though they are aware that this will lead to a diminution of fish stocks. This is because they know that if they do not take the fish someone else will. Why, then, should they be the ones to lose out?
>
> (Connelly and Smith, 2003, pp.125–6)

This relates also to groups within a society. For example, higher socio-economic groups are, statistically, multiple car owners with high annual mileage rates, generating demand for more roads rather than public transport (DoT, 2004). They are, directly and indirectly, larger consumers of finite resources and producers of higher levels of atmospheric pollution than poorer families. Yet successive governments have been very nervous about constraining the car use of some groups to achieve sustainable development targets, because of the potential political impact.

2.4.6 Change at different levels

In the face of these challenges, how can those promoting public health incorporate sustainable development into their everyday work? Box 2.4 considers action at a number of different levels.

Box 2.4 Examples of the potential for environmental health promoting action at different levels

Consumer action: 'green' purchasing, fitting double glazing

Citizen action: joining a pressure group, starting a local campaign, growing vegetables

Household action: recycling, monitoring and reducing energy use

Community action: setting up a recycling project, establishing a skills-exchange scheme

Professional action: giving greater priority to green issues within health promotion work, supporting local green initiatives, harnessing external resources from national or local campaigns

Local authority action: traffic restraint policies, energy-saving advice, setting and enforcing targets, enabling public participation in environmental priority setting

Organisational action: assessing the potential for energy saving in transport, cleaning, heating and lighting

National and international action: setting policy frameworks and targets, monitoring targets, enforcing regulations and inspection, providing resources to encourage change at lower levels.

Thinking point: is there potential within your own public health work for sustainable development action?

Perhaps the most obvious way in which anybody can take action is as a consumer and a citizen. There is keen public interest in purchasing green products, from washing-up liquid and free-range eggs to recycled goods and products made from wood grown in sustainable forests. Household and citizen action on green issues is much easier now; for example, through recycling bottles and paper, reusing materials, growing vegetables and saving energy. Many councils now operate sophisticated collection and recycling policies.

Environmental action can form part of working for health with families and communities. For example, the Communities Plan (ODPM, 2005a) included engaging local neighbourhoods in carrying out improvements to parks and cycling and walking routes to encourage green transport. These resources and projects, or similar resources produced by pressure groups and campaigns, could be adapted for use with local communities.

Sustainable development is a broad concept, and part of public health work is to turn it into a practical tool. Initiatives such as setting up a fruit and vegetable co-operative on a poor housing estate might be given a green dimension if local people could be helped to gain access to allotments and contribute their own produce.

Local authorities have a key role in environmental public health and all those involved in promoting public health may also have a role here. Neighbourhood renewal schemes, communities for health programmes and health improvement plans are among the local initiatives that can help to address sustainable development issues, and that offer scope for local action. However, there are likely to be tensions between the role of local authorities in developing sustainable communities and their need for economic development, as a study of regeneration in East Sheffield highlighted (Greig and Parry, 2002).

In the health sector, the NHS has introduced recycling and other measures, including green transport plans (Hookham, 1995). There is still much to do: *Choosing Health* (DoH, 2004) reported that of twenty-five billion passenger kilometres travelled in 2001, twenty-one billion (81 per cent) were by car and van. Some trusts have taken more radical measures, such as introducing cycle lease schemes, extending and subsidising bus access schemes and restricting staff living very near to the hospital from using their cars (Jones, 1995).

Conclusion

Healthy public policy is broad ranging, and its development is influenced by a variety of different factors at the international, national, regional and local levels. This chapter has shown how the development of national policy is informed by these different priorities and continues to change and evolve over time. Welfare services are crucial in underpinning health, and social policy research has played a key part in shaping and changing welfare state policies. In order to influence the factors that influence health, those engaged in promoting public health need to understand the impact of policy and welfare provision outside the health sector. The continuing debates about public and private provision, issues of choice and markers of inequality in social policy are not merely academic but ideological, and are reflected in everyday policy decisions and outcomes, as demonstrated in the two case-studies in housing and children's policies included in this chapter.

The call for sustainable development has become more prominent in multidisciplinary public health. At one level this requires action by international agencies and national governments to lay down a framework for guidance and regulation. At the local level, public health practitioners need to act in a flexible way, identifying and seizing opportunities as citizens, consumers and professionals. The rhetoric of sustainability is loud and clear. What is still needed is much more evidence of how it can be created. Healthy public policy can be highly effective; however, its implementation has been piecemeal. Although there is a need to develop the evidence base, evidence is available on interventions that are known to work. Progress requires political commitment and a change in values. These issues are developed further in the next chapter, which examines the making and changing of healthy public policy.

References

Baggott, R. (2000) *Public Health: Policy and Politics*, Basingstoke, Macmillan.

Bauld, L., Judge, K., Barnes, M., Benzeval, M., Mackenzie, M. and Sullivan, H. (2005) 'Promoting social change: the experience of Health Action Zones in England', *Journal of Social Policy*, vol. 34, no. 3 pp. 427–45.

Beattie, A. (1991) 'Knowledge and control in health promotion: a test case for social policy and social theory' in Gabe, J., Calnan, M. and Bury, M. (eds) *The Sociology of the Health Service*, London, Routledge.

Best, R. (1995) 'The housing dimension' in Benzeval, M., Judge, K. and Whitehead, M. (eds) *Tackling Inequalities in Health: An Agenda for Action*, London, King's Fund.

Bines, W. (1994) *The Health of Single, Homeless People*, Housing Research Finding No. 128, York, University of York, Centre for Housing Policy.

Blair, T. (1998) *The Third Way*, London, Fabian Society.

Blair, T. (1999) *Beveridge Lecture* [online], http://www.bris.ac.uk/poverty/Publication_files/Tony%20Blair%20Child%20Poverty%20Speech.doc (Accessed 2 March 2007).

Borrie Commission (1994) *Social Justice: Strategies for National Renewal – The Report of the Commission on Social Justice*, London, Vintage.

Caplan, R. (1993) 'The importance of social theory for health promotion: from description to reflexivity', *Health Promotion International*, vol. 8, no. 2, pp. 147–57.

Carson, R. (1965) *Silent Spring*, Harmondsworth, Penguin.

Collins, T. (1997) 'Models of health: pervasive, persuasive and politically charged' in Sidell, M., Jones, L., Peberdy, A. and Katz, J. (eds) *Debates and Dilemmas in Promoting Health: A Reader*, Basingstoke, Macmillan/Milton Keynes, The Open University.

Connelly, J. and Smith, G. (2003) *Politics and the Environment: From Theory to Practice* (2nd edn), London, Routledge.

Davies, A. and Jones, L. (1996) 'Health and environmental constraints: listening to children's views', *Health Education Journal*, vol. 55, pp. 363–74.

Department for Education and Skills (DfES) (2004) *Every Child Matters: Next Steps*, London, The Stationery Office.

Department for Transport (DoT) (2004) *Walking and Cycling: An Action Plan*, London, The Stationery Office.

Department of Health (DoH) (1999) *Saving Lives: Our Healthier Nation*, London, The Stationery Office.

Department of Health (DoH) (2002) *Tackling Health Inequalities: 2002 Cross-Cutting Review*, London, The Stationery Office.

Department of Health (DoH) (2004) *Choosing Health: Making Healthier Choices Easier*, London, The Stationery Office.

Department of Health (DoH) (2005) *Delivering Choosing Health: Making Healthy Choices Easier*, London, The Stationery Office.

Department of Health and Social Security (DHSS) (1976) *Prevention and Health: Everybody's Business*, London, HMSO.

Department of Health, Social Services and Public Safety (DHSSPS) (1996) *Health and Well-being*, Belfast, Department of Health, Social Services and Public Safety.

Department of Health, Social Services and Public Safety (DHSSPS) (1997) *Well into 2000*, Belfast, Department of Health, Social Services and Public Safety.

Department of Health, Social Services and Public Safety (DHSSPS) (2002) *Investing for Health,* Belfast, Department of Health, Social Services and Public Safety.

Department of Trade and Industry (DTI) (2004) *Environment and Health Action Plan, 2004–2010*, London, The Stationery Office.

Dobson, A. (1991) *The Green Reader*, London, Andre Deutsch.

Donkin, A., Goldblatt, P. and Lynch, K. (2002) 'Inequalities in life expectancy by social class, 1972–1999', *Health Statistics Quarterly*, vol. 15, pp. 5–15.

Draper, P. (1991) *Health through Public Policy: The Greening of Public Health*, London, Green Print.

Earle, S., Lloyd, C.E., Sidell, M. and Spurr, S. (eds) (2007) *Theory and Research in Promoting Public Health*, London, Sage/Milton Keynes, The Open University.

Friends of the Earth (FoE) (2004) *Poverty, Justice and the Environment*, London, Friends of the Earth; also available online at http://www.foe.co.uk/resource/factsheets/poverty_justice_environment.pdf (Accessed (2 March 2007).

Giddens, A. (1998) *The Third Way*, Cambridge, Polity.

Glendinning, C. and Millar, J. (eds) (1987) *Women and Poverty in Britain*, Brighton, Harvester Wheatsheaf.

Gordon, D., Adelman, L., Ashworth, K., Bradshaw, J., Levitas, R., Middleton, S., Pantazis, C., Patsios, D., Payne, S., Townsend, P. and Williams, J. (2000) *Poverty and Social Exclusion in Britain*, York, Joseph Rowntree Foundation.

Green, D.G. (1992) *Equalising People*, London, Institute of Economic Affairs, Health and Welfare Unit.

Greer, S.L. (2001) *Divergence and Devolution*, London, The Nuffield Trust.

Greer, S.L. (2006) 'The politics of health-policy divergence' in Adams, J. and Schmueker, K. (eds) *Devolution in Practice 2006*, Newcastle, Institute for Public Policy Research.

Greig, S. and Parry, N. (2000) 'Local communities and sustainable regeneration in the East End of Sheffield', in Adams, L., Amos, M. and Munro, J. (eds) *Promoting Health: Politics and Practice*, London, Sage.

Hazell, R. and Jervis, P. (1998) *Devolution and Health*, Nuffield Trust Series No. 3, London, Nuffield Trust.

Hills, J. (2004) *Inequality and the State*, Oxford, Oxford University Press.

Hills, J. and Lelkes, O. (1999) 'Social security, selective individualism and patchwork redistribution' in Jowell, R., Curtice, J., Park, A. and Thomson, K. (eds) *British Social Attitudes: The 16th Report*, Aldershot, Ashgate.

Hookham, J. (1995) 'Air quality, the commercial vehicle and company car fleets', *Greenhouse*, no. 5, Institute of Earth Sciences, Oxford.

Jochelson, K. (2005) *Nanny or Steward? The Role of Government in Public Health*, London, King's Fund.

Joffe, M. and Mindell, J. (2004) 'A tentative step towards healthy public policy', *Journal of Epidemiology and Community Health*, vol. 58, no. 12, pp. 966–8.

Jones, L. (1995) *Transport and Health: The Next Move*, Policy Statement on Transport No. 2, Association for Public Health.

Jones, L. (2002) 'The social policy contribution to health promotion' in Jones, L., Sidell, M. and Douglas, J. (eds) *The Challenge of Promoting Health: Exploration and Action* (2nd edn), Basingstoke, Palgrave Macmillan/Milton Keynes, The Open University.

Kickbusch, I. (1989) 'Healthy Cities: a working project and a growing movement', *Health Promotion*, vol. 4, no. 2, pp. 77–82.

Lewis, G., Gerwitz, S. and Clarke, J. (2000) *Rethinking Social Policy*, London, Sage.

Lindblom, C.E. (1975) 'Still muddling, not yet through', *Public Administration Review*, vol. 39, no. 6, pp. 517–26.

Malpass, P. (1985) *Housing Policy in Britain*, London, Macmillan.

Milburn, A. (2001) 'Breaking the link between poverty and ill-health', speech delivered to the Long-Term Medical Conditions Alliance conference, 28 February, London, Royal College of Physicians.

Milio, N. (1987) 'Making healthy public policy – developing the science by learning the art: an ecological framework for policy studies', *Health Promotion*, vol. 2, no. 3, pp. 263–74.

Milio, N. (2001) 'Glossary: healthy public policy', *Journal of Epidemiology and Community Health*, vol. 55, no. 9, pp. 622–3.

Millar, J. and Gardiner, K. (2004) *Low Pay, Household Resources and Poverty*, York, Joseph Rowntree Foundation.

Mullins, D. and Murie, A. (2003) *Housing Policy in Britain*, Basingstoke, Palgrave Macmillan.

Murray, C. (1994) *Underclass: The Crisis Deepens*, London, Institute of Economic Affairs, Health and Welfare Unit.

Naidoo, J. and Wills, J. (2000) *Health Promotion: Foundation for Practice* (2nd edn), Edinburgh, Baillière Tindall.

Nazroo, J. (1997) *The Health of Britain's Ethnic Minorities*, London, Policy Studies Institute.

Office of the Deputy Prime Minister (ODPM) (2005b) *Sustainable Communities: Homes for All*, London, Office of the Deputy Prime Minister.

Office of the Deputy Prime Minister (ODPM) (2005a) *Making it Happen in Neighbourhoods: The National Strategy for Neighbourhood Renewal Four Years On*, London, Office of the Deputy Prime Minister.

Palmer, G., Carr, J. and Kenway, P. (2004) *Monitoring Poverty and Social Exclusion in Scotland 2004*, York, Joseph Rowntree Foundation.

Powell, M. (ed.) (2002) *Evaluating Labour's New Welfare Reforms*, Bristol, Policy.

Review of Public Administration (2006) *Review of Public Administration Implementation* [online], http://www.rpani.gov.uk (Accessed 15 January 2007).

Scottish Executive (1999) *Review of the Public Health Function in Scotland*, Edinburgh, The Stationery Office.

Scottish Office (1998) *Working Together for a Healthier Scotland: A Consultative Document*, Edinburgh, The Stationery Office.

Scottish Office (1999) *Towards a Healthier Scotland*, Edinburgh, The Stationery Office.

Scottish Office (2003a) *Improving Health in Scotland: The Challenge*, Edinburgh, The Stationery Office.

Scottish Office (2003b) *Partnership for Care*, Edinburgh, The Stationery Office.

Strachan, D. (1988) 'Damp housing and childhood asthma: validation of reporting symptoms', *British Medical Journal*, vol. 297, pp. 1223–6.

Sure Start (2007) [online], http://www.surestart.gov.uk (Accessed 15 January 2007).

Tones, K. and Green, J. (2004) *Health Promotion: Planning and Strategies*, London, Sage.

Townsend, P. (1979) *Poverty in the UK*, Harmondsworth, Penguin.

UK Public Health Association (UKPHA) (2005) 'To choose or not to choose?', *Report: Newsletter of the UK Public Health Association*, no. 17, p. 1.

United Nations (UN) (2002) *World Summit on Sustainable Development, Johannesburg*, New York, United Nations.

United Nations (UN) World Commission on Environment and Development (1987) *Our Common Future* (The Brundtland Report), Oxford, Oxford University Press.

United Nations (UN) World Conference on Environment and Development (UNCED) (1993) *Agenda 21* (Earth Summit, Rio de Janiero, Brazil), New York, United Nations Department of Economic and Social Affairs.

Wanless, D. (2002) *Securing our Future Health: Taking A Long Term View*, London, HM Treasury.

Wanless, D. (2004) *Securing Good Health for the Whole Population: Final Report*, London, HM Treasury.

Welsh Assembly Government (2000) *Better Health: Better Wales*, Cardiff, The Stationery Office.

Welsh Assembly Government (2003) *Wales: A Better Country*, Cardiff, The Stationery Office.

Welsh Assembly Government (2004a) *Health Challenge Wales* [online], http://.new.wales. gov.uk (Accessed 11 August 2006).

Welsh Assembly Government (2006) *Health Challenge Wales: Background* [online], http://new.wales.gov.uk/topics/health/improvement/hcw/background/; jsessionid=6DFC11781C573DF59945C4804D8A5170.www2?lang=en (Accessed 1 August 2006).

Welsh Office (1997) *Health Gain Targets for Wales* (DGM (97) 50), Cardiff, Welsh Office.

Welsh Office (1998) *Better Health, Better Wales: A Consultation Document*, Cardiff, Welsh Office.

World Health Organization (WHO) (1946) Preamble to the Constitution of the World Health Organization as adopted by the International Health Conference, New York, 19 June–22 July 1946; signed on 22 July 1946 by the representatives of 61 States (Official Records of the World Health Organization, no. 2, p. 100) and entered into force on 7 April 1948.

World Health Organization (WHO) (1985) *Targets for Health for All*, Copenhagen, World Health Organization Regional Office for Europe.

World Health Organization (WHO) (1986) *Ottawa Charter for Health Promotion*, Ottawa, World Health Organization.

World Health Organization (WHO) (1988) *Adelaide Recommendations on Health Public Policy*, Geneva, World Health Organization.

World Health Organization (WHO) (1991) *Sundsvall Statement on Supportive Environments for Health*, from the 3rd International Conference on Health Promotion, Sundsvall, Sweden, 9–15 June, Stockholm, World Health Organization.

World Health Organization (WHO) (1997) *The Jakarta Declaration on Leading Health Promotion into the 21st Century*, Geneva, World Health Organization.

World Health Organization (WHO) (1998) *Health for All in the Twenty-First Century* (A51/5), Geneva, World Health Organization.

World Health Organization (WHO) Europe (1999) *Health 21: The Health for All Policy Framework for the WHO European Region*, Copenhagen, World Health Organization Regional Office for Europe.

Chapter 3

Making and changing healthy public policy

Revised by Kythé Beaumont, Jenny Douglas and Tom Heller
from an original chapter by Linda Jones (2002)

Introduction

Chapters 1 and 2 explored the relationship between public health and public policy at a global level and focused on the development of healthy public policy in the UK. This chapter focuses more closely on the policy-making process. It discusses how policies are made and why issues are added to the policy agenda, and will guide you through some of the processes by which a certain number of policies achieve priority and become implemented in practice. After first recapping, in Section 3.1, on what is meant by the term 'policy', Section 3.2 then looks at who makes policy. Section 3.3 briefly explores different models of policy making, and Section 3.4 looks at influences on those models. Section 3.5 uses a case-study of controls on tobacco use to examine how conflicts of value and interests may affect policy change. This chapter suggests that people involved in public health work can influence policy decisions directly; for example, through lobbying and pressure group membership, and by the important role they play in policy implementation. However, in order to do so it is important to understand the nature of the policy-making process itself: what policy is and how it is made, influenced, implemented and changed.

3.1 Understanding policy

Chapter 1 explored the nature of policy in a global context and came up with various definitions of the term 'policy'. On the one hand, policy may be seen as 'the authoritative statements of intent about action', with the assumption that 'as government has the ultimate authority to act, it is their policies which become a focus for debate and action' (Allsop, 1995). On the other hand, and just as plausibly, it can be argued that policy is the consequence of the actions taken by individuals in the process of implementation (Barrett and Fudge, 1981). The first definition emphasises that policy is deliberate, systematic and usually government led; the second highlights the potential for anyone at any level to be involved. It reminds us that 'policy' does not refer just to the latest government pronouncement, but also how it is put into practice and its intended and unintended consequences.

However, policies and policy making are not value free. It has been argued that a policy 'consists of a web of decisions and actions that allocate ... values' (Easton, 1953, p. 130). In an influential work on the politics of policy making, Easton highlighted the central importance of values. Values are those aspects which people regard as important, and they may be reflected in physical or symbolic goods and services. Policy, Easton suggested, is about 'the authoritative allocation of values' (Easton, 1953, p.136); in other words, is about the ability of those in positions of influence, at any level in or outside formal government, to sanction or withhold approval in relation to particular goods and services. For example, many surveys, such as the MORI poll (Ipsos MORI, 2006), have demonstrated that people in the UK attach great importance to retaining a national health service. Whichever health policies are enacted, politicians from all the major parties almost always make claims that they will make the National Health Service (NHS) more effective and give better value for money.

3.2 Who makes policy?

Thinking point: who is involved in making health policy?

As noted in Chapters 1 and 2, there is a difference between healthy public policy and health policy. Box 1.4 in Chapter 1 stated that 'healthy public policy' refers to placing 'health on the agenda of policy-makers in all sectors and at all levels, directing them to be aware of the health consequences of their decisions and to accept their responsibilities for health' (WHO, 1986, p. 2). In other words, it incorporates a broad range of policy across the entire spectrum, all of which may have an impact on health. 'Health policy' refers to the actions of governments that relate specifically to health and the healthcare services.

In terms of health policies, Ham (2004) has explored the relative influence of the Department of Health in England and the wider policy community in decision making. Although many of the organisational changes in healthcare have allegedly been introduced in order to give greater autonomy to hospital trusts and general practitioners, in fact policy is determined and delivered from the centre, as can be seen in the centralising role of the departments of health of the four nations of the UK and in the dominance of central government – for example, with regard to increasing the role of the private sector in healthcare provision. But the system is neither homogeneous nor even particularly well co-ordinated, and the personnel charged with bringing about change are themselves changing all the time: (fairly) transient politicians, generalist career administrators, and civil servants with a professional background may all have different interests to pursue.

Since 1999, certain elements of power have been devolved in Scotland, Wales and Northern Ireland. At the time of writing, the Scottish Parliament has greater powers than the Welsh Assembly, because of its ability to enact primary legislation. Scotland has a devolved legislature made up of the Scottish Executive, responsible for handling Scotland's day-to-day affairs, and the Scottish Parliament. The Scottish Executive is responsible for health, education, crime, housing and economic development. The UK government retains responsibility for employment, fiscal and economic policy, taxation, social security benefits, and pensions. In Wales, the Welsh Cabinet is the main decision-making body within the Assembly, and is responsible for education, environmental issues, local government finance, health and social services, rural affairs, culture and sport. In October 2002, devolution in Northern Ireland was suspended and powers previously held by the Northern Ireland Executive reverted to the Northern Ireland Office – including policy relating to health, social services and public safety. The different models of devolution have led to different NHS structures within the UK.

In addition to the national Departments of Health, the official policy community includes NHS bodies such as strategic health authorities and primary care trusts in England and Wales, health boards in Scotland, and combined health and social care boards in Northern Ireland. In recent years, the official health community responsible for policy development has been joined by a number of quasi-independent advisory bodies such as the National Institute for Health and Clinical Excellence (NICE) which is responsible for 'providing national guidance on promoting good health and preventing and treating ill health' (NICE, 2007).

At the next tier, powerful stakeholder or pressure groups have developed to pursue their sectional interests and attempt to influence policy as much as they are able. Examples of professional groups that will work to ensure their point of view is heard whenever policy is being developed include the British Medical Association (BMA, 2007) and the Royal College of Nursing (RCN, 2007). Single-issue pressure groups remain largely outside the official 'corridors of power' and will attempt to influence policy through a mixture of public pressure, criticism of official action and the use of research when this can be assembled. An example of this is Action on Smoking and Health (ASH, 2007), which attempts to develop increasingly rigorous policies to restrict the sale and use of tobacco. Commercial organisations will also attempt to influence policy in such a way as to promote their own interests. Much of this activity may be carried out behind the scenes, by lobbying or the formation of various alliances through sponsorship or hospitality initiatives. FOREST (2007), which campaigns on behalf of people who use tobacco, is an example of a commercial interest that has attempted to lobby for policies inimical to public health policy. This subject will be explored later in this chapter.

From time to time, specific issues are addressed by quasi-independent bodies in an attempt to balance the different views of all these disparate interest groups. Examples of this type of investigative body include Royal Commissions and inquiries such as the Acheson Inquiry into inequalities in health (Acheson, 1998), or the public inquiry, led by Professor Hugh Pennington, into the 2005 E. coli outbreak in Wales (E.coli Public Inquiry, 2006). The findings of such inquiries may be included, to greater or lesser extents, within future health-related policy directives.

The Healthcare Commission (formerly the Commission for Healthcare Audit and Inspection) is an independent body, set up to promote and drive improvement in the quality of healthcare and public health in England and Wales (Healthcare Commission, 2007). It has considerable influence, particularly in England.

In addition to all these official, quasi-official or established groups, there remains a role for campaigning or single-issue groups, which can become suddenly quite important players in the policy-making world. Activism at a local level can, on occasion, influence or subvert the best-laid official plans, and it is at this level that some public health practitioners might be able to act. An example of such activism is the 'Chuck Snacks off the Checkout!' campaign led by Parents Jury – a pressure group demanding healthy food for children. This campaign calls for supermarkets to stop appealingly displaying sweets and savoury snacks by the exit tills to encourage children (and adults) into last-minute buying (Food Commission, 2005).

Thinking point: are government policies always implemented as planned?

Although governments make plans and state intentions in legislation or regulation, this is only one part of the policy process. As they are implemented, policies become adapted and transformed into something rather different by the actions, inactions and priorities of other people. Indeed, Allsop (1995) suggests that what governments decide to do and what actually gets done are important to consider when making sense of the policy-making process.

It could be claimed that policy is action and that decisions are not always the way in which policy comes into being. A particular set of actions may be taken at grass-roots level to deal with a crisis – say, excessive pressure on community nursing staff during an influenza epidemic – and these become the accepted way of working. Management, which can see the benefits of the change, might then ratify the actions through formal decisions at a later stage, or the actions might simply become a part of what new entrants learn, when coming into the area, from those who have been in the job for some time. It would appear to be important to 'balance a decisional "top-down" perspective on policy with an action oriented "bottom-up" perspective. Actions as well as decisions may therefore be said to be the proper focus of policy analysis' (Ham, 2004, p. 115).

There are several stages in the making of a policy, and many opportunities for policy to change. A decision is not a policy, nor even an action, and the subsequent translation of a decision into action shifts the focus to other players. The people who make decisions in an attempt to create a policy are rarely the same as those who will implement the decisions. Ham (2004, p. 114) has commented that 'a decision network, often of considerable complexity, may therefore be involved in producing action and a web of decisions may form part of the network'. Conversely, policy makers rarely operate with a blank sheet. They are influenced and constrained by earlier decisions from other policy sectors as well as their own (Walt, 1994).

Some health-related policies appear to be driven by ideological imperatives that may override almost all other concerns and considerations. In recent times within the NHS, it appears that there has been an ideological thrust towards competition or 'contestability', which has the effect of increasing the involvement of the private sector in the NHS. This fits in well with similar New Labour initiatives in education, housing and many other government-controlled sectors that appear indistinguishable from previous Conservative policies. The theory is that the NHS and other state monopolies will benefit from the cut and thrust of the marketplace. With one part of the NHS competing against other parts, and against the private sector health providers, the NHS as a whole will become more efficient and provide more of what the general public wants, while at the same time becoming more cost-effective. Unfortunately, many of these initiatives have been introduced for ideological reasons and without much debate, and certainly without evidence that they will actually improve services or provide the much-heralded 'value for money'. Two specific areas in which policy of this type has been enacted are the introduction of independent sector treatment centres (ITCs) (Ruane, 2005), and the use of the private finance initiative (PFI) to build new hospital units (Pollock et al., 1999). ITCs were introduced as part of a programme of capital investment designed to perform elective (non-essential) surgery on a 'Fordist' model (a model based on standardised mass production). The private providers are guaranteed preferential contracts for certain operations, such as hip replacements, a fixed income that has the effect of putting additional financial pressure on cash-starved NHS facilities. Similarly, the way in which the private finance initiative has been introduced will ensure that the NHS is paying above the odds for the capital building for long into the future (Pollock et al., 1999).

Policies almost always change over time as other policies impact on them, as personnel change, and as political developments require changes of direction. The policy change in England and Wales over the use of Herceptin for breast cancer treatment is an example of this. As Allen has commented:

> the call by the health secretary, Patricia Hewitt, for local health trusts not to deny patients with early-stage breast cancer the drug Herceptin on cost grounds alone – even though it is licensed to treat only the advanced stage of the disease – has provoked legal challenges by women who have been refused the drug.
>
> (Allen, 2006)

After a high-profile campaign and positive clinical trials, NICE issued guidelines on the use of Herceptin for women with early stage HER2-positive breast cancer (NICE, 2006).

In 2006, the Scottish Medicines Consortium also issued guidelines on the use of Herceptin for patients with early stage breast cancer. Women in Northern Ireland have had access to the drug – where clinically appropriate – since 2005.

Policy analysts have also highlighted the importance of studying non-decision making, inaction and resistance, arguing that a focus on decision making has ignored the importance of 'more routine activities leading to policy maintenance and even inertia' (Ham, 2004, p. 114). An example of non-decision making is the inability of the relevant authorities and partners to decide on new hospital provision in Paddington, West London. Despite initial clinical need, the plan for the development of the Paddington Health Campus Scheme collapsed. The National Audit Office found several reasons for this, including the high costs, the lack of suitable land and the lack of strategic support (National Audit Office, 2006).

Thinking point: how might policies be sabotaged at the implementation stage?

You may be able to think of policies that people have attempted to implement and which were effectively sabotaged by the refusal to respond to others, often key people within an organisation, but perhaps quite junior members of the workforce. Sometimes situations arise where the outward form of a policy is implemented, but the intention of the policy is undermined or ignored.

3.3 The policy-making process

> Process refers to the way in which policies are initiated, developed
> or formulated, negotiated, communicated implemented and
> evaluated.
>
> (Buse et al., 2005, p. 13)

There have been many attempts to describe how policy is made, but most
analysts use a process approach in which four main stages are delineated:

1 agenda setting: problem identification and issue recognition
2 policy formulation: setting of alternatives, forecasting, appraisal,
   cost–benefit analysis
3 policy choice and implementation
4 evaluation.

(Adapted from Barker, 1996; Buse et al., 2005)

However, there is little agreement on how far this process is put into
operation as a set of deliberate, linear, systematic steps proceeding from
identification of a problem, to appraisal of options, to implementation and,
finally, to evaluation.

Two main perspectives prevail in the policy making process: a *rational
view* and an *incremental view*.

3.3.1 A rational view

The 'rational' view of policy making is often linked to the work of
Simon (1957) on decision making in organisations. This view would
suggest that policy makers start by identifying a problem and, using
guiding objectives and values, analyse the various alternatives for
dealing with it. Having assessed the various options and their relative
political and resource costs, policy makers choose the option that
maximises their objectives and values. But there is considerable
scepticism about whether this approach is feasible. In the first place,
problems are not discrete and cannot necessarily be dealt with in
isolation. For example, securing better primary care services or more
effective health promotion services is bound up with resource questions
about secondary care.

Second, policy makers may be less concerned about finding a rational
solution than a politically acceptable one. They are not likely to be wholly
objective in their assessment. Ideological considerations – for example,
about the superiority of 'free market' solutions and the wisdom of
deregulation – may mean that some policy options are ignored. Even if a
problem is relatively uncontentious, policy makers are unlikely to have
the time to gather and weigh up all the evidence. In relation to some

problems – for instance, global environmental concerns – conflicting evidence may mean that it might be impossible to be sure about what needs to be done.

Third, the rational view of policy making is dependent on 'expert' advice and available evidence. It suggests that if conclusive evidence is not available, an objective decision cannot be made. Finally, past decisions will influence the range of policy options available.

To summarise, the rational model assumes:

- accurate problem identification and isolation of the problem
- clear explication of goals, values and objectives
- identification of all the alternatives for addressing the issue
- rational and objective appraisal of each alternative
- selection of the most appropriate alternative to attain the goal.

(Adapted from Tones and Green, 2004, p. 185; Buse et al., 2005, p. 40)

3.3.2 An incremental view

Proponents of incrementalism have criticised the rational view as unrealistic and have argued that most policy change happens in a much more disjointed and piecemeal way. According to Buse et al. (2005, p. 14), for example, 'Policy making is seldom a rational process – it is iterative and affected by interests ... Many people agree with Lindblom (1959) that the policy process is one which policy makers "muddle through".' Lindblom (1959) used the phrase 'muddling through' – or 'incrementalism' – to describe much of policy analysis and change. He drew attention to incremental change, the inability to make clear decisions and the preference of most players to analyse policy problems one at a time, and to make minor adjustments rather than explore the whole policy framework. The features of incrementalism can be defined as:

- a blurring of the distinction between objectives and implementation, with objectives not clearly thought through
- appraisal of only a limited range of policy options
- a restricted analysis of these options and their consequences
- policy choice based on consensus rather than on systematic cost–benefit analysis
- acceptance of the remedial, incremental and temporary nature of any change.

This draws attention to the practical difficulties involved in any policy change: the weight of vested interests, organisational inertia and the problems of implementation that this raises. For example, Klein (1983) noted the policy inertia of the UK health service, which he argued arose from its occupational complexity and the distribution of power between the medical profession, the health authorities and the Department of Health. At times when more radical policy initiatives have been attempted, the outcomes have not always been very lasting or substantial (Harrison et al., 1990).

This happened in the late 1980s, when a radical analysis of UK healthcare resulted in attempts to carry through comprehensive rather than incremental policy change: the outcomes were not as dramatic as expected. The projected working of the internal market in healthcare was initially undermined by long-standing relationships between hospitals, health authorities and family doctors.

Critics of incrementalism argue that it is, at root, a conservative analysis – suggesting that it is acceptable to make small adjustments. This may be appropriate in a society in which there is a high degree of social stability, but it cannot adequately explain how more dramatic change can take place.

To summarise, the incremental view is characterised by:

- lack of a clear distinction between goals and the means of achieving them
- consideration of a restricted number of alternatives
- identification of the major consequences rather than all consequences
- no ideal policy option – the best option is the one that policy makers agree is the most appropriate
- achieving small changes to existing policy, rather than major change.

(Adapted from Tones and Green, 2004, p. 186, after Walt, 1994;
Buse et al., 2005, p. 42)

3.3.3 Mixed scanning

Thinking point: is one perspective more applicable than the other to policy making in health?

Both perspectives may be necessary. The rational view is really describing an ideal model of policy making – how it ought to be made – whereas the incremental view is describing what actually happens in the policy process and how policy is made in the real world (Buse et al., 2005, p. 41). The incremental view recognises that all the evidence may not be available, and usually the small adjustments made do not affect the status quo and can be easily adjusted in another direction. In 1967, Etzioni proposed mixed scanning as a compromise between a rational view and an incremental view. This still has resonance today. In this way, policy makers:

> concern themselves not just with everyday operational details, but also devote some of their energy to scanning the environment, both near and distant, for issues which might demand attention ... For fundamental decisions, policy makers should consider all the main alternatives for such choices, trying to eliminate those options which reveal crippling objections.
>
> (Collingridge and Douglas, 1984, pp. 362–3)

Critics of mixed scanning argue that, in reality, it adds nothing to incrementalism as policy makers do not have 'predictive powers' to be able scan problems on the horizon, and major decisions are still dependent on 'expert evidence' on which to make rational decisions (Collingridge and Douglas, 1984, pp. 362–3).

The role of evidence in policy making is of crucial importance. Health policy in practice continues to provide a mixture of those policies for which there is clear research evidence to substantiate change, and those for which other factors, such as ideology or political and economic imperatives, achieve dominance.

3.4 Influences on policy making

Governments have considerable power to set agendas and create policies, but an incrementalist perspective would suggest there are certain boundaries on policy change, created by the implications of past decisions, political pressures and the complexities of policy making itself. In addition, there is the question of how much influence can be exerted by the wider public, as opposed to the more influential members of the 'policy-making community'. An exploration of two models of policy making – pluralist (also known as consensus) and conflict – offers some answers to these questions.

3.4.1 A pluralist/consensus model

Figure 3.1 shows a simple model of policy making which begins to identify some of the main processes and stages. It is a systems theory or 'pluralist' approach; that is, it explores political activity as a series of processes which must be kept in balance, and it draws on biological frameworks to furnish the idea of interaction and interdependence (Easton, 1965). It pays attention to some central aspects of the policy process: the pressures on the political system from the wider environment and the feedback loop from outputs to inputs.

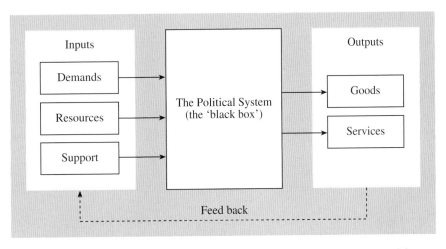

Figure 3.1   A simple systems approach to policy making (Source: adapted from Jones, 2002, p. 132, Figure 7.1)

'Demands' refer to pressures exerted by groups and individuals at all levels for some kind of change; for example, better services for people with AIDS/HIV. 'Resources' refer to natural, financial or human resources that enable governments to respond to demands. For example, a lack of people trained effectively in multidisciplinary public health work may mean that health targets will not be met. 'Support' refers to the extent to which the political system counts on wider public support to sustain it. If demands for action are overwhelming or if support for politicians, the constitution or policies dwindles because of a failure to meet demands, then the system becomes unstable. If outputs are not acceptable this creates greater pressures at the 'inputs' end of the process. Easton (1965) argues that, as a response, the political system will adapt and restabilise through policy or personnel changes. In the UK this is ultimately resolved by a general election, but before this happens, governments with very slender majorities may change their policies in order to maximise support.

On the other hand, it is clear that policy change is not that simple, and there are limits to this model. Easton's analysis is underpinned by a 'pluralist', essentially consensual conception of policy making. In other words, it assumes that all the players in the policy-making process are able to exert some influence and make their needs and demands felt. It assumes that the state is more or less even handed in the way it manages demands, balancing conflicting values and different interest groups. Others have drawn attention to the deficiencies in this analysis and have argued that only some powerful or insider groups may influence policy making; other groups may find their needs ignored (Earle et al., 2007). Not every group has the ability to articulate their needs; it is those groups better able to define their needs, express them in forms acceptable to professionals and then to muster support from influential groups to have those needs met that will be successful in changing policy.

Thinking point: can you think of any groups that currently find it difficult to influence policy making?

Marginalised groups in current policy making would include those people who are homeless or unemployed. Many are not on electoral rolls and cannot express their needs; coming together to press for change is very difficult. Governments can argue that there is no evidence of support for policy change and therefore no need to act, or, as in the case of unemployed people, it may cut their benefit and entitlements. Others are also unable to make their voices heard: those in prison, for example, or those with mental health problems.

3.4.2 A conflict model

Almost all public health issues have traditionally involved competing interests, and policy has been determined through greater or lesser conflict between these interest groups. For example, the tobacco industry, as will be discussed later, has interests that are not compatible with those groups concerned to stop the harmful effects of smoking. Most of the ways in which the health of the public could be improved will potentially involve the restriction or curtailment of the activities of some other sectional interest: for example, road safety involves control over vehicular road users; the nation's nutritional intake will not be improved without some form of restriction over the ways in which harmful foods are produced, advertised and marketed. It is out of these tensions and struggles between competing interests that public health policy emerges. The shape of a policy will necessarily reflect the comparative strengths of the various combatant groups. A 'conflict' model of public health policy development therefore exposes the limits of the pluralist/consensual model and argues that the realpolitik of policy making can be fraught with complexity and political manoeuvrings.

Health promotion and public health interests from the 1960s to the mid-1980s were characterised by a focus on the (possibly harmful) behaviours of individuals. The health education message was predominately aimed at individuals who were exhorted to stop smoking, to eat sensibly and to indulge only in safe sexual practices. Conflict during that time was largely channelled into individualised concerns.

With the development of what has come to be known as the 'new public health era' (Ashton and Seymour, 1988; Baum, 1998), public health has deliberately entered the political arena. This new political realism was apparent at all levels of public health activity. The World Health Organization (WHO) policies, especially the Alma Ata Declaration of Health for All (WHO, 1978) and the Ottawa Charter (WHO, 1986), which have been discussed earlier in this book, led the way for public health to enter explicitly political waters. At national and local levels it also became increasingly apparent that health-enhancing policies were inherently political, and the necessary conflicts with powerful interest groups would have to be engaged with. The new public health movement prided itself on its involvement in those political spheres that could have an effect on the health of the nation.

There are many interest groups that would like to be involved in the shaping of public health policy; for example, professional organisations, health workers and their unions, commercial interests, and consumer groups. Rather in the same way that the influence of such groups grows and then recedes in wider society, these various interests have greater or lesser involvement in the determination of health policy at various historical stages. For example, the power of trade unions has diminished since the days of 'beer and sandwiches' at Downing Street, and they seem considerably marginalised in contemporary political life. Similarly, their influence on recent public health policy has shrunk such that their ability to influence the shape of major health 'reforms' is hard to ascertain.

The power and influence of some other specific interest groups, such as the medical profession, has similarly ebbed and flowed. The medical profession has historically been involved in the conflicts that have arisen in the production of public health policies. Although the interests of the entire medical profession can hardly be characterised as a homogeneous entity, it could be considered that they represent what has come to be known as the 'medical model'. This focus on disease and illness has, on occasion, spilt over into the public health arena. For example, the Health of the Nation strategy in England (DoH, 1992) seems to have been heavily influenced by a medical agenda. The targets set were concerned largely with disease reduction rather than with more holistic or community-oriented goals. More recently, it could be argued that the power of the medical profession in determining public health policy has been serious eroded. Successive reorganisations of the NHS have left public health practitioners within health authorities and primary care organisations increasingly unsure of their role. Their specific public health functions have been largely subsumed into more general managerial tasks, and individual directors of public health have been unable to create a power base from which to exert their authority. David Hunter, a professor of health policy and management, takes the view that: 'Since the New Labour government was first elected in 1997, four major NHS "redisorganisations" have occurred, culminating in the changes currently weakening the service further and which are arguably the most far reaching in its history' (Hunter, 2006, p. 503).

In the 1970s, 'corporatism' was a marked feature of policy making (Cawson, 1982). Corporatism highlighted the incorporation of the most powerful interest groups, such as trade unions and employers' groups, into policy making. From being outsiders influencing policy and making demands, some groups became insiders, enmeshed in the policy process. In the 1980s, when managerialism became the vogue in the UK health sector, hospital doctors were generally successful at protecting their own conditions of service and privileges (Cox, 1991). Only in the 1990s, as the internal market system came more fully into effect via the purchaser–provider split and fund holding, did doctors find their influence challenged to a greater extent by managers. Managers (and to some extent politicians) became more influential in health policy making, and the increasing involvement of a health sector market has signalled a change of priorities, further reducing medical power over decision making.

Conflict theorists draw attention to the 'closure' that can be created by powerful insider groups. In other words, politicians and officials may tend to create their own agenda and not respond to outside demands (Ham, 2004). Politicians – for example, those at the Department of Health and those even nearer to central government – remain critically involved in the overall direction of public health policy. The role of these politicians is to create the environment in which their policies will be accepted without excessive conflict. For this reason, they have used various reorganisations and restructuring processes to decrease the power of many of the interest groups (including public health doctors), which may previously have been involved in the creation of public health policy (Ham, 2004).

There is considerable evidence of this in relation to the direction of recent health policies. For example, there is not much evidence that the shift to the creation of a market system in the UK NHS was the result of demands for change coming from within the health sector itself or from the wider public. Indeed, the 'crisis' of healthcare could be considered to be a cash crisis arising from under-funding, rather than a management or organisational crisis. This 'crisis', however, has been used as a rationale for the introduction of 'market forces' and private sector initiatives into the NHS.

It has been suggested that the notion of 'bounded pluralism' may best describe this conflict between policy-making levels and agendas (Hall, 1975). With this approach, insider or elite groups may be able to screen out sensitive issues at national level and use the state to serve their own ideological interests, but this is compatible with accepting more open debate about less politically dangerous issues. Analysts have identified mainly economic issues as the 'high' politics over which the political elite keeps control, whereas in particular policy fields there may be quite wide debate (Walt, 1994).

The next section is based on a case-study that relates to the introduction of tobacco policy. This is an example where the conflict model can easily be applied. However, it is also an illustration of the way in which conflict and potential conflict have been exported, away from the central, ideological areas of particular government concern. Central government has become adept at reorganising the structures of the NHS to remove or incorporate potential arenas of conflict and restrict the power of those, previously influential, groups that might challenge the policy imperatives that they themselves have determined.

3.5 A case-study of smoking policy

The development of smoking policy in the UK represents an example of the way in which public health policy is determined, over time, by the battle between various competing interests. Some of the interest groups involved in smoking-related policy making can be clearly observed in their effort to impose their views on government, while other factors remain less visible, but possibly equally influential.

Thinking point: which interest groups do you think are the major players in the struggle to influence government opinion in relation to tobacco-controlling legislation?

Obviously, there is a direct conflict between people representing the sectional interests of the tobacco industry and those involved in attempting to improve the health of the nation. In some respects, it is the task of governmental policy makers to draw up legislation that balances these various interest groups. The incremental introduction of tobacco-controlling legislation could be seen to represent changes in the balance of forces between competing groups. And, of course, the political complexion of the government makes a difference. Each government in turn will tend to be influenced by those arguments that reinforce its own political ideology. Thus, during times of greater centralised government control over individual behaviour, public health arguments will tend to dominate legislative changes. Those governments with an ideological stance favouring 'individual freedoms' and laissez-faire attitudes towards the control of financial markets in particular will allow the tobacco industry more freedom to pursue its own goals.

Virginia Berridge (2003) has described a chronology that relates to smoking policy in the UK since the Second World War. In the first phase, during the 1950s and 1960s, there remained a cultural acceptance of smoking and, although initial epidemiological evidence was emerging that demonstrated the harmful nature of tobacco, the government remained uncertain about turning this research work into policy. During this phase, the tobacco industry was especially active in its attempts to undermine the 'science' behind the links between tobacco smoking and illhealth. During the second phase, the 1970s, the government became more convinced of public health benefits of tobacco control and based its policies on the reduction of harm from smoking and the development of voluntary agreements between government and industry. During this phase, a more activist stance was being taken by some public health advocates who were determined to paint the tobacco industry as villains whom they considered to be aided by a largely sympathetic media.

From the 1980s, the concept of 'passive smoking' emerged as a major force that contributed to the strengthening of government resolve to introduce tighter controls over the harmful effects of tobacco smoking, particularly in the workplace environment and public places.

Figure 3.2 shows some of the most important policy developments that reflect the way in which successive governments have attempted to control the harmful effects of tobacco consumption.

Figure 3.2 UK government action on smoking and health: a summary	
1965	Television advertising of cigarettes banned
1971	First voluntary agreement with tobacco companies not to sponsor sports events aimed at those aged under eighteen Requirement for cigarette packets and all advertising to carry health warnings
1977	Government circular advising health authorities on tobacco control
1985	Voluntary agreement on stopping advertising in teenage magazines
1986	Poster advertisements visible from schools banned
1991	50 per cent voluntary reduction in shop front advertising Shop front advertising to carry health warnings
1992	Health of the Nation sets target for one-third reduction in adult smoking by the year 2000 European directive that all tobacco products must be labelled 'tobacco seriously damages your health'
1993	All NHS premises to introduce no-smoking policies Revised GP contract targets health checks and support for those wishing to quit smoking
1996	Voluntary ban on shop front advertising of tobacco products and requirement to display 'no sales to under 16s' in retail premises
1998	*Smoking Kills* (DoH, 1998) – a White Paper on tobacco
1999	*Saving Lives: Our Healthier Nation* (DoH, 1999) sets out targets for the reduction of cancer and coronary heart disease and stroke by 2010
2003	All forms of tobacco advertising and promotion banned in the UK with the exception of limited advertising at point of sale Tobacco sponsorship of domestic sporting events banned
2004	Republic of Ireland full ban on smoking in public places
2005	*Choosing Health Delivery Plans* (DoH, 2005) – ban on tobacco sponsorship of international events such as Formula One motor racing All estates of Welsh Assembly become smoke free
2006	Scotland full ban on smoking in public places
2007	Full ban on smoking in public places: Northern Ireland from April Wales from April England from July

3.5.1 Wider policy concerns

The ways in which governments are able to act in order to control tobacco consumption are not confined to specific public health legislation such as those measures outlined in Figure 3.2. Policy in other fields will also influence the amount of tobacco that is used within society. For example, the taxation that is added to tobacco products seems to be crucial in determining the amount of tobacco that is consumed. Figure 3.3 shows that, as the total price of cigarettes increases, people are more inclined to give up their habit, and young people especially seem to be deterred from establishing a habit (Jha and Chaloupka, 1999). As Joossens and Raw have noted: 'According to the World Bank, price increases are the most effectiveand cost effective tobacco control measure, especially for youngpeople and others on low incomes, who are highly price responsive. A price rise of 10% decreases consumption by about 4% in high-incomecountries' (Joossens and Raw, 2006, p. 247).

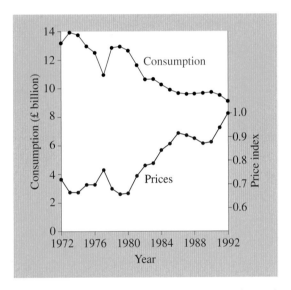

Figure 3.3   Relation between consumption (pounds sterling billion at 1992 prices) and real price (1992 index = 1.0, used here as the comparator) of cigarettes in Britain during 1972–92 (Source: Townsend et al., 1994, Figure 1)

However, for governments this is not a simple issue and they will be keen not to alienate significant sectors of their electorate by imposing punitive taxation. In addition, geographical variations between different countries in the price of tobacco products may lead to the emergence of smuggling (Wiltshire et al., 2001), and even to the growth of organised crime involved in the international movements of tobacco products (Jamrozik, 2006).

Research in fields other than public health can also be used to help influence government policy with regard to tobacco-controlling legislation. For example, the fear that considerable job losses would be involved in the decline of the British tobacco industry has been countered effectively by economic research that has demonstrated that job losses in the tobacco industry have been largely attributable to automation (Joffe and Mindell, 2004). Additionally, because cigarette production is not labour intensive, money spent by ex-smokers on their new pursuits generates more employment than that previously required to make cigarettes. Buck et al. (1995) estimate that a 40 per cent reduction in tobacco consumption would create about 150,000 jobs in the UK.

3.5.2 Behind the scenes

The development of government policies designed to restrict the consumption of tobacco products could be considered to be reasonably rational and incremental, with sociological and epidemiological research findings apparently leading to new, increasingly restrictive legislation. However, behind the scenes the various interest groups are continuing to engage in a wide range of activities designed to influence smoking behaviour directly and government legislation in particular.

Thinking point: in what ways do you think the tobacco industry acts in order to slow down or subvert government activity that may introduce tobacco-control policies?

The tobacco industry

The tobacco industry continues to use considerable imagination and immense economic power in order to undermine the efforts of those who would wish to control tobacco consumption for public health reasons. Various tobacco company records have come into the public domain through whistleblowers and, more recently, as a result of litigation (Lee et al., 2004). These documents revealed a long history of attempts by the tobacco industry to cast doubt on the links between their products and illhealth: 'The documents revealed '*decades of deceit*' (Ciresi et al., 1999), including the tobacco industry's awareness and manipulation of nicotine addiction, overt targeting of young people and women, involvement in smuggling and extensive and often covert efforts to undermine tobacco control across the globe' (Lee et al., 2004, p. 394, emphasis added). This subversive tobacco industry activity has continued in recent years when the link between passive smoking and disease continues to be challenged, perhaps because of its central importance in the public health debate (Muggli et al., 2003).

As controls are introduced over more overt forms of tobacco advertising, the industry has become increasingly skilful at exploiting loopholes and creating associations between healthy products and tobacco-related brand names.

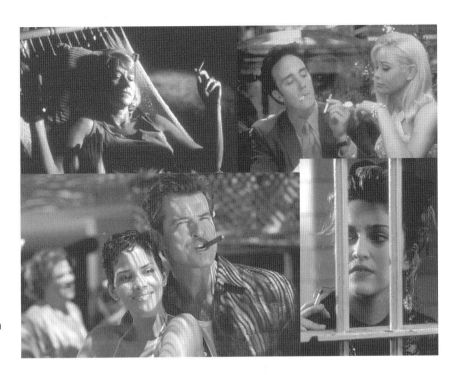

Figure 3.4 Smoking seems prevalent in Hollywood films and remains associated with wholesome activities and 'clean' actors

Health activists

In response to the continued activities by the powerful tobacco companies, health activists have needed to be imaginative and resourceful in their attempts to influence both public opinion and those people responsible for legislation and health policy development. In the 1970s and 1980s, when cigarette advertising was largely conducted on outside advertising hoardings, several influential campaigns (see Figure 3.5), were led by a group of Australian doctors calling themselves 'BUGA-UP' (Billboard Utilising Graffitists Against Unhealthy Promotions). Adbusters (Figure 3.6) have a wider agenda and as part of their campaign 'to advance the new social activist movement of the information age', they have developed a series of spoof advertisements on a range of issues including tobacco use (Adbusters, 2007).

More recently, national and international health campaigns have become increasingly sophisticated in their enterprises, and campaigning groups such as Action on Smoking and Health (ASH, 2007) have developed a wide range of activities that are aimed at members of the general public as well as health promotion activists. They also target their action towards health policy makers in an attempt to ensure that existing legislation is implemented and, wherever necessary, sponsor new legislation to counteract tobacco company initiatives that continue to promote increasing consumption.

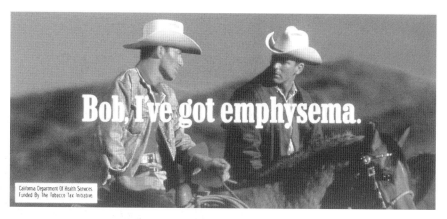

Figure 3.5   The 'BUGA-UP' paint bombers from Australia were instrumental in bringing important anti-smoking health messages to the fore

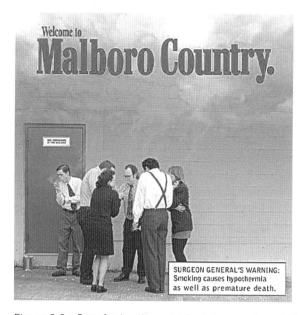

Figure 3.6   Spoof advertisement for tobacco, from Adbusters

3.5.3 Social differentials and tobacco control policies

Figure 3.7 shows the social class distribution of cigarette smoking in the UK and the changes that occurred during the years between 1973 and 1993.

Thinking point: what social features do you think are demonstrated by the data presented in Figure 3.7?

People from the poorest social groupings appear to smoke much more than those people who come from more affluent groups. In addition, the reduction in smoking prevalence over the years 1973 to 1993 occurred to the greatest extent in the more affluent groups.

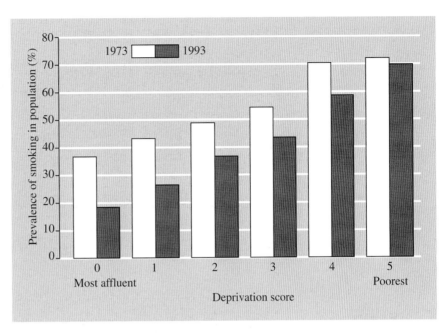

Figure 3.7   Cigarette smoking by deprivation level in Great Britain. Data from General Household Survey (Source: Edwards, 2004, p. 217)

Policies designed to reduce the consumption of tobacco products would appear to be most effective if they are aimed at people from the least affluent groups within society (Wanless, 2003). However, Graham et al. point out that, in addition to any policies designed to change smoking habits, attention will have to be paid to the social inequalities that may be responsible for the high levels of smoking: 'However, it is possible that improved messages and more interventions are not enough [to encourage lower socio-economic groups to stop smoking]: that the barriers lie in the social disadvantages to which recipients are exposed' (Graham et al., 2006, p. ii11).

3.5.4 International activity and tobacco regulation

The success of governmental control policies to restrict tobacco consumption in developed countries, such as the UK, has led tobacco companies to redouble their efforts to increase their sales in developing countries (Sebrié and Glanz, 2006). This has resulted in a rise in sales of cigarettes in developing countries and other emerging markets such as China, Uzbekistan (Gilmore et al., 2006) and Mexico (Samet et al., 2006), which in turn leads to an increase in health inequalities between rich and poor countries. Figure 3.8 shows the predicted number of deaths attributed to smoking in the developed and the developing world. As Sebrié and Glanz (2006, p. 313) have observed: 'Unlike mosquitoes, another vector of worldwide disease, the tobacco companies quickly transfer the information and strategies they learn in one part of the world to others.'

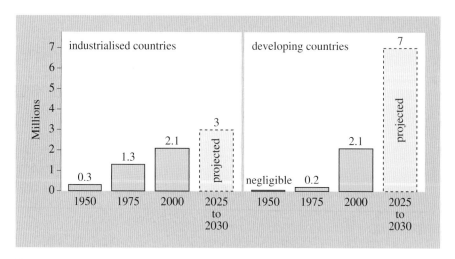

Figure 3.8   Past and future: annual deaths due to tobacco, estimated, worldwide (1950–2030 projected) (Source: MacKay and Eriksen, 2002 p. 36)

Thinking point: how do you think internationally co-ordinated policy could help to curb tobacco consumption?

The Framework Convention on Tobacco Control

The tobacco industry has become increasing adept at sidestepping controls and restrictions on advertising and promotion, as well as countering other public health controls over their activities (Sebrié and Glanz, 2006). Tobacco advertising that targets women and children in developing countries has been increasing, as has the use of tobacco logos on other products such as clothes, shop fronts and computer games – a practice called 'brand stretching'. In order to create international policies and controls that might be able to protect individual nations from the power of multinational tobacco companies, the World Health Organization has been responsible for the development of the WHO Framework Convention on Tobacco Control (FCTC) (WHO, 2003).

The Framework Convention on Tobacco Control (FCTC) is the first global health treaty and came into force in February 2005. Participation in the FCTC process has been strongly supported by many governments and by 180 non-governmental organisations (NGOs). By June 2004, 131 countries had signed the treaty and twenty-one had ratified it, but, crucially, not the USA. This fits a wider pattern. At the time of writing, the USA had signed but not ratified a range of treaties, including the Convention on the Rights of the Child, the Convention on Biological Diversity, the Kyoto Protocol, the International Criminal Court, and the

Convention on the Elimination of all Forms of Discrimination Against Women. Box 3.1 looks at the process involved in creating the FCTC.

Box 3.1 The process of creating the Framework Convention on Tobacco Control

The process of creating the FCTC was an attempt to tackle powerful vested interests within the tobacco industry as well as the International Tobacco Growers' Association. In May 2003, the text of the FCTC was agreed after almost four years of negotiation by the member states of the World Health Organization.

The process of deciding on the wording of the treaty was predictably polarised, with 'Big Tobacco' (industry) pitted against public health activists and scientists – while both sides attempted to influence the negotiating position of member states. Whereas the text of the FCTC provides the basis for national legislation among ratifying countries, the process highlights the important role that global civil society can play in international health forums, as well as its limits. Carter (2002) describes some of the ways in which the tobacco industry attempted to destroy the treaty 'from the inside', while other NGOs (see, for example, Infact, 2004) have criticised the persistent way in which the USA government, appearing to act on behalf of the vested interests of the tobacco industry, attempted to weaken the treaty at all stages of the negotiation. Interested NGOs with 'consultative status' at the WHO participated formally, but in a circumscribed manner (i.e. no voting), in the negotiation process – although were able to use this status to lobby official delegations.

The WHO hosted public hearings in relation to the Convention at which many civil society organisations provided testimony and written statements, while others, such as the Campaign for Tobacco Free Kids and ASH, provided an educative function (see, for example, White, 2004). These campaigning groups organised seminars, prepared briefings for delegates on technical aspects of the Convention and issued a daily news bulletin on the proceedings. In addition, the NGO campaigning groups acted as the public health conscience during the negotiations.

For example, some NGOs drew attention to the obstructionist positions of some member states and industry tactics – often in a colourful manner, such as that shown in Figure 3.10, illustrating the 'Orchid Awards' which were given to the delegation deemed to have made the most positive contribution on the previous day, and the 'Dirty Ashtray' award given to the most destructive. Individuals working for civil society organisations were, on some occasions, able to participate directly in the negotiations through their inclusion in national delegations. Over the course of the negotiations, global civil society organizations became a more powerful lobbying force through the formation of a Framework Convention Alliance which sought to improve communication between groups directly involved in systematically outreaching to smaller groups in developing countries. The Alliance thus provided a bridge to national level actions which involved lobbying, letter writing, policy discussions, advocacy campaigns and press conferences before and after meetings.

(Adapted from Collin et al., 2002)

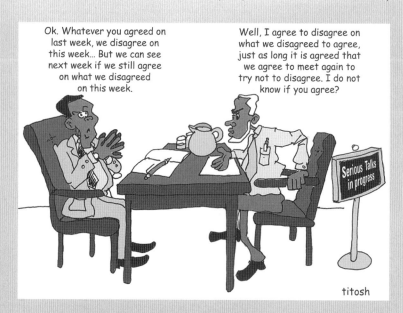

Figure 3.9   The process that led to the Framework Convention on Tobacco Control was a good example of the conflict model of public health policy making

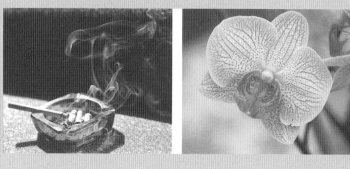

Figure 3.10   The Orchid Awards

Conclusion

Public health policy is not only about decision taking and policy enactment. It is also about making change, and this involves policy implementation. Several differing models and views influence the policy-making process.

The case-study on smoking policy has shown how public health policy development can be complex and political, with several stakeholders holding conflicting positions.

Public health practitioners can play a significant part in the policy process through joining pressure groups and campaigns, through their membership of professional bodies which educate policy making, help to set agendas and lobby for change, and through exercising their rights as citizens.

People involved in promoting public health, whether they are professional or lay, and whether they work within or outside the health sector, can have considerable influence on the later stages of the policy-making process – in particular on implementation, evaluation and policy review. The enactment of policy does not mean that it is necessarily translated into action. Quite often this requires the commitment of people in the organisation to push the policy through and make it work. Looking for opportunities to endorse and support policies promoting public health, and to modify policies that might damage health, can be part of any multidisciplinary public health practitioner's role. Forging partnerships for health and collaborating with other practitioners to achieve change can further extend success. Settings are also key to the success of policy implementation. This will be explored further in the next chapter, which will look at organisational development and settings for promoting healthy public policy.

References

Acheson, D. (1998) *Independent Inquiry into Inequalities and Health* (The Acheson Report), London, The Stationery Office.

Action on Smoking and Health (ASH) (2007) [online], http://www.ash.org.uk/ (Accessed 9 January 2007).

Adbusters (2007) *About Adbusters: The Media Foundation* [online], http://adbusters.org/network/about_us.php (Accessed 9 January 2007).

Allen, J. (2006) 'Rationing is only rational', *Guardian Unlimited*, 25 April [online], http://www.guardian.co.uk/medicine/story/0,,1761029,00.html#article_continue (Accessed 9 January 2007).

Allsop, J. (1995) *Health Policy and the NHS: Towards 2000*, London, Longman.

Ashton, J. and Seymour, H. (1988) *The New Public Health*, Buckingham, Open University Press.

Barker, C. (1996) *The Health Care Policy Process*, London, Sage.

Barrett, S. and Fudge, C. (eds) (1981) *Policy and Action: Essays on the Implementation of Public Policy*, London, Methuen.

Baum, F. (1998) *The New Public Health: An Australian Perspective*, Melbourne, Oxford University Press.

Berridge, V. (2003) 'Post-war smoking policy in the UK and the redefinition of public health', *Twentieth Century British History*, vol. 14, no. 1, pp. 61–82.

British Medical Association (BMA) (2007) [online], http://www.bma.org.uk/homepage.nsf (Accessed 9 January 2007).

Buck, D., Godfrey, C., Raw, M. and Sutton, M. (1995) *Tobacco and Jobs*, York, University of York, The Society for the Study of Addiction and the Centre for Health Economics.

Buse, K., Mays, N. and Walt, G. (2005) *Making Health Policy*, Maidenhead, Open University Press.

Carter, S. (2002) 'Mongoven, Biscoe & Duchin: destroying tobacco control activism from the inside', *Tobacco Control*, vol. 11, no. 2, pp. 112–18.

Cawson, A. (1982) *Corporatism and Welfare: Social Policy and State Intervention in Britain,* London, Heinemann.

Ciresi, M., Walburn, R. and Sutton, T. (1999) 'Decades of deceit: document discovery in the Minnesota Tobacco Litigation', *William Mitchell Law Review*, vol. 25, pp. 477–566.

Collin, J., Lee, K. and Bisell, K. (2002) 'The framework convention on tobacco control: the politics of global health governance', *Third World Quarterly*, vol. 23, no. 2, pp. 265–82.

Collingridge, D. and Douglas, J. (1984) 'Three models of policymaking: expert advice in the control of environmental lead', *Social Studies of Science*, vol. 14, no. 3, pp. 343–70.

Cox, D. (1991) 'Health service management – a sociological view: Griffiths and the non-negotiated order of the hospital' in Gabe, J., Calnan, M. and Bury, M. (eds) *The Sociology of the Health Service*, London, Routledge.

Department of Health (DoH) (1992) *The Health of the Nation: A Strategy for Health in England*, London, HMSO.

Department of Health (DoH) (1998) *Smoking Kills*, London, The Stationery Office.

Department of Health (DoH) (1999) *Saving Lives: Our Healthier Nation*, London, The Stationery Office.

Department of Health (DoH) (2005) *Choosing Health Delivery Plans*, London, The Stationery Office.

E.coli Public Inquiry (2006) [online], http://www.ecoliinquirywales.org/ (Accessed 9 January 2007).

Earle, S., Lloyd, C.E., Sidell, M. and Spurr, S. (eds) (2007) *Theory and Research in Promoting Public Health*, London, Sage/Milton Keynes, The Open University.

Easton, D. (1953) *The Political System*: *An Inquiry into the State of Political Science*, New York, Knopf.

Easton, D. (1965) *A Systems Analysis of Political Life*, New York, Wiley.

Edwards, R. (2004) 'The problem of tobacco smoking', *British Medical Journal*, vol. 328, pp. 217–19.

Etzioni, A. (1967) 'Mixed scanning: a "third approach" to decision making', *Public Administration Review*, vol. 27, no. 5, pp. 385–92.

Ewles, L. and Simnett, I. (2003) *Promoting Health: A Practical Guide* (5th edn), Edinburgh, Baillière Tindall.

Food Commission (2005) *Checkouts Still Failing the Junk Test* [online], http://www.foodcomm.org.uk/latest_chucksnacks_jan05.htm (Accessed 9 January 2007).

FOREST (2007) [online], http://www.forestonline.org/output/Page1.asp (Accessed 9 January 2007).

Gilmore, A., Collin, J. and McKee, M. (2006) 'British American tobacco's erosion of health legislation in Uzbekistan', *British Medical Journal*, vol. 332, pp. 355–8.

Graham, H., Inskip, H.M., Francis, B. and Harman, J. (2006) 'Pathways of disadvantage and smoking careers: evidence and policy implications', *Journal of Epidemiology and Community Health*, vol. 60 (Suppl. II), pp. ii7–ii12.

Hall, P. (1975) *Change, Choice and Conflict in Social Policy*, London, Heinemann.

Ham, C. (2004) *Health Policy in Britain: The Politics and Organisation of the National Health Service* (5th edn), London, Palgrave Macmillan.

Harrison, S., Hunter, D.J. and Pollitt, C. (1990) *The Dynamics of British Health Policy*, London, Unwin.

Healthcare Commission (2007) [online], http://www.healthcarecommission.org.uk (Accessed 9 January 2007).

Hunter, D.J. (2006) Review, 'The New NHS: a guide', *British Medical Journal*, vol. 333, p. 503.

Infact (2004) *NGOs Call For Decisive Action to Ensure Strong Implementation of Global Tobacco Treaty* [online], http://www.infact.org/062104iwg.html (Accessed 9 January 2007).

Ipsos MORI (2006) *What State Are We In?* [online], http://www.ipsos-mori.com/publications/bp/what-state-are-we-in.shtml (Accessed 20 February 2007).

Jamrozik, K. (2006) 'Policy priorities for tobacco control' *British Medical Journal*, vol. 328, pp. 1007–9.

Jha, P. and Chaloupka, F.J. (1999) *Curbing the Epidemic: Governments and the Economics of Tobacco Control.* Washington, DC, The World Bank.

Joffe, M. and Mindell, J. (2004) 'A tentative step towards healthy public policy', *Journal of Epidemiology and Community Health*, vol. 58, no. 12, pp. 966–8.

Jones, L. (2002) 'Making and changing public policy' in Jones, L., Sidell, M. and Douglas, J. (eds) *The Challenge of Promoting Health: Exploration and Action* (2nd edn), Basingstoke, Palgrave Macmillan/Milton Keynes, The Open University.

Joossens, L. and Raw, M. (2006) 'The tobacco control scale: a new scale to measure country activity', *Tobacco Control*, vol. 15, pp. 247–53.

Klein, R. (1983) *The Politics of the National Health Service*, London, Longman.

Lee, K., Gilmore, A. and Collin, J. (2004) 'Looking inside the tobacco industry: revealing insights from the Guilford Depository', *Addiction*, vol. 99, no. 4, pp. 394–7.

Lindblom, C. (1959) 'The science of muddling through', *Public Administration Review*, vol. 19, no. 2, pp. 79–88.

Lindblom, C. (1979) 'Still muddling, not yet through', *Public Administration Review*, vol. 39, no. 6, pp. 517–26.

MacKay, J. and Eriksen, M. (2002) *The Tobacco Atlas*, Geneva, World Health Organization.

Muggli, M., Hurt, R. and Blanke, D. (2003) 'Science for hire: a tobacco industry strategy to influence public opinion on second-hand smoke', *Nicotine and Tobacco Research*, vol. 5, no. 3, pp. 303–14.

National Audit Office (2006) *The Department of Health: The Paddington Health Campus Scheme*, London, The Stationery Office; also available online at http://www.nao.org.uk/publications/nao_reports/05-06/05061045.pdf (Accessed 2 March 2007).

National Institute for Health and Clinical Excellence (NICE) (2006) *2006/038 NICE Issues Final Guidance on Trastuzumab* [online], http://www.nice.org.uk/page.aspx?o=354932 (Accessed 4 September 2006).

National Institute for Health and Clinical Excellence (NICE) (2007) *Welcome to the National Institute for Health and Clinical Excellence* [online], http://www.nice.org.uk (Accessed 9 January 2007).

Pollock, A., Dunnigan, M., Gaffney, D., Price, D. and Shaul, J. (1999) 'The private finance initiative: planning the "new" NHS: downsizing for the 21st century', *British Medical Journal*, vol. 319, pp. 179–84.

Royal College of Nursing (2007) [online], http://www.rcn.org.uk (Accessed 9 January 2007).

Ruane, S. (2005) 'Evolution of independent sector treatment centres and their impact on the NHS' in Politics of Health Group, *UK Health Watch 2005: The Experience of Health in an Unequal Society*, London, Politics of Health Group; also available online at http://www.pohg.org.uk/support/downloads/ukhealthwatch-2005.pdf (Accessed 25 February 2007).

Samet, J., Wipfli, H., Perez-Padilla, R. and Yach, D. (2006) 'Mexico and the tobacco industry: doing the wrong thing for the right reason?', *British Medical Journal*, vol. 332, pp. 353–4.

Sebrié, E. and Glanz, S. (2006) 'The tobacco industry in developing countries', *British Medical Journal*, vol. 332, pp. 313–4.

Simon, H.A. (1957) *Administrative Behaviour* (2nd edn), New York, Macmillan.

Tones, K. and Green, J. (2004) *Health Promotion: Planning and Strategies*, London, Sage.

Townsend, J., Roderick, P. and Cooper, J. (1994) 'Cigarette smoking by socioeconomic group. Sex and age; effects of price, income and health publicity', *British Medical Journal*, vol. 309, pp. 923–7.

Walt, G. (1994) *Health Policy: An Introduction to Process and Power*, London, Zed.

Wanless, D. (2003) *Securing Good Health for the Whole Population: Population Health Trends*, London, HM Treasury.

White, A. (2004) 'Controlling big tobacco: the winning campaign for a global tobacco control treaty', *Multinational Monitor*, vol. 25, nos 1/2 [online], http://www.multinationalmonitor.com/mm2004/04jan-feb/jan-feb04corp1.html (Accessed 9 January 2007).

Wiltshire, S., Bancroft, A., Amos, A. and Parry, O. (2001) '"They're doing people a service" – qualitative study of smoking, smuggling and social deprivation', *British Medical Journal*, vol. 323, pp. 203–7.

World Health Organization (WHO) (1978) *Alma Ata Declaration*, Geneva, World Health Organization.

World Health Organization (WHO) (1986) *Ottawa Charter for Health Promotion*, Ottawa, World Health Organization.

World Health Organization (WHO) (2003) *Framework Convention on Tobacco Control*, Geneva, World Health Organization; also available online at http://www.who.int/ tobacco/framework/en/ (Accessed 9 January 2007).

Chapter 4

Organisations and settings for promoting public health

Mark Dooris and David J. Hunter

Introduction

Promoting public health in settings and organisations, such as schools and workplaces, is an important, though often neglected, area. Yet, organisations can be a significant and productive focus for public health planning and delivery. Social systems – whether they are organisations, settings or whole communities – are able to deliver messages to individuals that can either reinforce or oppose health promotion messages. More importantly, however, they can have an impact on the determinants of health.

Syme (1996), among others, believes there is an urgent need for a paradigm shift in the conceptual framework and problem-solving strategies of public health. Above all, a paradigm shift must recognise that most health risks and the determinants of health are systemic and located within complex, dynamic and interactive social relationships which themselves are determined by social institutions and organisations, including families, communities, schools and workplaces. Such a change of paradigm requires the health of a population to be seen as integral to the impact of social systems on individuals, communities and societies. Crucially, the determinants of health are mediated through social systems, but are determined by social relationships within those systems. Within such diverse relationships, the exercise of power is a major feature since whoever, in a given situation, possesses the greater positional power determines the outcome. So, for example, the overall weakness of, and low priority attached to, occupational health in organisations, including the National Health Service (NHS), demonstrates the low value attached to it in terms of its contribution to developing a healthy workforce. Within many organisations public health is not accorded a high priority because it is not regarded as core business.

This chapter explores the role of organisations and settings in promoting public health. Building on previous chapters on global and national policies for public health, Section 4.1 provides an overview of what has become known as the 'settings approach'. In Section 4.2 the specific examples of prison, hospital and workplace settings are used to illuminate the development of the settings approach in relation to current policy and practice, which is then addressed in Section 4.3. The settings approach refers, basically, to the way in which organisations, such as schools, workplaces or hospitals, can promote the health and wellbeing of those involved in or affected by these organisations. This inevitably requires change and development within organisations. These issues are explored in Sections 4.4 and 4.5, together with the skills required to facilitate such change and development. The final section addresses some key contemporary issues and dilemmas for further debate.

4.1 The settings approach

A range of terminology has been used in relation to 'settings', as discussed by Whitelaw et al. (2001) and Tones and Green (2004). This includes 'settings for health', 'the settings approach', 'the settings-based approach', 'health-promoting settings' and 'healthy settings', alongside broader terms such as 'organisational development for health' and 'investment for health'. Although it is possible to identify semantic differences between terms such as 'health-promoting settings' and 'healthy settings' – the former more clearly suggesting a commitment to ensuring that the setting takes account of its external health impacts – they have increasingly been used interchangeably. In this chapter, the terms 'settings approach', 'settings' and 'organisations' are mainly used.

Thinking point: why is it important to focus on organisations and settings in promoting public health?

At a basic level, it has long been recognised that settings such as workplaces and schools provide an opportunity to target health messages and interventions at a specific audience. In this way, settings – together with population groups and health topics or problems – make up the matrix used to organise health education programmes concerned with encouraging individual health-related behaviour change. However, what has become known as the 'settings approach' moves beyond this mechanistic view of the carrying out of health education *in* a setting, recognising more broadly that the places and contexts in which people live their lives are crucially important in determining health and wellbeing.

The rationale for the settings approach is based on a recognition that health is largely determined outside of 'health' services and that effective health improvement requires investment in the social systems in which people spend their time and live their lives. The settings approach is seen as an important way of investing for health at a local level, with health being seen as an asset for and an outcome of the development and effective functioning of organisations (Grossman and Scala, 1993; Dooris et al., 1998).

The settings approach has developed since the mid-1980s to become a key element of public health strategy at local, national and international levels. In tracing the origins and evolution of the approach, it is important to recognise the role of international- and national-level policy drivers.

4.1.1 International-level policy context and development

The settings approach has its roots within the World Health Organization (WHO) Health for All strategy (WHO, 1980, 1981) and, more specifically, the Ottawa Charter for Health Promotion, which stated that: 'Health is created and lived by people within the settings of their everyday life; where they learn, work, play and love' (WHO, 1986, p. iii). As Kickbusch (1996) has reflected, the Ottawa Charter resulted in the settings approach becoming the starting point for the WHO's lead health promotion programmes, with a commitment to: 'shifting the focus from the deficit model of disease to the health potentials inherent in the social and institutional settings of everyday life ... [and] pioneer[ing] strategies that strengthened both sense of place and sense of self' (Kickbusch, 1996, p. 5).

Although it is important to acknowledge that most settings exist primarily for purposes not directly related to 'health', the WHO *Health Promotion Glossary* (WHO, 1998a) suggests that a 'setting for health' is:

> The place or social context in which people engage in daily activities in which environmental, organisational and personal factors interact to affect health and wellbeing. A setting is also where people actively use and shape the environment and thus create or solve problems relating to health. Settings can normally be identified as having physical boundaries, a range of people with defined roles, and an organisational structure.
>
> (WHO, 1998a, p. 19)

By the end of the 1990s, there were national and international programmes and networks covering settings as diverse as regions, cities, islands, schools, hospitals, workplaces, prisons and universities. This paved the way for settings to be included within the WHO *Health Promotion Glossary* (WHO, 1998a) and incorporated under Target 13 of the WHO's new European Health for All Policy Framework, Health 21 – which stated that 'by the year 2015, people in the region should have greater opportunities to live in healthy physical and social environments at home, at school, at the workplace and in the local community' (WHO, 1998b, p. 100). Although the *Bangkok Charter for Health Promotion in a Globalized World* (WHO, 2005a) does not give as high profile an endorsement to the settings approach as the Ottawa Charter and the *Jakarta Declaration on Leading*

Health Promotion into the 21st Century (WHO, 1997a), it highlights the role of settings in developing strategies for health promotion, the need for government to prioritise an integrated policy approach and to commit to working across settings, and the impact of the private sector on local settings. Box 4.1 gives an example of a 'Healthy Islands' development in the Western Pacific.

Box 4.1 Healthy Islands: Western Pacific

A vision for the development of Healthy Islands was first articulated in the Yanuca Declaration (WHO, 1995a), a response by the health ministers of fourteen Pacific island nations to the WHO Western Pacific Region's health policy framework, *New Horizons in Health* (WHO, 1995b). Reflecting a holistic and ecological model of health promotion, Healthy Islands are understood to be places where:

- children are nurtured in body and mind
- environments invite learning and leisure
- people work and age in dignity
- ecological balance is a source of pride
- the ocean which sustains us is protected.

(WHO, 2005b, p. 7)

Inspiring a range of diverse projects, this initial concept of Healthy Islands provided a potent catalyst for change, based on a commitment to community empowerment, capacity building and cultural sensitivity. In the 1997 Rarotonga Agreement (WHO, 1997b), ministers reaffirmed their commitment to the pursuit of Healthy Islands and outlined an emerging framework, whereby health promotion and health protection strategies, along with topic-specific programmes in the areas of environmental management (community action, and policy and infrastructure development) are co-ordinated both across the overarching island setting and within smaller settings, such as villages, schools, workplaces and markets.

More recent developments have sought to respond to the specific internal and external challenges (e.g. AIDS, global warming, pollution) facing Pacific island communities in the twenty-first century, which themselves reflect their vulnerability to environmental and socio-economic change. Importantly, these developments have taken place within the framework provided by Healthy Islands – with an emphasis on creating supportive environments through the implementation of healthy settings initiatives; on policy development at village, city, district and island nation levels; and on education, training and workforce development (Galea et al., 2000).

4.1.2 National-level policy context and development

Within England, settings received some legitimation in the early 1990s through the Conservative Government's strategy for health as set out in *The Health of the Nation* (DoH, 1992), which encouraged joint action in a range of settings where people live and work. The Labour Government's Green Paper, *Our Healthier Nation* (DoH, 1998), indicated a strong endorsement of the approach. Although this explicit commitment was weakened in *Saving Lives*, the subsequent White Paper (DoH, 1999), there was still an acknowledgement of the value of the approach for improving health and reducing inequalities – with specific reference to healthy schools, healthy workplaces and healthy neighbourhoods. More recently, although the English White Paper *Choosing Health: Making Healthy Choices Easier* (DoH, 2004a) makes no explicit commitment to the settings approach as a whole, there is a strong recognition of the importance for health settings in which people live, learn, work and play. Box 4.2 summarises the concept of 'Healthy Schools'.

Box 4.2 Healthy Schools: England

The concept of the health-promoting school was developed by the WHO in the 1980s, and the European Network of Health Promoting Schools (ENHPS) was launched in 1992 by the WHO's European Regional Office, the Council of Europe and the European Commission. The ENHPS is a strategic programme for the European Region. It is supported by the Council of Europe, the European Commission and WHO/Europe. It seeks to integrate the policy and practice of the health-promoting school into the wider health and education sectors. It works at three levels: school, national and international.

In England, the government's commitment to promoting health among young people resulted in the establishment, in 1998, of the National Healthy Schools Programme. Based on the premise that healthier children perform better academically and that education plays an important role in promoting health, the programme has four strategic aims:

1   to support children and young people in developing healthy behaviours

2   to help raise pupil achievement

3   to help reduce health inequalities

4   to help promote social inclusion.

National Healthy School status (DoH, 2005b) requires schools to meet criteria in four core themes, using a whole-school approach:

1   personal, social and health education (including sex and relationship education and drug education)

2   healthy eating

3   physical activity

4   emotional health and wellbeing.

Using the school improvement process of consultation, needs identification, target setting, action, monitoring and evaluation, this whole-school approach requires schools to consider the following aspects when implementing healthy schools themes: leadership, management and change; policy development; curriculum; teaching and learning; school culture and environment; pupil voice; staff development, health and welfare; partnership with parents/carers and local communities; and assessing, recording and reporting pupils' achievement.

Schools are supported in the process by their local healthy schools programme, co-ordinated by a partnership between the primary care trust (PCT) and local authority, which receives annual funding from the DoH and DfES to support their work.

The government's commitment has more recently been reinforced by the inclusion within *Choosing Health* (DoH, 2004a) of a national target for half of all schools in England to be healthy schools by December 2006, with the remaining schools working towards becoming healthy schools by 2009.

In addition, the importance of the programme is highlighted in the *Five Year Strategy for Children and Learners* (DfES, 2004b), the *National Service Framework for Children, Young People and Maternity Services* (DoH, 2004b) and *Every Child Matters* (DfES, 2004a).

As well as a strong focus on the government-led Healthy Schools Programme, there is a discussion in *Choosing Health* (DoH, 2004a) on early years settings, a new commitment to support healthy colleges and universities, chapters on 'A health-promoting NHS', mention of health in prisons, and a focus on communities for health. The issue of 'work and health' has long been on the public health agenda. In order to contextualise the concept of the settings approach, the next section explores three different settings for health.

4.2 Promoting public health in organisations and settings

This section illustrates the potential of the settings approach for promoting public health by focusing on three contrasting settings: prisons, hospitals and workplaces.

4.2.1 Healthy prisons

The criminal justice system offers significant opportunities for improving health and tackling inequalities, not least because a high proportion of prisoners come from socially excluded sections of society, many with poorer health than the population at large, and a history of unhealthy lifestyles and little contact with health services (Social Exclusion Unit, 2002, 2004; DoH, 2004a). It is therefore important, from the perspective of both human rights and public health, that both time in custody and the resettlement process back into the wider community are used positively to prevent disease and to promote health and wellbeing.

In 1996, the WHO Regional Office for Europe established its Health in Prisons Project (HIPP), intended to follow the settings approach as previously developed in relation to cities, schools and hospitals (Gatherer et al., 2005). The HIPP aims to encourage innovation in prison health, to promote stronger links with public health, and to improve the health of prisoners, staff, visitors, prisoners' families and local communities. It functions by networking key stakeholders, creating and disseminating knowledge and expertise, and working to influence prison health policies and programmes in member countries. Membership of the HIPP requires a national-level ministerial commitment with appropriate resourcing, and at the time of writing there are thirty-four member countries.

The WHO Collaborating Centre for the HIPP is based at the Department of Health in England, which has been instrumental in encouraging national-level policy development to support a settings approach within prisons. In 2002, the government published *Health Promoting Prisons: A Shared Approach* (DoH, 2002). Grounded in the concept of decency and recognising that prisons should be safe, secure, reforming and health promoting, this endorsed a 'whole-prison' approach comprising three main components:

1   policies that promote health (e.g. smoking policy)
2   an environment that is actively supportive of health (e.g. as part of the developing agenda around decency in prisons)
3   prevention, health education and other health promotion initiatives.

The document paved the way for *Prison Service Order (PSO) 3200 on Health Promotion* (HM Prison Service, 2003), which prioritised mental health, smoking, healthy eating, healthy lifestyles (including sex and relationships, and active living) and drug and other substance misuse.

The subsequent publication of the new public health White Paper, *Choosing Health: Making Healthy Choices Easier* (DoH, 2004a) further strengthened the prison health improvement agenda, within the context of a major reconfiguration of prison healthcare that saw the transfer of healthcare commissioning from the Prison Service to the NHS. Box 4.3 gives an example of an initiative developed as a result of that change.

Box 4.3 A Regional Healthy Prisons Co-ordinator

The North West is the only English region to have appointed a Regional Healthy Prisons Co-ordinator, with joint funding from the Department of Health and the Prison Service (Baybutt et al., 2006). Between 2004 and 2006, all sixteen prisons in the North West worked closely with the co-ordinator, who was based within the Healthy Settings Development Unit at the University of Central Lancashire, to develop robust locally agreed action plans that include activity in each of the key priority areas of PSO 3200 on Health Promotion (HM Prison Service, 2003) and ensure that this is aligned with key national targets.

The co-ordinator played a pivotal role in nurturing this emerging agenda and developing a whole prison approach to health improvement, by providing the interface between NHS PCTs and the Prison Service, and supporting the development of local partnerships to integrate health across the prison setting. The facilitation of networking and the consequent sharing of good practice and public health expertise have been key drivers in delivering a 'joined-up' approach to public health across the sixteen North West prisons and their local partnerships.

A crucial part of the performance management process will be the demonstration of how prisons are meeting their targets. Some establishments have chosen to use existing structures, reflecting how prison health in its broadest sense is being integrated throughout their local PCT's health planning processes. Others have chosen more creative ways to gather evidence and illustrate how health is inextricably linked to all areas of the prison environment and how they are engaged in the broader NHS (e.g. using a portfolio). Moving beyond healthcare to identify public health roles and responsibilities has proved an effective means of developing a whole prison approach to health improvement in North West prisons. Health promotion action plans from all sixteen prisons will be monitored by the Regional Offender Development Team at the North West Prisons Area Office, on behalf of the strategic health authority, providing a clear reporting structure for whole-prison health across the region.

4.2.2 Healthy hospitals

Although primarily focused on treatment and care, hospitals have the potential to promote health: as major institutions, they can reach large numbers of service users, staff and visitors; as centres of modern medicine, research and education, they can influence professional practice; as producers of large amounts of waste, they can contribute to the reduction of environmental pollution; and as large-scale consumers, they can develop socially and environmentally responsible procurement and institutional management practices.

In 1988, the WHO Regional Office for Europe launched the Health Promoting Hospitals (HPH) Project, with the goal of reorienting healthcare institutions to integrate health promotion, disease prevention and rehabilitation services (WHO, 2006). Since the initiation of a pilot programme in 1993, more than 700 hospitals in twenty-five European countries and worldwide have joined the international network. The HPH concept reflects the principles and strategies of the Ottawa Charter (WHO, 1986).

The HPH Project aims to facilitate change in order to promote total quality management of hospitals, supporting countries to:

- change the culture of hospital care towards interdisciplinary working and transparent decision making, with active involvement of patients and partners
- evaluate health promotion activities in the healthcare setting and build an evidence base
- incorporate standards and indicators for health promotion in existing quality management systems.

The WHO Collaborating Centre for Health Promotion in Hospitals and Health Care has been established at the Ludwig Boltzmann Institute in Vienna, to support the development of hospitals and other healthcare institutions in Europe and other regions of the world into healthy and health promoting settings and organisations (WHO, 2007). The WHO Collaborating Centre for Evidence-based Health Promotion in Hospitals, based at Bispebjerg University Hospital in Copenhagen, provides the secretariat for the HPH Project and international network (Clinical Unit of Health Promotion, 2006).

Within England, the role of secondary care in delivering public health has been highlighted by a number of key documents, including *Improving Working Lives Standard* (DoH, 2000); *Standards for Better Health* (DoH, 2004c), which includes public health as one of its domains; and *Choosing Health* (DoH, 2004a), which, as mentioned in Section 4.1.2 above, has a chapter entitled 'A health-promoting NHS', and highlights a smoke-free NHS, action in relation to cancer, respiratory disease and coronary heart disease, and the development of corporate social responsibility. A range of healthcare settings are now adopting the settings approach, some formally signed up to the English Network of Health Promoting Hospitals and Trusts, which is part of WHO's International Network of Health Promoting Hospitals. To join the Health Promoting Hospitals (HPH) network, hospitals and trusts must:

- endorse the Ottawa Charter (WHO, 1986) and Vienna Recommendations for Health Promoting Hospitals (1997)
- provide a letter of intent signed by the chief executive
- use the WHO *Standards for Health Promotion in Hospitals* toolkit (WHO, 2004) to undertake a self-assessment and identify priorities
- submit data on projects and actions
- develop a smoke-free setting.

Box 4.4 describes the first English HPH.

Box 4.4 Lancashire Teaching Hospitals Foundation Trust

Lancashire Teaching Hospitals Foundation Trust became England's pilot HPH in 1992. In accordance with the WHO criteria, seven sub-projects were initially identified, addressing the seven key perspectives of patients, healthcare staff, the organisation and the community/environment:

1   food and health

2   health at work

3   HPH in the community

4   storage, collection, transport and disposal of domestic and clinical waste

5   management of post-coronary patients

6   prevention of accidents in children

7   a young people's information service.

At the end of the pilot phase in 1997, the intervention studies were evaluated and most integrated into core services. A programme of work towards a smoke-free hospital followed in 1998, achieving the objective of smoke-free buildings and grounds in 2000. With the resurgence of public health as a political imperative, and government-level acknowledgement of the wider social and environmental determinants of health, the trust has been able to broaden its role as an HPH – progressing the corporate social responsibility agenda and using the *Standards for Health Promotion in Hospitals* toolkit (WHO, 2004) to undertake a self-assessment and develop action plans that reflect local and national priorities. With a whole-system emphasis on the development of healthy public policies and the joining up of services, the HPH increasingly functions as a health catalyst, providing evidenced opportunities for health gain across the setting – for staff, patients, visitors and the wider community.

The HPH approach encourages people to think and do things differently, and challenges traditional systems of work. With a rising incidence of chronic diseases, the integration of health promotion is recognised to be an important factor for sustained health, quality of life and efficiency of service provision. For example, protocols to facilitate early identification and referral have been developed on the basis of evidence that smoking and excessive alcohol consumption increase the risk of complications in surgery. This work has highlighted a lack of community resource and so has also been valuable in providing data to support increased capacity at the point where it will most benefit the community.

4.2.3 Healthy workplaces

There is a hard and convincing economic argument underlying calls to employers to take the health of employees seriously. In his report on public health, the government's adviser, Derek Wanless (2004, p. 162), stated that: 'Employers have much to gain from considering the revenue implications of preventative health for their businesses'. The cost of sick leave and incapacity benefit is considerable and growing, working out at an average of £476 per worker (in 2002). Wanless concluded that companies in both the public and private sectors could benefit from investment in their employees' health and, in particular, in preventing illhealth. Engagement in the health of staff fosters not only improvements in staff turnover and workplace absence, but contributes to long-term health gains for the population.

Taking the workplace, for example, as a setting for health (or illhealth), it is known that the social organisation of work, management styles and social relationships in the workplace all matter (Wilkinson and Marmot, 2003). Stress at work plays an important role in contributing to the large social status differences in health, sickness absence and premature death. Studies show, too, that health suffers when people have little opportunity to use their skills and lack decision-making authority (see, for example, Wilkinson, 2006, pp. 74–6). Having little control over one's work is particularly strongly related to an increased risk of low back pain, sickness absence and cardiovascular disease. Work demands can play a role in determining state of health, especially when linked to control and its presence or absence. Jobs with both high demand and low control carry special risks.

The presence, or otherwise, of rewards for the effort put into work is associated with increased cardiovascular risk. Rewards need not comprise only money, although this is not unimportant. Status and self-esteem are also critically important. If people are appreciated and thanked for their efforts, this can have a positive impact on their health.

Although the UK's economic success has been put down in large part to its flexible, and often low-paid, labour market, such a market can have an adverse impact on the health of the workforce that is subject to short-term contracts and risky employment opportunities. In such a context, receiving appropriate rewards that have a positive impact on health may be harder to come by. A feature of good management is to ensure that appropriate rewards – in terms of money, status and self-esteem – are available to all employees.

Job insecurity, which can be a feature of a flexible labour market and short-term contracts, can act as a chronic stressor which increases sickness absence and places additional demands on health services. People generally feel much happier if they know their job is secure (Layard, 2003). Despite this, frequent calls from powerful business leaders suggest that we cannot afford to offer job security and that flexibility is the only option in a global competitive economy. But, as Layard points out, is there not something strangely paradoxical in not being able to afford security now that we are richer when we could afford it when we were poorer? Similarly, reduced working hours can be beneficial in achieving a better work/life balance that can promote better health. Again, the UK government is ambivalent on this issue, preferring to opt out of the European standard working time directive on the grounds that such matters should be for individual decision.

The policy implications of these findings are considerable if the objective is to improve health for all and narrow inequalities between social groups. Most important, there need be no trade-off between health and productivity at work. A virtuous circle can be established, with improved conditions of work leading to a healthier workforce which, in turn, will lead to improved productivity and hence to opportunities to create even healthier and more productive workplaces.

Appropriate involvement in decision making is likely to benefit employees at all levels of an organisation. This means introducing mechanisms that would allow employees to influence the design and improvement of their work environment. Through such means, employees would have more control, greater variety, and increased opportunities and space for development at work.

Workplace health requires having in place appropriate health services, with people trained in the early detection of mental health problems and physical signs of stress, which can have an impact on an employee's physical as well as mental health state. Companies need to employ occupational health visitors or public health practitioners who can carry out such functions. Box 4.5 discusses three kinds of healthy workplace initiatives, and illustrates these with five examples.

Box 4.5 Healthy workplace initiatives

Engaging employers and employees in improving their health can result in a happier, more contented and more productive workforce. For example, in one company an integrated health management programme provides all employees with access to personalised advice and information through an online service. Information covers four key areas: stress and how to manage it, nutrition, sleep and exercise. Anonymised data is used to provide feedback to the company on health issues. Initial results have been positive. The widespread introduction of such programmes could help institutionalise health promotion in the workplace.

There is a need to provide services to people where they tend to congregate. For example, one health centre ran a 'MOT' clinic for men, next to the railway station between 5.30 pm and 8 pm (when the health centre itself was not open). Almost seventy men attended for blood pressure, cholesterol and diabetes tests, as well as body mass index assessment.

There is also a need to encourage increased physical activity. For instance, the Everyday Sport campaign was launched in June 2004 to encourage people in the north-east of England to become more active. The region has some of the lowest levels of participation in physical activity and sport in the country. Citizens were encouraged to do a little more activity each day in a way that suited them. Staff tackled lazy lifestyles by getting involved in a range of activities, including speed walks at lunchtime, office games and team activities after work.

Designing offices with fitness in mind is another mechanism whereby employees can be encouraged to become healthier. In the Broadgate Centre in the City of London, architects have designed office buildings to encourage employees to walk while they are at work. Meeting rooms, canteens and car parks are being located at appreciable distance from desks so workers have to expend energy getting to them. One government department has introduced changes to help promote a healthy workplace, including stair

> prompts to encourage staff to take the stairs; provision of pedometers; investment in new bike racks and shower facilities to encourage cycling to work; and healthier options in the canteen and vending machines.
>
> (Adapted from Wanless, 2004, p. 162; DoH, 2004a, Chapter 7)

4.2.4 Wider policy and practice implications

If public health and health promotion represent a mediating strategy between people and their environments, synthesising personal choice and social responsibility in health, then this has important implications for the management and organisational dynamics within a social system or health setting regardless of whether it is a school, hospital, university, prison or workplace. In this way, health promotion can be viewed as an intervention in social and organisational systems to improve health.

Through such means, public health can be taken out of the ghetto into which many believe it has become trapped. It was a former Secretary of State for Health, Alan Milburn, who gave a lecture to the London School of Economics and Political Science (LSE) in 2000, in which he said:

> For too long the overarching label 'public health' has served to bundle together functions and occupations in a way that actually marginalises them from the NHS and other health partners ... 'Public health' understood as the epidemiological analysis of the patterns and causes of population health and ill-health gets confused with 'public health' understood as population-level health promotion, which in turn gets confused with 'public health' understood as health professionals trained in medicine.
>
> (Milburn, 2000)

What most developed countries have is a *healthcare* system rather than a *health* system. Whereas a social system and set of agencies exist to manage illness, there is no equivalent for managing health. As Harrison puts it: 'health is an unincorporated cloud that hovers amorphously, part of all other social systems – education, agriculture, politics, etc.' (Harrison, 1999, p. 130).

Thinking point:　what implications does this have for public health?

If everything else other than the healthcare system primarily contributes to health improvement, then the principal function of public health and health promotion is to develop social system interventions that build systems for health into other established social structures. Health therefore becomes an integrative goal of the organisation regardless of whether that organisation is a workplace, school or business.

In his report mentioned in Section 4.2.3 above, specifically on public health, Wanless (2004) concluded that for all the health policy statements that had appeared over the previous thirty years or so, the results remained disappointing. There was a serious implementation gap between the rhetoric and the reality and the NHS remained a sickness rather than a health service. He saw addressing this imbalance as the main challenge to government. There was no need for new policy. Rather, the effort should be devoted to achieving change and implementing effective interventions to improve health.

The White Paper, *Choosing Health*, which appeared in 2004 and was accompanied a few months later, in 2005, by a delivery plan, reflected Wanless's counsel (DoH, 2004a; DoH, 2005a). It stressed the importance of managing change and developing new approaches to improving health, and working with new organisations in the public and private sectors. The White Paper acknowledged that, traditionally, and largely reflecting their training, public health practitioners have been skilled at acquiring knowledge and handling epidemiological information about the state of health of their communities, but they have been less skilled at applying this knowledge and at effecting change in local settings.

As a result of these criticisms, it is now accepted that public health practitioners, and all those whose actions impact on health, need new skills and competences to enable them not merely to collect the evidence on what is (and is not) effective by way of interventions to improve health, but also to act on this evidence by creating the conditions in their organisations and social systems to ensure that action follows (see, for example, DoH, 2007; Hunter, 2007). In short, those working in public health, regardless of whether it is in the NHS, local government, the voluntary sector or private companies, need to become effective change agents and be in a position to apply organisational development skills.

The political and policy context in which public health and those practising it find themselves is both complex and dynamic. Expectations are running high and yet there are few role models available to those engaged in public health to help bring about change. They will need to be very clear and focused about what they want to achieve now and in the future, and how they intend to get there.

Public health organisations need to become learning organisations, devising their own route map as they navigate their way through muddy or uncharted waters. A range of skills will be required, especially those around commissioning and partnership working across different organisations. Many of these are new to those working in public health. Such a way of comprehending the role of public health and health promotion has implications for its leadership and skills base. Public health practitioners should be primarily skilled in organisational development and change management. Health is the goal, but change management is the means by which this can be achieved.

In general, public health practitioners and others engaged in promoting health are poorly prepared and equipped to function in a way that is likely to bring about significant improvements in health. In the light of this, organisational development (OD) and change management (CM) are vital tools to enable public health organisations find the solutions that will work for them in achieving their goals.

4.3 Organisational development and change management

In this brief review of organisational development and change management, the emphasis is on helping you to understand the concepts used and to assess the benefits of new ideas and insights.

4.3.1 What is organisational development?

There is considerable mystique surrounding organisational development, which is unhelpful. The term is interpreted in different ways by different practitioners, some seeing it as a comprehensive organisation-wide development programme with particular underpinning principles and common approaches, while others use it more loosely to describe any development programme within an organisation that is designed to meet organisational objectives as well as personal ones. Although OD encompasses a huge area of management theory and practice, it is not as complicated as it can seem and is largely basic common sense, though no less important for that.

OD is a field of applied behavioural science which seeks to develop the principles and practice of managing change and improving effectiveness in organisations. It has been defined as: 'a set of behavioural science-based theories, values, strategies and techniques aimed at the planned change of organizational work setting for the purpose of enhancing individual development and improving organizational performance, through the alteration of organizational members' on-the-job behaviours' (Porras and Robertson, 1992, p. 723).

Transforming organisations, and the services they provide, requires a whole-organisation perspective and OD can help achieve this. Successful OD requires that chief executives, senior managers and political leaders all need to be at the forefront of the change process, setting the challenge, defining the goals and shaping the approach (ODPM, 2005).

Depending on the type of organisational change sought, initiatives may be targeted directly at individuals in order to secure specific behaviour change, or they may be directed at a group or at organisational level. In an OD resource document for local government, it is claimed that OD favours dealing with causes over symptoms, working with whole systems rather than parts of them, changes in culture over changes in behaviour, and change *of* a system over changes *in* a system (ODPM, 2005).

Consistent with this conception of organisations as complex interrelated systems, affected by their environment, by their leaders and by the systems and processes that staff adopt to provide services, four dimensions are particularly important for public health. These constitute a framework within which to locate the various components that need to be addressed. The four dimensions are:

1 **environment and context:** to provide insights into, and understanding of, the policies and politics surrounding the development of public health and tackling health inequalities across the NHS, local government, the independent sector, and so on

2 **cultural change:** to ensure that the underlying core beliefs and values of the organisation support the open, constructive reflection required for effective public health organisations to bring about change

3 **skills development:** to ensure that people have the repertoire of skills needed to undertake the work, and the capacity and capability to deploy them effectively

4 **structural development of systems and processes:** necessary to co-ordinate and ensure that the work is executed efficiently and optimally.

Organisations often make the mistake of concentrating their energies and efforts on developing the organisational structures required: that is, putting form before function, as has happened with increasing regularity in the NHS since 1974 (Webster, 2002; Hunter 2005; Blackler, 2006). But arguably, of greater importance is work to establish trust, good communication and good relationships between all members of the public health team. For this to happen successfully, effective OD requires good leadership and adequate resources.

Within each of the four dimensions noted above are a number of specific examples where OD can make a useful contribution. Two dimensions – cultural change and skills development in the context of leadership for health improvement – are considered further in Section 4.5 after change management has been introduced below.

4.3.2 What is change management?

The literature on change management is large and not easy to access for various reasons. A major problem in the CM field is the prevalence of fads and fashions and the dominance of gurus who prescribe courses of action without any basis in evidence. Good empirical studies are relatively rare and mainly single-site case reports. The nature of the evidence in the field of CM may differ from that which is relevant and useful in the clinical arena.

Clarifying the nature of change is important. Sometimes it is deliberate, a product of conscious reasoning and actions. This type of change is called planned change. In contrast, change sometimes occurs in a seemingly spontaneous and unplanned way. This type of change is known as emergent change. The importance of these two interpretations of change is that change is rarely fixed or linear in nature, but contains an important emergent element. The theory of complex adaptive systems accepts that, although organisational change can be planned to a degree, it can never be fully isolated from the effects of serendipity, uncertainty, ambivalence and chance (Dawson, 1996). A complex adaptive system has been defined as '[a] collection of individual agents with freedom to act in ways that are not always totally predictable, and whose actions are interconnected so that one agent's actions change the context for other agents' (Plsek and Greenhalgh 2001, p. 625). An example of such a system is almost any collection of human beings.

Change can also be episodic or continuous. Episodic change might involve the replacement of one programme or strategy with another. Continuous change, on the other hand, is ongoing, evolving, incremental and cumulative. Constant adaptation is a feature of continuous change.

In addition, change may be developmental, transitional and transformational. Developmental change may be planned or emergent, as discussed above. Transitional change seeks to achieve a known desired state that is different from the existing one. It is episodic, planned or radical, and is the basis of much of the organisational change literature. It involves unfreezing the existing organisational equilibrium, moving to a new position or state, and then refreezing in a new equilibrium position. Finally, transformational change is radical in nature and requires a shift, or step change, in the assumptions made by the organisation and its members. Transformation can result in an organisation that differs significantly in terms of structure, processes, culture and strategy.

The impression often given is that organisational change is, or can be, a rational, controlled and orderly process. In practice, however, change can be chaotic and unexpected, often involving shifting goals and discontinuous activities. It is therefore perhaps best seen in context and best understood in relation to the complex dynamic systems within which it occurs. Whole-systems thinking endeavours to embrace the complexity of change in complex organisations, such as health services, and involves taking into account all the many influences that contribute to a particular outcome or state. So, for example, achieving improved health entails not simply a focus on health services (a downstream emphasis), but a focus on all the socio-economic and environmental factors that go to shape health (an upstream emphasis). Public health is a particularly good example of a complex activity since it spans so many organisational settings, all of which have an impact on health even if this is not necessarily their core purpose. For this reason, systems thinking is perhaps best suited to a consideration of change management in public health.

4.4 How can public health be promoted in organisations and settings?

The relationship between public health, organisational development and change management is ambivalent. It may be that inappropriate models of management have been unhelpfully applied to the public health task, which is intrinsically complex, involving as it does many agencies and professional groups, and the exercise of influence over systems where direct control is either weak or absent.

The notion of public health management is helpful here (Alderslade and Hunter, 1994; Hunter, 2002, 2003). It involves mobilising society's resources to improve the health of populations – an example of whole-systems thinking as mentioned above. Public health management seeks to integrate the twin approaches of knowledge and action so that public health knowledge can be harnessed to action through the deployment of appropriate management and planning skills. These skills are rooted in an open-systems approach to management.

Open-system theories do not view organisations strictly as mechanical models. Organisations are viewed instead as systems that are 'loosely coupled', both internally and externally. Internally, the organisation's structural elements, activities and members may be only loosely connected to each other, and therefore semi-autonomous in their behaviour. It poses difficulties in achieving concerted action among organisational groups. Externally, the organisation is subject to, but not completely determined by, the constraints and uncertainties in its environment.

Drawing on an open-systems approach, public health management demands skills other than those generally to be found in public health. Relevant skills for such work require being able to assess whether investment in health has been made, and whether an infrastructure for health promotion has been constructed within the formal or informal fabric of the organisation or social system. Success factors may include:

*   written roles/job descriptions that include health responsibilities
*   evidence of health-related infrastructures, such as policy on health or health inequalities audits or impact assessments that are embedded in core business

- the establishment of formal health committees
- changes in values/policies within the organisation, such as a shift to reduced working hours, flexible working practices and job sharing.

Importantly, public health in this context is not confined to the specialty of public health or to public health practitioners working in the NHS. There are people working in many disciplines whose activities and work are central to improving health, but who would not consider themselves public health practitioners or call themselves such. They might include teachers, town planners, and architects.

There are many obstacles in the way of creating successful health-promoting organisations and settings. The majority of these barriers to change have their roots in culture and in leadership skills, and these notions are themselves related. Successful leaders, especially those of a transformational persuasion, are able to change the culture within their organisations. Each dimension – culture and leadership – is considered in turn below, in order to assess its contribution to promoting public health successfully.

4.4.1 Making sense of culture

Culture matters yet is hard to define. Change can often be stifled by culture. Culture constitutes the informal social aspects of an organisation that influence how people think, what they regard as important, and how they behave and interact at work (Mannion et al., 2005). Organisational culture has been defined by Schein as:

> a pattern of basic assumptions – invented, discovered, or developed by a given group as it learns to cope with its problems of external adaptation and internal integration – that has worked well enough to be considered valid and, therefore, to be taught to new members as the correct way to perceive, think, and feel in relation to those problems.
>
> (Schein, 1985, p. 9)

Culture is, therefore, not merely that which is observable in social life, but also the shared cognitive and symbolic context within which a society or institution can be understood. For example, a biomedical (in contrast to a social) understanding of health and illness dominates the majority of organisations concerned with the delivery of healthcare, and therefore exerts significant influence, possibly covertly rather than overtly.

Thinking point: how far do you agree that a biomedical conception of health is deeply ingrained in healthcare organisations?

Whenever there is any mention of health, it is the medical model that is either invoked or implied. In the context of public health, however, which is concerned with populations as well as individuals and with a whole-systems perspective in regard to the determinants of health, a biomedical perspective is inappropriate. Such a bias is in keeping with the dominance of a medical culture that pervades not only healthcare organisations, but often public conceptions more generally of what constitutes health. There are many successful examples of organisations that have demonstrated a corporate social responsibility for health by seeking to improve the environment in which individuals make their healthy choices, but they still tend to be the exception.

If organisations are to take public health seriously, then they need to change their culture accordingly, using OD and CM tools to assist in bringing about the necessary shift. Work on cultural change suggests that while it is relatively easy to change certain artefacts, such as language, mission statements and particular systems, the deeper assumptions governing behaviour may be more difficult to shift and have the potential to negate, attenuate or redirect the change effort (Harris and Ogbonna, 2002). Indeed, such difficulties seem to underlie the conclusion in the Wanless report on public health that despite 'numerous policy initiatives being directed towards public health they have not succeeded in rebalancing health policy away from the short-term imperatives of health care' (Wanless, 2004, p. 6).

Although there is much talk of culture change, there is little practical guidance available on how to deliver it on the ground. Most recently, in the context of public health and health improvement, the government has been attracted to what social marketing can offer by way of reinforcing positive messages about health aimed not just at individuals and behavioural change at this level, but also at organisations and social mores more generally. A central characteristic of leadership is culture change, with leaders acting as catalysts for change.

4.4.2 Leadership for health

As mentioned earlier, the discipline of public health has had twin intellectual approaches – knowledge and action – which have gone together. However, in practice there has been a tension between knowledge and action, with many practitioners in public health and health promotion focusing on the former rather than the latter (Nutbeam and Wise, 2002). Notions such as public health management (Hunter, 2002) and leadership for health improvement seek to integrate the two approaches so that public health knowledge can be harnessed to action through the deployment of appropriate management and planning skills.

Public health leadership, which includes an ability to manage, demands skills other than those generally to be found in public health, which focus on analysing health problems in a population. Nutbeam and Wise state: 'Influencing health behaviour in populations and influencing the structural and environmental determinants of health requires public health specialists to have substantial knowledge and skills in the behavioural, social and political sciences' (Nutbeam and Wise, 2002, p. 1883).

The emphasis on interventions also highlights the need for a different style of leadership. Those leading public health are expected to respond to the multisectoral nature of health problems and serve a variety of agencies over which they may have little direct control or authority. Working in a multisectoral arena to develop healthy alliances requires strengthening capacity, which has been acknowledged by the Chief Medical Officer for England in a review of the public health function (DoH, 2001). Strengthening multidisciplinary public health, together with strengthening leadership and management development, not only in the NHS but also in local government, were key themes of the review. The review concluded that public health leadership 'requires a facilitative, influencing style that can make use of horizontal networks in addition to vertical "command and control" networks. Advocacy, political skills and commitment are also important' (DoH, 2001, p. 32).

The focus on alliance building across a range of diverse organisations and professions, as well as the public, will make heavy demands on the public health workforce and will require well-honed political and managerial skills in addition to the traditional scientific skills associated with public health. It is a particularly difficult synthesis to achieve, not because of the range of skills required, but because they come from two quite distinct paradigms. Whereas the traditional basis of public health medicine belongs to the positivist, biomedical view of scientific inquiry, the political and managerial skills base comes from an intuitive, contextual orientation grounded in the way in which organisations work. The tradition is sociological and anthropological rather than biomedical. This may explain why public health specialists often find rational, linear 'scientific management' theories more immediately appealing than theories of a less 'rational' and more behavioural persuasion, where uncertainty, complexity, paradox and ambiguity all figure prominently.

Leadership for health improvement demands knowledge and management skills of the highest order (Hannaway et al., 2005). Leaders must be able to adopt a strategic approach and be able to describe and understand the health experience of populations, and analyse the factors affecting health. To achieve change, skills in leadership and political action are necessary.

Because managers have to operate in a multiprofessional, multi-agency environment and be able to achieve multisectoral change, operating on the margins of their own organisations becomes a prerequisite.

In taking forward this multisectoral approach to a health agenda, a number of key processes are involved:

- **building alliances and networks with non-health service organisations:** relationships will be based on influence rather than on direction and control

- **market management:** having a strategic framework based on health improvement, and the capacity to work within alliances, and possessing good market-relevant information

- **giving attention to organisational fitness for purpose:** this means moving away from functional departments and towards a blending of skills in task forces and in project-managed initiatives – such a team approach will be looser and more fluid than conventional functional departments with their hierarchies and multiple layers of management.

The leadership of such complex work will demand, among other things, communication skills, interpersonal skills, understanding of organisational behaviour, intellect, analytical skills, planning skills, accounting skills, and an understanding of how the system works. Another way of framing the leadership challenge is to view it as comprising three knowledge domains which bring together both the hard and soft elements of the management function. These three domains are:

1   **leadership:** the art of getting things done by enabling others to do more than they could or would do otherwise

2   **improvement science:** the study and practice of enhancing the performance of processes and systems of work

3   **health improvement systems:** the practical realities and future possibilities of the way in which health improvement is experienced by staff and communities.

Strengthening the health improvement system means that organisations are better placed to focus on addressing the health needs of their whole populations. Through a system-wide approach focusing on people and communities, a health improvement system orientation empowers individual organisations to address health inequalities within their populations. It is easy to list the ingredients required for organisations to promote health both in themselves and in the communities in which they are located, but many organisations find great difficulty in refocusing their goals and purpose on health promotion. They may give credence to such a notion in the rhetoric they espouse, but fail to live up to it in practice because they remain entrenched in the way the business is transacted. The next section explores some of the problems and pitfalls in creating healthy organisations and settings.

4.5 Facing the challenges

Creating healthy organisations and settings is a complex enterprise and the potential difficulties need to be faced. In this section, three challenges are addressed: first, those relating to organisational and geographical boundaries; second, issues of power and inequalities; and third, the question of evidence of effectiveness of healthy settings.

4.5.1 Joining up organisations and settings

Health issues do not necessarily 'respect' organisational or geographical boundaries, and a particular problem manifest in one setting may have its roots in a different setting (e.g. bullying in schools may have its roots in neighbourhood relationships). People's lives straddle a range of different organisations and settings, both concurrently and consecutively. For instance, a person's time might be divided between home, work and leisure pursuits, and they will also interact with and be influenced indirectly by other settings; or someone might spend a length of time in prison before resettlement into the community, or an extended stay in hospital before moving back to home and work. Organisations and settings also operate at different levels and may therefore be located within the context of another, like Russian dolls. Galea et al. (2000) discuss this, suggesting that a distinction should be made between different levels of what they term 'elemental' and 'contextual' settings. For example, an organisation such as a hospital or a school will be situated within a particular neighbourhood, which is within a larger town or city, which in turn is within a district, region or island. It is therefore vital that settings initiatives reject the tendency to operate on parallel tramlines and begin to network 'horizontally' as well as 'vertically' – making links with other settings, seeking to understand more fully the synergies or contradictions between them, and maximising their potential contribution to public health beyond their own boundaries by exploring 'joined-up' delivery through mechanisms such as local strategic partnerships (Dooris, 2004). In England, the Labour Government's establishment of area-based initiatives such as Health Action Zones, Healthy Living Centres and regeneration programmes provided important opportunities for experimentation and for the development of integrated settings-based approaches.

4.5.2 Power and inequalities within organisations and settings

Green et al. (2000) highlight a range of issues related to power and inequalities. They suggest, first, that health promotion has too often ignored issues relating to power and may have inadvertently 'played into existing power relations and alliances' (p. 24) by aligning itself with management and thereby marginalising or alienating less powerful groups (e.g. workers, students or patients). As Dooris (2001, p. 59) has argued, 'it is important to build senior management commitment while developing broad-based ownership ... The politics of this dual process can be extremely challenging'. The issue of power relations is also relevant to more complex area-based settings initiatives, such as healthy cities, which involve a range of stakeholders from public, private, voluntary and community sectors (Costongs and Springett, 1997), and to joint working between settings.

A second issue highlighted by Green et al. relates to who spends time in which settings – and who is left out. Although the settings approach moves beyond a view of settings as places with 'captive audiences', it is obviously pertinent from an inequalities perspective to consider who benefits and who loses out. It is, therefore, of concern that – with a few exceptions such as prisons – 'the settings in which one is to find the unemployed, the homeless, the disenfranchised youth, the illegal immigrants, and so forth are not as well defined' (Green et al., 2000, p. 25). Poland et al. (2000) echo Kickbusch (1997) in arguing for the approach to respond by embracing 'non-traditional' settings.

A third issue discussed by Green et al. concerns the relationship of settings initiatives to other approaches and macro-policy. A criticism of the settings approach has been that is has tended to fragment action to promote public health and divert attention from the underlying determinants of health. It is therefore important that healthy settings initiatives look upwards and outwards, focusing on the organisational structures, policies and practices that will create supportive environments and make a difference (St Leger, 1997), while at the same time explicitly addressing broader social, economic and political contextual factors (Baum, 2002). In this respect, Dooris (2004, p. 46) has argued that the approach has the potential to be 'a springboard for broad-based corporate citizenship, developing organizational and individual awareness of the wider impacts of institutional practice at local, national and global levels'. This area is explored further in a more recent article on corporate citizenship and public health (Dooris, 2006b).

4.5.3 Evidence and evaluation

In terms of effectiveness, the settings approach is widely seen to have a range of benefits (Dooris, 2003). It encourages exploration of connections between people, behaviours and environments; it enables examination of the interplay between health issues and programmes; it allows the relationships between different population groups in a setting to be addressed; it encourages multi-stakeholder ownership of health; and it provides a coherent framework within which to work, making it possible to see the bigger picture and contribute to 'joined-up' holistic public health. However, although recent evaluation and evidence reviews have included a focus on settings (International Union for Health Promotion and Education, 2000; Rootman et al., 2001), it can be argued that: 'The settings approach has been legitimated more through an act of faith than through rigorous research and evaluation studies ... much more attention needs to be given to building the evidence and learning from it' (St Leger, 1997, p. 100).

In addition to the general difficulties faced by public health and health promotion in responding to the demand for evidence, it can be argued that a number of specific challenges make it difficult to undertake consistent, rigorous evaluation and to build a convincing evidence base for the settings approach (Dooris, 2006).

Thinking point: can you think of reasons why it may be difficult to evaluate the settings approach?

First, the way in which funding for evaluation is made available and, more generally, the way in which the evidence base for public health and health promotion is constructed, tends to reflect a continuing focus on specific diseases and single-risk factor interventions rather than on settings. Second, the diversity of both conceptual understandings and real-life practice brought together under the banner of the settings approach presents obvious difficulties in generating a substantive body of research that allows comparability and transferability; these might include the complexity of the decision-making process in a given setting and its contextual nature, which would make generalising from a specific setting possibly difficult to do with any confidence. Third, it is very complex to evaluate the settings approach as defined above – characterised by integrating health within the cultures, structures, processes and routine life of organisational and other settings, and by adopting an ecological perspective that prioritises systems thinking. This requires an approach to evaluation and evidence that is not linear and reductionist, but instead acknowledges the interrelationships, interactions and synergies within and between settings: with regard to different groups of the population, different components of the system and different 'health' issues. These challenges have resulted in and further reinforced an ongoing tendency to evaluate only discrete projects in settings, and have militated against the generation of credible evidence of effectiveness for the settings approach as a whole – in terms of synergy and 'added value'.

Conclusion

Public health goes far beyond the confines of healthcare although even within health service organisations it struggles for its voice to be heard. Health-promoting settings need to be created through change strategies, using organisational development and change management tools to help ensure healthier goods and services and cleaner, safer and more enjoyable environments. Transforming organisations and the services and support they provide effectively requires a whole-organisation perspective, and OD is an approach that helps to achieve this. An important aspect of successful OD and CM is that chief executives, senior managers and political leaders all need to be at the forefront of the change process, setting the challenge, defining the goals and shaping the approach.

However, as this chapter has shown, there are many obstacles to the adoption of healthy public policies, which may result from the powerful influence of culture as well as from competing professional conceptions of health. There exists an imbalance of power between the medical profession, which occupies a dominant position not only in healthcare systems but in society at large, and other healthcare professions, many of which subscribe to a social model of health which in turn puts a premium on health-promoting strategies.

The Ottawa Charter for Health Promotion (WHO, 1986) provides a useful conceptual framework comprising the elements of a health-promoting policy. To support the successful implementation of such a policy within a range of organisations and settings which impact on health at both individual and population levels, OD and CM tools provide ways of shifting cultural impediments to change and of putting in place appropriate leadership. But neither provides an easy option for achieving change. Shifting culture in particular is painstaking and difficult work. Developing effective leadership is also challenging and carries the risk that the effective leader will indeed bring about change while in that position in a particular organisation or setting, but this change may not be sufficiently embedded to withstand the departure of that person. Change champions have great strengths, but these are often also their weaknesses.

References

Alderslade, R. and Hunter D.J. (1994) 'Commissioning and public health', *Journal of Management and Medicine*, vol. 8, no. 6, pp. 9–10.

Baum, F. (2002) *The New Public Health* (2nd edn), Oxford, Oxford University Press.

Baybutt, M., Hayton, P. and Dooris, M. (2006) 'Prisons in England and Wales: an important public health opportunity?' in Douglas, J., Earle, S., Handsley, S., Lloyd, C.E. and Spurr, S. (eds) (2007) *A Reader in Promoting Public Health: Challenge and Controversy*, London, Sage/Milton Keynes, The Open University.

Blackler, F. (2006) 'Chief executives and the modernisation of the English National Health Service', *Leadership*, vol. 2, no. 1, pp. 5–30.

Clinical Unit of Health Promotion (2006) [online], http://clinicalhealthpromotion.dk/ (Accessed 9 January 2007).

Costongs, C. and Springett, J. (1997) 'Joint working and the production of a city health plan: the Liverpool experience', *Health Promotion International*, vol. 12, no. 1, pp. 9–19.

Dawson, S.J.N.D. (1996) *Analysing Organisations*, Basingstoke, Macmillan.

Department for Education and Skills (DfES) (2004a) *Every Child Matters*, London, The Stationery Office.

Department for Education and Skills (DfES) (2004b) *Five Year Strategy for Children and Learners*, London, The Stationery Office.

Department of Health (DoH) (1992) *The Health of the Nation: A Strategy for Health in England*, London, HMSO.

Department of Health (DoH) (1998) *Our Healthier Nation*, London, The Stationery Office.

Department of Health (DoH) (1999) *Saving Lives: Our Healthier Nation*, London, The Stationery Office.

Department of Health (DoH) (2000) *Improving Working Lives Standard*, London, The Stationery Office.

Department of Health (DoH) (2001) *The Report of the Chief Medical Officer's Project to Strengthen the Public Health Function*, London, The Stationery Office.

Department of Health (DoH) (2002) *Health Promoting Prisons: A Shared Approach*, London, The Stationery Office.

Department of Health (DoH) (2004a) *Choosing Health: Making Healthy Choices Easier*, London, The Stationery Office; also available online at http://www.dh.gov.uk/ PublicationsAndStatistics/Publications/PublicationsPolicyAndGuidance/ PublicationsPAmpGBrowsableDocument/fs/en?CONTENT_ID= 4097491&MULTIPAGE_ID=4916860&chk=cfOsph (Accessed 14 March 2007).

Department of Health (DoH) (2004b) *National Service Framework for Children, Young People and Maternity Services: Executive Summary*, London, The Stationery Office.

Department of Health (DoH) (2004c) *Standards for Better Health*, London, The Stationery Office.

Department of Health (DoH) (2005a) *Delivering Choosing Health: Making Healthier Choices Easier*, London, The Stationery Office.

Department of Health (DoH) (2005b) *National Healthy School Status: A Guide for Schools*, London, The Stationery Office.

Department of Health (DoH) (2007) *Commissioning Framework for Health and Well-Being*, London, The Stationery Office.

Dooris, M. (2001) 'The "health promoting university": a critical exploration of theory and practice', *Health Education*, vol. 101, no. 2, pp. 51–60.

Dooris, M. (2003) 'Health settings: theory and practice' in Dooris, M. and Hobbs, A. (eds) *Healthy Settings in England's North West: Report of Conference*, Preston, University of Central Lancashire.

Dooris, M. (2004) 'Joining up settings for health: a valuable investment for strategic partnerships?', *Critical Public Health*, vol. 14, no. 1, pp. 37–49.

Dooris, M. (2006) 'Healthy settings: challenges to generating evidence of effectiveness', *Health Promotion International*, vol. 21, no. 1, pp. 55–65.

Dooris, M. (2006b) 'The challenge of developing corporate citizenship for sustainable public health: An exploration of the issues with reference to the experience of north west England', *Critical Public Health*, Vol. 16, no. 4, pp. 331–343.

Dooris, M., Dowding, G., Thompson, J. and Wynne, C. (1998) 'The settings-based approach to health promotion' in Tsouros, A., Dowding, G., Thompson, J. and Dooris, M. (eds) *Health Promoting Universities: Concept, Experience and Framework for Action*, Copenhagen, World Health Organization Regional Office for Europe.

Galea, G., Powis, B. and Tamplin, S. (2000) 'Healthy islands in the Western Pacific – international settings development', *Health Promotion International*, vol. 15, no. 2, pp. 169–78.

Gatherer, A., Moller, L. and Hayton, P. (2005) 'WHO European Health in Prisons Project after ten years: persistent barriers and achievements', *American Journal of Public Health*, vol. 95, no. 10, pp. 1696–700.

Green, L., Poland, B. and Rootman, I. (2000) 'The settings approach to health promotion' in Poland, B., Green, L. and Rootman, I. (eds) *Settings for Health Promotion: Linking Theory and Practice*, London, Sage.

Grossman, R. and Scala, K. (1993) *Health Promotion and Organisational Development: Developing Settings for Health*, Copenhagen, World Health Organization Regional Office for Europe.

Hannaway, C., Plsek, P. and Hunter, D.J. (2005) *The Framework for the Leadership for Health Improvement Programme*, York, North East Yorkshire and Northern Lincolnshire Strategic Health Authority.

Harris, L.C. and Ogbonna, E. (2002) 'The unintended consequences of culture interventions: a study of unexpected outcomes', *British Journal of Management*, vol. 13, pp. 31–49.

Harrison, D. (1999) 'Social system intervention' in Perkins, E.R., Simnett, I. and Wreight, L. (eds) *Evidence-Based Health Promotion*, Chichester, Wiley.

HM Prison Service (2003) *Prison Service Order (PSO) 3200 on Health Promotion*, London, HM Prison Service.

Hunter, D.J. (2002) *Public Health Management: Making It a World Concern*, Report of World Health Organization/University of Durham meeting, Geneva, World Health Organization.

Hunter, D.J. (2003) *Public Health Policy*, Cambridge, Polity.

Hunter, D.J. (ed.) (2005) 'Theme: the National Health Service 1980–2005', *Public Money and Management*, vol. 25, no. 4.

Hunter, D.J. (ed.) (2007) *Managing for Health*, London, Routledge.

International Union for Health Promotion and Education (2000) *The Evidence of Health Promotion Effectiveness: Shaping Public Health in a New Europe. Part Two: Evidence Book*, Brussels, ECSC-EC-EAEC.

Kickbusch, I. (1996) 'Tribute to Aaron Antonovsky – "what creates health?"', *Health Promotion International*, vol. 11, no. 1, pp. 5–6.

Kickbusch, I. (1997) 'Think health: what makes the difference?', *Health Promotion International*, vol. 12, no. 4, pp. 265–72.

Layard, R. (2003) *What Would Make a Happier Society?*, Lecture, Monograph, London School of Economics/Centre for Economic Performance [online], http://cep.lse.ac.uk/events/lectures/layard/RL050303.pdf (Accessed 12 March 2007).

Mannion, R., Davies, H.T.O. and Marshall, M.N. (2005) *Cultures for Performance in Health Care*, Maidenhead, Open University Press.

Milburn, A. (2000) *A Healthier Nation and a Healthier Economy: The Contribution of a Modern NHS*, Lecture to the London School of Economics and Political Science, [online], http://www.dh.gov.uk/NewsHome/Speeches/SpeechesList/SpeechesArticle/fs/en?CONTENT_ID=4000761&chk=XE0Hp4 (Accessed 12 March 2007).

Nutbeam, D. and Wise, M. (2002) 'Structures and strategies for public health intervention' in Detels, R., McEwen, J., Beaglehole, R. and Tanaka, H. (eds) *Oxford Textbook of Public Health, Volume 3: The Practice of Public Health* (4th edn), Oxford, Oxford University Press.

Office of the Deputy Prime Minister (ODPM) (2005) *An Organisational Development Resource Document for Local Government*, London, Office of the Deputy Prime Minister.

Plsek, P. and Greenhalgh, T. (2001) 'The challenge of complexity in health care', *British Medical Journal*, vol. 323, pp. 625–8.

Poland, B., Green, L. and Rootman, I. (2000) 'Reflections on settings for health promotion' in Poland, B., Green, L. and Rootman, I. (eds) *Settings for Health Promotion: Linking Theory and Practice*, London, Sage.

Porras, J. and Robertson, P. (1992) 'Organisation development' in Dunnette, M. and Hough, L. (eds) *Handbook of Industrial and Organisational Psychology, 3*, Palo Alto, CA, Consulting Psychologists Press.

Rootman, I., Goodstadt, M., Hyndman, B., McQueen, D., Potvin, L., Springett, J. and Ziglio, E. (eds) (2001) *Evaluation in Health Promotion: Principles and Perspectives*, Copenhagen, World Health Organization Regional Office for Europe.

Schein, E.H. (1985) *Organizational Culture and Leadership*, San Francisco, CA, Jossey-Bass.

Social Exclusion Unit (SEU) (2002) *Reducing Re-Offending By Ex-Prisoners*, London, Social Exclusion Unit.

Social Exclusion Unit (SEU) (2004) *Mental Health and Social Exclusion*, London, Office of the Deputy Prime Minister.

St Leger, L. (1997) 'Health promoting settings: from Ottawa to Jakarta', *Health Promotion International*, vol. 12, no. 2, pp. 99–101.

Syme, S.L. (1996) 'To prevent disease: the need for a new approach' in Blane, D., Brunner, E. and Wilkinson, R. (eds) *Health and Social Organisation: Towards a Health Policy for the 21st Century*, London, Routledge.

Tones, K. and Green, J. (2004) *Health Promotion: Planning and Strategies*, London, Sage.

Vienna Recommendations for Health Promoting Hospitals (1997) [online], http://www.euro.who.int/document//IHB/hphviennarecom.pdf (Accessed 12 March 2007).

Wanless, D. (2004) *Securing Good Health for the Whole Population: Final Report*, London, HM Treasury.

Webster, C. (2002) *The National Health Service: A Political History*, Oxford, Oxford University Press.

Whitelaw, S., Baxendale, A., Bryce, C., Machardy, L., Young, I. and Witney, E. (2001) 'Settings based health promotion: a review', *Health Promotion International*, vol. 16, no. 4, pp. 339–53.

Wilkinson, R. and Marmot, M. (eds) (2003) *Social Determinants of Health: The Solid Facts* (2nd edn), Copenhagen, World Health Organization.

Wilkinson, R.G. (2006) *The Impact of Inequality*, London, Routledge.

World Health Organization (WHO) (1980) *European Regional Strategy for Health for All by the Year 2000*, Copenhagen, World Health Organization Regional Office for Europe.

World Health Organization (WHO) (1981) *Global Strategy for Health for All by the Year 2000*, Geneva, World Health Organization.

World Health Organization (WHO) (1986) 'Ottawa Charter for Health Promotion', *Health Promotion International*, vol. 1, no. 4, pp. iii–v.

World Health Organization (WHO) (1995a) *Yanuca Island Declaration*, Manila, World Health Organization Regional Office for the Western Pacific.

World Health Organization (WHO) (1995b) *New Horizons in Health*, Manila, World Health Organization Regional Office for the Western Pacific.

World Health Organization (WHO) (1997a) *The Jakarta Declaration on Leading Health Promotion into the 21st Century*, Geneva, World Health Organization.

World Health Organization (WHO) (1997b) *The Rarotonga Agreement: Towards Healthy Islands*, Manila, World Health Organization Regional Office for the Western Pacific.

World Health Organization (WHO) (1998a) *Health Promotion Glossary*, Geneva, World Health Organization.

World Health Organization (WHO) (1998b) *Health 21 – The Health for All Policy for the WHO European Region – 21 Targets for the 21st Century*, Copenhagen, World Health Organization Regional Office for Europe.

World Health Organization (WHO) (2004) *Standards for Health Promotion in Hospitals: Self-Assessment Tool for Pilot Implementation*, Copenhagen, World Health Organization Regional Office for Europe; also available online at http://www.euro.who.int/document/E85054.pdf (Accessed 12 March 2007).

World Health Organization (WHO) (2005a) *Bangkok Charter for Health Promotion in a Globalized World*, Geneva, World Health Organization.

World Health Organization (WHO) (2005b) *Samoa Commitment – Achieving Healthy Islands: Conclusions and Recommendations*, Manila, World Health Organization Regional Office for the Western Pacific.

World Health Organization (WHO) (2006) *Health Promoting Hospitals* [online], http://www.euro.who.int/healthpromohosp/20060815_1 (Accessed 12 March 2007).

World Health Organization (WHO) (2007) [online], http://www.hph-hc.cc/ (Accessed 9 January 2007).

Chapter 5

Partnerships and alliances for health

John Kenneth Davies and Pam Foley

Introduction

Partnerships and alliances are frequently necessary to achieve the goals of modern multidisciplinary public health and they are fundamental to implementing an integrated healthy public policy. Public health policy reflects the need to promote health through alliances involving a wide range of organisations, and not through the health services alone. Although some aspects of the conceptual and knowledge base of public health have perhaps been dominated by an individually focused, biomedical paradigm of health, and the health sector has been seen as the main stakeholder through its emphasis on individual treatment services (Baggott, 2000), it is clear that the health sector alone cannot tackle the complex determinants that underpin the distribution of health. New and more effective approaches to healthy public policy are based on participation, collaboration, co-operation and empowerment through the mechanism of partnership working.

This chapter will describe and discuss the rapid growth in partnership working for health, and examine definitions, explanations and challenges using both national and international examples. It starts by considering different definitions of partnerships before moving on to outline, in Section 5.2, some of the national and international developments in policies related to partnerships. The final section focuses on the implementation and evaluation of partnerships and alliances in a local, national and global context.

5.1 Defining partnerships

Many policies and strategies indicate that the only way for inequalities in health to be addressed, and comprehensive health improvement interventions implemented successfully, is through partnerships with other individuals and organisations. The term 'intersectoral collaboration' is often used to reflect this switch and was defined by the World Health Organization (WHO) as:

> a recognized relationship between part or parts of different sectors of society which has been formed to take action on an issue to achieve health outcomes or intermediate health outcomes in a way which is more effective, efficient or sustainable than might be achieved by the health sector acting alone.
>
> (WHO, 1998, pp. 14–15)

Thinking point: why do many people, both lay and professional, choose to work in partnership?

People may decide to try to work in partnership for a variety of reasons, and the formation of this process can come from the private or the public sectors. One reason might be that partnership is thought to be a good way of making things happen and achieving change. For example, partnership working may be thought to be most effective at implementing outreach work that addresses social exclusion, and therefore of increasing the likelihood of locally appropriate practices and services being provided; or a public sector organisation may need private resources. To some, it may seem obvious that, with many agencies working on common ground, partnerships between them will lead to more effective work. For a recent example, see Box 5.1.

Box 5.1   SWISH: sex workers' outreach project

SWISH (Sex Workers into Sexual Health) is an outreach project run by the Terrence Higgins Trust. The project is funded by the Drug Action Team and Community Safety Project, providing HIV, hepatitis, sexual health and safer sex information, direct services, advocacy and support to women working in both indoor and outdoor sex work. The project was set up in consultation with local community and neighbourhood groups, and collaborates with a range of partner agencies; these include: the Community Drugs Team, The Magistrates Court, the Police Service, the Probation Service and healthcare service providers. By working in partnership, the project has achieved an increase in women accessing the service, a decrease in homelessness and a 25 per cent decrease in complaints to the police.

(Adapted from renewal.net, 2006)

Notwithstanding the demonstrable advantages of working in partnership, developing collaborations, alliances and partnerships is not straightforward. The development of partnerships needs consensus building and commitment as partnerships can be very time consuming and fraught with difficulties. In order to understand the possible benefits of partnership working, it is important to explore health as a holistic concept and take account of mental and social as well as physical aspects. This reflects the shift away from individually and biomedically defined health problems to encapsulate a socio-ecological perspective of health and wellbeing (see Earle et al., 2007). This shift highlights the importance of socio-structural factors and relationships: in other words, social processes in health development and a concern with intersectoral action outside the health sector alone.

By the late 1990s, a new partnership culture had surfaced in the UK, but the concepts of alliances, partnership and partnership working remained difficult to define in precise terms (Audit Commission, 1998). It can be difficult to separate partnerships in practical terms from other forms of interorganisational relationships (Powell and Glendinning, 2002). The concepts of partnership and partnership working are contested as they have different meanings in different contexts: 'Partnership means many things to many people. Indeed it is not clearly defined precisely because its ambiguity can be politically attractive. It is difficult to be opposed to partnerships ... There is no single easily transferable model of partnership' (Roberts et al., 1995, p. 7).

As you saw in previous chapters in this book, partnerships can be developed globally, internationally: between the WHO, for example, and its member governments. The goal of the Global Alliance for Vaccines and Immunization, for instance, is to promote the immunisation of all the world's children. Box 5.2 provides an example of partnership working at a global level.

Box 5.2 The Global Alliance for Vaccines and Immunization (GAVI)

Vaccination provides enormous benefits to public health at very low cost. However, approximately one in four children are not vaccinated and two to three million children die from vaccine-preventable diseases each year. The GAVI alliance is a public/private global public health partnership which provides partners with a forum to develop policies, strategies and priorities for immunisation. The alliance includes governments, the World Health Organization, UNICEF, the Bill & Melinda Gates Foundation, non-governmental organisations, research institutes and vaccine manufacturers.

> The GAVI takes proposals from national governments to implement their immunisation programmes. It also plays a role in advocacy, as well as in finding and implementing best practice.
>
> (Adapted from GAVI, 2006)

The structure of the alliance is illustrated in Figure 5.1.

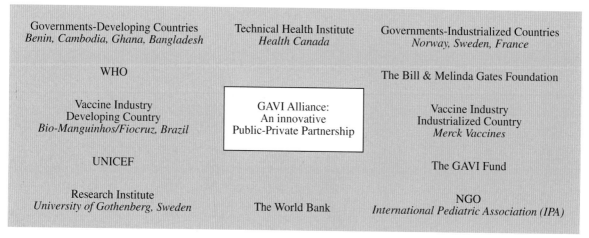

Figure 5.1   GAVI Alliance: an innovative public/private partnership (Source: GAVI, 2006)

Alliances such as that shown in Figure 5.1 can combine financial and organisational components in order to try to overcome huge global challenges. Partnerships can be formed nationally – for example, between the UK central government and the devolved Scottish Executive and the Welsh Assembly; or locally – for example, between statutory and voluntary agencies in the health and local authority spheres. They can also develop between statutory and voluntary agencies and the communities they serve, and, finally, between individuals. There is a vast number of stakeholders in multidisciplinary public health who are potential partners based in various sectors and operating at various levels.

Numerous attempts have been made to produce a definition of partnerships. Some authors stress the importance of identifying common goals and objectives: 'Partnerships are formal structures of relationships among individuals or groups, all of which are banded together for a common purpose' (Peckham, 2003, p. 61). Others reflect this in terms of a focus on health outcomes: '[a partnership is] a voluntary agreement between two or more partners to work cooperatively towards a set of shared health outcomes' (Gillies, 1998, p. 10, adapted from WHO, 1998).

The following definition is useful as it emphasises the values underlying health promotion: '[a partnership is] a mutually beneficial relationship that is transparent and accountable and based on agreed ethical principles, mutual understanding, respect and trust' (Japhet and Hulme, 2004, p. 120). A definition put forward by Barnes and Prior (2000) highlighted, alongside the mobilisation of those with common interests to work towards benefits that are not achievable by single agencies alone, another important feature: evaluation.

Thinking point: does partnership working incorporate a particular set of underlying values or principles?

Within the broad concept of partnerships that can be identified working across all aspects of the political spectrum, there remains a need for clarity on agreed definitions and parameters, especially related to their underlying values and ideology. Successful partnership working has to reflect values and principles such as those related to participatory democracy and equality, as well as collaboration, participation, joint ownership, empowerment and equity. While it is important to understand ideological and practical differences at political, cultural and technical levels, there is a continuing need to ensure that partnership working is based on common key values and principles.

Partnership working can be focused on issues, target groups or localities and can occur at a number of levels (Hudson, 1987; Rummery and Glendinning, 1997; Exworthy and Powell, 2000; Peckham, 2003). When referring specifically to partnerships for health promotion, the WHO both stresses their intersectoral nature and endorses the importance of clearly defined goals:

> Such partnerships may form a part of intersectoral collaboration for health, or be based on alliances for health promotion. Such partnerships may be limited by the pursuit of a clearly defined goal – such as the successful development and introduction of legislation; or may be on-going, covering a broad range of issues and initiatives. Increasingly health promotion is exploring partnerships between the public sector, civil society and the private sector.
>
> (WHO, 1998, p. 17)

However, a lack of a precise definition can be seen as being beneficial as it provides:

> a form of organisational governance whose flexibility, responsiveness and adaptability is ideally suited to the demands of contemporary society (Glendinning and Clarke, 2000) ... so that collaborative activities can reflect local circumstances, needs and agreed joint objectives and remain appropriate to the expertise and levels of trust of local partners.
>
> (Glendinning, 2002, p. 117)

Gillies highlights the effectiveness of partnerships by referring to action at both population and individual levels: 'Alliance or partnership initiatives to promote health across sectors, across lay and professional boundaries and between public, private and non-governmental agencies, do work. They work in tackling the broader determinants of health and well-being in populations in a sustainable manner, as well as in promoting individual health-related behaviour change' (Gillies, 1998, p. 99). An example of this is given in Box 5.3.

Box 5.3 Prison health and healthcare services

Prison Health is a partnership between the Department of Health and the Prison Service. This partnership aims to improve the standard of healthcare in prisons by ensuring that those living securely have the same access to healthcare services as the general public. Budgetary responsibility for prison health has been given to the Department of Health, and primary care trusts have full commissioning responsibilities. The Prison Health Work Programme includes dental services, harm minimisation, promoting health, and mental health and pharmacy services.

(Adapted from DoH, 2006)

The framework given in Figure 5.2, offered by Peckham (2003), gives you an opportunity to examine, analyse and perhaps categorise the partnerships and alliances of which you might have had experience.

Figure 5.2 A framework for partnership working (Source: Peckham, 2003, p. 61, Box 4.1)

Isolation	No partnership exists and agencies or individuals work in isolation from each other
Encounter	Some interagency and interprofessional contact, but this is informal, ad hoc and marginal to the goals of the separate organizations
Communication	Separate organizations or professions do engage in joint working of a formal and structured nature, but this still tends to be marginal to separate organizational goals or individual roles, and needs to be able to demonstrate how such activity will help achieve these respective goals or fulfil individual work roles
Collaboration	Separate agencies recognize that joint working is central to their mainstream activities; this implies a trusting relationship in which organizations are seen to be reliable partners
Integration	A situation where the degree of collaboration is so high that the separate organizations no longer see their separate identity as significant and may be willing to contemplate the creation of a unitary organization

Of course, partnerships and alliances change over time. They can evolve and strengthen towards integration or they can unravel, perhaps leading to different partnerships being formed, but a drive to form and maintain alliances and partnerships for public health, in the foreseeable future, is likely to remain.

5.2 Developing partnerships: the policies

The WHO Jakarta Declaration (1997) sought specifically to consolidate and expand partnerships for health:

> Health promotion requires partnerships for health and social development between the different sectors at all levels of governance and society. Existing partnerships need to be strengthened and the potential for new partnerships must be explored.

> Partnerships offer mutual benefit for health through the sharing of expertise, skills and resources. Each partnership must be transparent and accountable and be based on agreed ethical principles, mutual understanding and respect.

> (WHO, 1997, p. 4)

The importance of partnerships was further affirmed in the Bangkok Charter for Health Promotion (WHO, 2005), which reinforced the recommendation that partnerships empower communities to improve health and promote health equality and should be at the core of global and national developments. Within the European Union (EU), partnership working lies at the heart of a range of policy directives and activities, including the Health and Social Inclusion Programme, the European Lisbon Social Model, Narrowing the Health Gap/Public Health Programme, the work of the EU Public Health Forum and a wide range of recommended public/ private partnership initiatives. The EU has the goal of placing health at the centre of European policymaking under the theme of Partnerships for Health (Byrne, 2004). Partnership working for health is also a favoured contemporary strategy that is firmly on the agenda at national level in terms of policy directives, conference topics and recommended good practice. It forms an underlying theme that runs through key government health policy papers in the four countries of the UK, for example. The Labour governments in the UK, since coming to power in 1997, have emphasised partnerships and collaboration as a cross-cutting theme in all its policies, reflecting this as the core element of its political philosophy of the 'Third Way'. Within the British context, the government view is that successful partnership working involves developing common aims and appropriate staff skills, and facilitating a partnership culture. Agencies such as the

Department of Health have expressed their objectives in these terms: 'Successful partnership working is built on organisations moving together to address common goals: on developing in their staff the skills necessary to work in an entirely new way – across boundaries, in multidisciplinary teams, and in a culture in which learning and good practice are shared' (DoH, 1999, p. 123).

This approach has dominated, in particular, recent government policies to tackle growing social and health inequalities. Current policies reflect the need to halt growing inequalities in health by tackling health determinants, which are now well documented (see Marmott and Wilkinson, 2005) and are one of the principal justifications for developing partnerships for health. This is due to there being evidence from the literature that partnership working for health, when implemented properly, leads to better health processes and health outcomes (Gray, 1985, 1989; Gillies, 1998; Taket and White, 2000; de Leeuw and Skovgaard, 2005). Rather belatedly, policies have embraced a wider social model of health, with an emphasis on intersectoral and partnership working: the model that has been advocated for at least two decades by the WHO. Since it came to power, the Labour Government has encouraged a practical partnership culture by initiating a plethora of new approaches to public health development in an attempt to address continuing inequalities in health.

The continuing importance of partnership working for health is also reflected in its current popularity as a conference theme. For example, 'Partnerships for Health' was the theme of the 2005 UK Community Practitioners and Health Visitors Association Annual Conference and also the 2005 European Health Forum Gastein, the annual European health policy conference held in Austria. At a global level, partnership working for health forms the seventh of the United Nations' Millennium Development Goals (MDGs) and lies at the heart of its strategy (see Figure 1.2 in Chapter 1). The establishment of effective global partnerships for development is seen as essential for the achievement of all other MDGs. Agenda 21, the United Nations' comprehensive plan of action for sustainable development, stresses the importance of civil society working in partnership to make sustainable development happen. Agenda 21 identifies the nine major groups that must work in partnership for sustainable development, recognising the importance of strengthening their role (see Box 5.4).

Box 5.4 Civil society working in partnership

- Women's participation in political and economic decision making is seen as vital to success.
- Non-governmental organisations play a role in influencing, developing and implementing sustainable policies.

- Business and industry play a role in local, regional, national and international economic development and prosperity.

- Children and youth will contribute to the future success of sustainable development programmes and should be encouraged to participate.

- Local authorities must work in partnership to tackle local problems and develop local solutions.

- Scientific and technological communities must communicate effectively with the general public, and make an open and effective contribution to policy making.

- Indigenous people should be enabled to participate fully in sustainability, recognising their traditional knowledge of their lands, natural resources and environments.

- Workers and trade unions should support and practise opportunities for sustainable development.

- Farmers should be enabled to manage their resources in a sustainable way.

(Adapted from UNDESA, 2006)

5.2.1 Partnerships as the new model for local governance

Within the UK, partnerships have been seen as the new model for local governance and the changing relationship between 'the state, the market and civil society' (Heenan, 2004, p. 106). Partnership lies at the heart of New Labour's public service reform programme, for example, in relation to education and employment zones, public/private partnerships, health and social care trusts and children's trusts. Soon after the Labour Government's agenda for collaboration was launched, the Economic and Social Research Council (ESRC) commissioned a seminar series on 'Improving partnerships between health and local government' (see Snape and Taylor, 2004, for a full analysis of this work). Within the health and social services fields in the UK, it is widely assumed that it is best practice for statutory, voluntary and private sectors to collaborate together. Lucas and Lloyd note that:

> 'partnerships', 'collaboration', and 'working together' are terms found scattered liberally throughout the documentation of health promotion planning over the last 10 years or so ... It is self-evident that lasting benefits to health can only be obtained by co-operation between all statutory bodies, together with voluntary, community and commercial groups.

(Lucas and Lloyd, 2005, p. 18)

Yet they cite Nutbeam and Harris who observe that:

> there is increasing concern that the level of investment that is required in establishing and maintaining effective relationships may be greater than the benefits. For this reason it is important to develop a critical approach to deciding if, and how, these relationships should be developed and what it is that we hope will be achieved by them.
>
> (Nutbeam and Harris, 2004, p. 58)

Barnes and Prior (2000), in their analysis of the characteristics that appeal to New Labour governments, include 'partnership', or active 'joined-up' working, not only between the state and its various agencies, but also between the private and voluntary sectors, community organisations, user groups and individual members of the community. The concept of community lies at the heart of multidisciplinary public health, reflecting the importance of social capital and communitarianism. Community development is a key approach to facilitate the production of social capital and address issues of social justice. Partnership working at community level facilitates effective communication, community empowerment and the provision of social support (see Part II of this book for further elaboration of these concepts). The Local Government Act 2000, for example, had set a duty on local authorities to develop 'community strategies' to improve social, economic and environmental wellbeing, thereby providing a key context in which to tackle determinants of health. So, as Barnes et al. note: 'Almost all significant public policy proposals introduced since 1997 have, to a greater or lesser extent, required the forming of partnerships to secure the desired outcomes. Partnership has been at the heart of New Labour's redefinition of relationships between central and local government' (Barnes et al., 2005, p. 25). But Barnes et al. also point out that, although partnership working is nothing new, what is different is the scale of its implementation by the Labour governments since 1997.

Groups taking action in the public health arena can take many forms – healthy alliances, community coalitions, school and community partnerships, collaborative partnerships, strategic partnerships, action-oriented partnerships, community development through partnerships, community partnerships, community-provider partnerships, academic-practice partnerships, intersectoral partnerships and public/private partnerships: all these can be found liberally scattered through health and social care.

Thinking point: of those groups working for health of which you have had experience, do most work autonomously, collaboratively or in partnership?

Alliances and collaborations have been demonstrated as being most effective where there is at least a partial coming together of interests and values, mutual respect for differences, stability, time to build trust and joint ownership of agendas, as well as resources of various kinds (Sullivan and Skelcher, 2002). Peckham (2003) concludes his review of partnerships by demonstrating that they are a fundamental concept underlining efforts to maintain and improve public health, and perceives this as both a strength and a weakness. The case is clearly made that inequalities in health, and the complex interaction of the determinants that influence them, need to be tackled by intersectoral approaches that can be achieved only by partnership working.

However, two key problems highlighted by Barnes et al. (2005) relate to the difficulty of defining precisely what New Labour actually means by 'partnership', and to the difficulty of being able to transfer the development of 'project-based partnerships' into mainstream public services (i.e. by influencing cultures, budgets and organisational structures, for example). Sullivan and Skelcher (2002) identified more than sixty different types of public policy partnership, and estimated that in 2001–2002 between £15 billion and £20 billion was being spent on sub-national partnership working, and that an estimated 75,000 partnership board places existed, compared with 23,000 elected councillors.

5.2.2 Partnerships in action: the case of Health Action Zones

Prominent among New Labour public health projects have been Health Action Zones (HAZs), large projects through which the strategy of *Our Healthier Nation* (DoH, 1998) could be delivered: 'HAZ was credited with preparing the ground for lasting partnership working in each area ... and in some cases providing a template for the development of Local Strategic Partnerships. It did this by providing the practical means of partnership engagement' (Barnes et al., 2005, p. 179).

In addition, HAZs were seen to create an awareness of the various factors that made partnerships work, and the barriers to them. They had sought to tackle conflicts before partnership working became possible and brought about a cultural shift. Several of the HAZs did bring services into the mainstream and develop partnerships; however, Barnes et al., in their evaluation of HAZs, have noted that: 'Building effective local partnerships is not possible without taking very seriously the strengthening of both individual and organizational capacity' (Barnes et al., 2005, p. 189).

In their final comments, Barnes et al. recommend that the effects of HAZs should not be seen in isolation, and they suggest the need for 'a critical review of the design, implementation and achievements of the many complex social interventions introduced in the United Kingdom in recent years' (Barnes et al., 2005, p. 196).

A central goal of HAZs and other similar projects was the eventual integration of their work into mainstream services and activities. Stewart and Purdue (2002) identified three levels of mainstreaming:

1 **mainstreaming projects:** obtaining funding to continue activities
2 **mainstreaming best practice:** examples of activities adapted into mainstream services, etc.
3 **mainstreaming policy:** adaptation and replication into the main policy arena.

Mainstreaming has to be occurring at these three levels for sustainable change to take place. In most, if not all, cases, existing power relationships are left intact. This has been seen by some commentators as a limitation of the Healthy Cities/settings approach which relies so heavily on effective partnership working. (You read about the Healthy Cities movement in Chapter 1; see also WHO, 2006.) The WHO European Healthy Cities Project provides another example of the settings approach to public health in action, based on the key foundation of partnership working. Established in 1987, it evolved from a project to an international movement. It is firmly based on the establishment of an intersectoral committee, which reinforces collaboration through both technical means and interpersonal relations. Cities have developed intersectoral steering committees with strong links to the political decision-making system. The movement's intention is to move from informal partnerships to formal intersectoral arrangements, and to 'mainstream' action for healthy urban development. However, de Leeuw and Skovgaard (2005), in their analysis of the European Healthy Cities Project, cite Tsouros and Draper (1993) when they state that some cities involved in the project have commented that implementing intersectoral collaboration 'is very hard indeed because it challenges traditional patterns of (public) organizations and management' (de Leeuw and Skovgaard, 2005, p. 1337). Referring to Goumans (1998), they highlight the failure of some Healthy City projects to move into the mainstream: 'In many cases multi-sectoral collaborations take the form of joint projects and actions only. Measures to install long-term, formal co-operations with the ultimate aim of developing innovative policies with lasting impact on the ways in which municipal authorities deal with, and prioritize, health-related issues are few in number' (p. 1337). They go on to state that in their view, after twenty years of the Healthy City Programme, real and effective partnerships were still not in place.

When making a critical examination of the role of government, the following negative issues can be highlighted or seen as problematic: increased fragmentation through a plethora of initiatives; establishment of a new type of 'market' (Hunter, 2003) which is short term, with a lack of integration; NHS bias towards disease/illhealth rather than towards maintaining and improving health; and the overlooking of the contribution of other agencies, especially local government. In practice, the medical model can still dominate, and this acts as a major barrier to ownership by partners outside the health sector, especially in local government and the voluntary sector. In practical terms, the vision of 'joined-up government' has not yet been achieved and departmentalism still rules.

From their experience of evaluating HAZs, Barnes et al. (2005) suggest that there are three requirements for achieving whole systems change:

1   to understand the cycle of change and its drivers and barriers at national and local level
2   to understand the context for any complex community-based initiative from initial strategic planning
3   to have a strong commitment to building evaluation and structures for mainstreaming.

Although it is always assumed that mainstreaming will best occur at national level, Barnes et al. (2005), citing Stewart and Purdue (2002), indicate that lessons from HAZs have been focused at the project level in the short term by securing continued funding. Barnes et al. found evidence that those projects more closely integrated within existing infrastructures were more likely to be effective in mainstreaming policy and practice at local level. They cited the examples of Leeds City Children's Strategy, which included innovative models of care using community-based paediatricians, and the CHD (coronary heart disease) Programme in Merseyside, which targeted deprived populations in order to tackle specific local needs. With specific regard to HAZs and their role in the enhancement of local capacity to tackle health inequalities, they found that 'in a range of ways the additional HAZ funding "oiled the wheels" of local partnership activities, for example, by supporting mainstream posts and service developments; through the work of the HAZ team; and, in some cases, by bringing into the local economy a range of different consultants and facilitators' (Barnes et al., 2005, p. 140).

Numerous government initiatives have dismantled and reorganised both traditional partnerships and newly established ones: for example, HAZs are, at the time of writing, being devolved to primary care trusts (PCTs) and local strategic partnerships (LSPs). Barnes et al. (2005) reported that following the government's decision to channel HAZ funds through PCTs, no specific guidance has been given to PCTs on the allocation of these funds. With the linking of HAZ work with LSPs and PCTs, Barnes et al. (2005, p. 136) felt that: 'some LSPs were believed to be at risk of "reinventing the wheel" particularly in relation to developing multi-agency partnerships and engaging communities'.

Judge and Bauld (2006) argue that there are essential lessons to be learned from the HAZ initiative, not least that HAZs set themselves impossibly ambitious goals, including radically reducing those major social problems that have resisted change for decades. Judge and Bauld advised on the importance of major social and health initiatives – such as the HAZs – learning from previous experience, and particularly from evaluations of initiatives that preceded the HAZs. Community-based initiatives also need to be able to measure change from clearly established baselines, and they need to collect data in common regarding outcomes and process; otherwise any judgement on effectiveness will be fatally flawed. Overall, Judge and Bauld point to an important turning away from a belief in 'big government' that directly fed into strategies such as HAZs:

> Too many users of policy research still expect clear answers about impact when a more realistic product of evaluations is that they contribute to a process of enlightenment about highly complex processes that are interpreted by different actors in multiple ways.
>
> [...]
>
> ... What has changed is that there appears to be a more sophisticated recognition of the complexity, pervasiveness and durability of the social problems that have to be confronted.
>
> (Judge and Bauld, 2006, pp. 342, 343)

Yet there remains a clear danger in the UK partnership experience of the public service culture, in particular the NHS culture, dominating in the public health arena. In reviewing the history of the UK experience (and noting variation among the four nations involved), the following changes in relation to partnership culture can be noted: a move away from the welfare state (i.e. statutory and voluntary organisations working alongside each other); through a market-led economy (i.e. a contract culture and consumer choice); to partnerships being forced to bid for funds, and to New Labour's 'Third Way' – that is, the encouragement of partnership-linked neighbourhood renewal (e.g. Sure Start, New Deal, Early Years); and, finally, to the proliferation of partnerships with little central focus (either national or local). As Stewart (2003, p. 191) has stated: 'The evidence of the past is of complexity in the arrangements for joint working both vertically between centre and periphery, and horizontally between organizations at the same level.'

Perhaps governments will rely on the introduction of local strategic partnerships to help to solve this latest challenge. Opportunities are offered by LSPs outside the health sector (Duggan, 2001), including the co-ordination of local neighbourhood strategies and linking with Healthy City initiatives. But the long-standing issue is that the role of local authorities in public health has been problematic since the NHS reorganisation in 1974, when community and public health services were institutionalised into the NHS medical model culture. The government policy paper *Shifting the Balance of Power within the NHS* (DoH, 2001b) highlighted regional accountability for public health. Regional Directors of Public Health were expected to facilitate the rolling out of the public health perspective to all relevant areas of regional policy and to utilise LSPs as a mechanism. Since LSPs lie outside NHS/health sector control, the health sector has tried to rectify this by issuing guidance from the DoH regarding strengthening links to LSPs through, for example, the disability White Paper (DoH, 2001c), the National Service Framework for Older People (DoH, 2001a), and children's services planning (Statutory Instrument, 2005).

Different directions for English public health have been proposed, but a major problem is that public health is still seen as part of the management structure of the NHS (with a narrow managerial agenda) (Hunter, 2003). An additional problem is the lead role being given to PCTs whose primary responsibilities and culture are not focused on public health. In practical terms, the governments of the four UK nations exert political pressure for early successes in particular by building partnership structures, which is not the same as partnership working (Mayo, 1997; Atkinson, 1999). As a result, most partnerships have failed to move into the 'mainstream' and to change core departmental/agency cultures, organisational structures, budgets and/or working practices.

Partnership formation, despite the problems, continues to be the response to a series of drivers (Mackintosh, 1992; Huxham, 1996; Hughes et al., 1998; Hudson et al., 1999; Savas, 2000). These are summarised by Barnes et al. (2005) as:

- a shared vision

- maximising the use of available resources

- tackling complexity in public policy

- maximising power and influence

- resolving conflict through partnerships.

Although these factors may be prioritised differently by different partners, they will be important in shaping the partnership that eventually develops, and they will continue to exert pressure on services and practitioners to set up, facilitate and evaluate alliances and partnerships.

5.3 Partnerships: implementation and evaluation

Partnerships are usually complicated systems operating in many layered environments. Figure 5.3 shows a model of public health provision.

The EUHPID (European Health Promotion Indicators Development) Health Development Model takes a social systems perspective in order to explore complex interactions (Bauer et al., 2006). In Figure 5.3, the left-hand side illustrates a salutogenesis approach, the right hand-side a pathogenesis

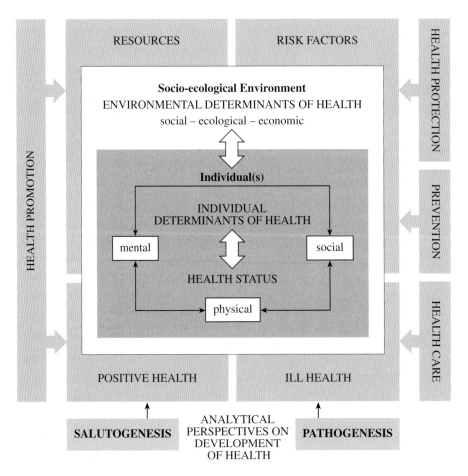

Figure 5.3 EUHPID Health Development Model: public health intervention approaches (Source: Bauer et al., 2006, p. 155, Figure 1)

approach (see Earle et al., 2007, for further details of these approaches). The model distinguishes three qualitatively different dimensions of health: physical, mental and social health. The arrows between these dimensions illustrate that they are highly interdependent.

Thinking point: what does this model highlight with regard to partnership working?

The model relates to the interaction between the physical, mental and social health of individuals, and demonstrates how health develops by interaction between individuals and their ecological/environmental health determinants. It also demonstrates that health development can be analysed from both salutogenic and pathogenic perspectives. This is of importance in helping us understand the centrality of partnership working in addressing the breadth of health-related issues and their interactivity.

Partnerships are very likely to remain core strategies to tackle the multidisciplinary nature of health and actively involve the multi-stakeholders involved. But building effective intersectoral collaboration is a difficult and complex process. It can include collaboration and community development, and both multidisciplinary and multiprofessional working as well as public/private working. With commitment, however, clear steps to successful partnerships are discernible. According to Fawcett et al. (1995) and Markwell (2003), these are:

- **Leadership and vision (know what you want)**

  Shared realistic vision

- **Effective leadership**

- **Common goals and clear objectives**

  Ensure appropriate resources are available

  Define the 'problem'

  Be aware of your organisation's strengths – what it can offer

  Be aware of organisational limitations – have realistic expectations

- **Preparation**

  Allocate appropriate time and resources

  Be committed and be aware of benefits

  Be aware of resource implications

  Be aware of political and socio-economic context

- **Building profile of potential partners**

  Undertake a SWOT ('strengths, weaknesses, opportunities and threats') analysis of various potential listed partners

  Be aware of contexts within which potential partners are working

  Ensure equality among partners

- **Approaching preferred partner**

  Clearly define roles/responsibilities

  Draw up a memorandum of agreement – time line, evaluation, exit strategy

  Ensure clear communication lines and channels

  Allocate time

  Ensure clear decision-making processes

- **Managing the partnership**

  Develop a clear strategy built on local needs and continuous dialogue

  Set policies, targets and delivery mechanisms

- **Manage process with flexibility**

  Maintain trust and sharing learning opportunities

  Share resources

  Pay appropriate or better rates

  Decide on action if partnership not working (including third party mediation)

- **Evaluation and review**

  Process evaluation of partnership

  Document outcomes/deliverables

  (Adapted from Fawcett et al., 1995; Markwell, 2003)

5.3.1 Benefits of successful partnerships

In considering the uptake of partnership working in UK public health, Peckham (2003) suggests that three broad strategies have been used: collaboration based on agreement between organisations/individuals, incentives such as funding and its more flexible use, and authoritarian approaches with a range of 'must-do' requirements – related, for example, to Health Action Zones, Sure Start programmes and local strategic partnerships (LSPs). Intersectoral collaboration, including public, private and voluntary sectors, can challenge the traditional patterns of management and organisation within the public sector. Each sector retains a unique role and responsibility. Yet intersectoral collaboration is a central building block for public health and health promotion action. A recent compendium describing a wide range of good practices from a number of European countries to tackle health inequalities, through intersectoral partnership working, is provided by EuroHealthNet (2004). Good practices include implementation methods such as appropriate education and training to build capacity and capability; the use of intercultural mediators; and the establishment of local initiatives to provide support to a wide range of stakeholders that generate social cohesion, a key to effective partnership working.

Thinking point: what are the real benefits of forming alliances and partnerships?

Among the benefits of successful partnerships are the sharing of responsibility, the increased access to funding for some partners, joint funding, increased information/knowledge, a higher profile representation for some partners, staff development, more effective and efficient use of resources, avoiding duplication of effort, and achieving a more comprehensive and coherent approach. However, as we have seen, ideological and practical issues at political, technical and cultural levels can act as bridges and barriers to effective partnership working. Situations which deter collaboration can arise from the self-interest of the organisation, when organisations strive to maximise their autonomy; professionalisation of issues of powerful groups; and conflicting values and priorities (Delaney, 1994). Many of these situations relate to power relationships. Some partnerships therefore collapse after a couple of meetings; others remain merely 'talking shops', or become inward looking and exclusive; yet others work with unclear or unrealistic goals, cannot make decisions, or are not flexible enough to consider various points of view.

One commonly erroneous assumption in partnership working is that all partners are equal and share equality of power. The inevitable importance of power and potential conflict in partnership working has been noted (HEBS, 2000). There is a series of pre-conditions that enable partnerships to be more effective. These include a clear definition of the issue/tangible problem, availability of community support, a common understanding of the 'problem' and a level of respect between partners, and a sharing of common ground. There needs to be an awareness of tensions between local/ national and national/international strategies and, consequently, different expectations of the stakeholders involved. For example, global health issues generate partnerships with the UN, WHO, UNICEF or UNAIDS at their centre, and can involve financial institutions such as the World Bank, multinational pharmaceutical and biotechnological companies, non-governmental health organisations, and philanthropists. An example of this is the WHO/WFME strategic partnership (see Box 5.5) to improve medical education, where educators across the world are working together to improve the human resources for health.

Box 5.5   WHO/WFME strategic partnership to improve medical education

WHO and the World Federation for Medical Education (WFME) propose a strategic partnership to pursue a long-term work plan – open to participation by all medical schools and other educational providers – intended to have a decisive impact on medical education in particular and ultimately on health professions education in general. The WHO/WFME work plan will benefit from the accumulated experience and assets of each partner and will result in:

- A shared database that will include up-to-date experience in implementing quality-improvement processes in medical schools

- Access, via the database, to information on specific schools and in particular to a description of their approach to quality improvement

- Promoting twinning between schools and other institutions in processes to foster innovative education

- Means to update the management of medical schools
- Identification and analysis, by WHO regions, of innovations in medical education in order to help define appropriate lines of work for each region
- Assistance to institutions or national/regional organizations and agencies in developing and implementing reform programmes or establishing recognition/accreditation systems
- A review of good practices in medical education that can serve as examples and as a source for further innovation.

The strategic partnership will also address other crucial questions that medical schools now face, such as improving their leadership function. Through a systematic dialogue, the partners will pursue the work plan and provide useful information to medical schools worldwide.

[...]

There is no single path towards improving the quality of medical education. Each region and country features different approaches that must be acknowledged, explored and brought to wider use. But to achieve significant and lasting results, institutions must be committed to an ongoing process of quality development. The WHO/WFME strategic partnership aims to foster this commitment.

(WFME, 2006)

Of course, such projects need to be monitored and evaluated to improve partnership workings and chances of success. Situations which help to facilitate alliance and partnership success relate to increased efficiency and quality, a survival strategy, pre-existing networks, and the ethos of the organisation (Delaney, 1994). Effective and authentic partnerships have better chances of succeeding when all partners have well-defined mission statements, organisational goals and a clear sense of purpose, and have established their own power and legitimacy; this may involve a period of conflict between powerful and marginalised partners. The provision of resources by marginalised partners is important if such resources remain in the autonomous control of these groups.

Taking a global perspective or approach to health involves finding out about which problems affect which populations, about who contributes to global health problems (e.g. unsafe commercial actions), and where nation states can offer experience and expertise (such as the case given in Box 5.6) in disease surveillance, health education and research, and essential medicines and vaccines to fight diseases and respond to global health priorities.

Box 5.6   The Global Partnership to Stop Tuberculosis

In 2001, the STOP TB partnership of 200 members, co-ordinated by the WHO, presented a comprehensive five-year global plan and budget to the World Bank. Although the international standard treatment for TB – the directly observed treatment short course (DOTS) – is one of the most effective public health interventions, only 25 per cent of those with TB received the treatment in 2000. While the WHO co-ordinates the development of the global strategy and policy for TB control, six working groups now cover the vital areas of the partnership's activities; namely, expanding the use of DOTS and DOTS Plus for the drug-resistant TB, and TB with HIV, and for TB drugs research, TB diagnostics and TB vaccination.

(Adapted from WHO, 2007)

So partnerships need to work towards recognition of the value and individual power of each partner, and work in a spirit of co-operation; they have to be amenable to change and have means to resolve potential conflict. The objectives and expectations of the partners need to be made clear, and written agreements are helpful to communicate objectives, roles and responsibilities, together with evaluation criteria. All stakeholders can develop and strengthen values related to respect and understanding of their fellow partners. All partners can be committed to strive for open-mindedness, patience, respect and sensitivity within partnering organisations.

5.3.2 Barriers to successful partnerships

Thinking point: what do you think might be some of the barriers to setting up effective partnerships?

Some of the potential barriers to effective partnership working are a lack of executive commitment, an imbalance in resources, differences in outlook and objectives, the exclusion of new partners, a failure to evaluate, a lack of necessary skills and/or shared goals, a lack of understanding of various organisational cultures, a lack of short-terms wins/lack of real achievement, and a lack of obvious benefits for each partner involved.

Numerous studies have explored partnership working (Mackintosh, 1992; Roberts et al., 1995; Hastings et al., 1996; Geddes, 1997; Harding, 1998; Lowndes and Skelcher, 1998) and highlight a lack of necessary evaluation and research. Research studies using quantitative methods and 'conventional' paradigm/methodology cannot be used. In assessing partnerships, objectives, targets, indicators/proxy indicators (including process as well as outcome indicators) are important. Therefore dedicated measurement instruments have to be developed (see Earle et al., 2007, for a consideration of both quantitative and qualitative methods in multidisciplinary public health and research). Bush and Mutch (2002) have developed an instrument called the Community Capacity Index (CCI). It seeks to identify the level and extent of existing capacity within a local network of groups and organisations in order to provide evidence about the capacity of a network. This is then compared against a series of indicators. These issues are identified by the community itself. One of the four domains studied in the CCI is 'network partnerships': that is, the capacity to identify groups and organisations with appropriate resources to launch a programme, and to deliver, maintain and sustain that programme. Another useful planning tool and series of case studies of partnerships or alliances for health in the UK is provided by Funnell et al. (1995).

Although Gillies (1998) makes a strong case for partnerships and intersectoral collaboration to tackle the determinants of health as well as individual health behaviour, she has called for a set of new 'social' indicators to measure the effects of health promotion. She also proposes the concept of 'social capital' as a potential framework for action. But further in-depth exploration is needed in order to adopt the social capital concept, and move from an illness/disease/problem-based approach to facilitate socio-ecological and salutogenic change. The production of such health promotion measurement indicators is being progressed in Europe by the EUHPID Project (Davies et al., 2004) as part of the planned further development of the ECHIM Project 2005–2008 (European Health Knowledge and Information System), for example. In this regard, key indicator sets are being focused on health promotion policy and practice (see HP-Source.net, 2003) and on integrated settings (workplaces, schools, hospitals, etc.), both areas being of key importance in understanding, planning and monitoring concepts of partnership working.

There is a pressing need to develop appropriate theories, models and measurement indicators that analyse effective partnership working for health. Although there are many positive reasons to build partnerships and alliances for health, a critical perspective is also needed, as there remains a dearth of research and theory building with regard to partnership development and intersectoral working in public health and health promotion. As Lucas and Lloyd (2005, p. 19) note: 'Regrettably, theoretical explanations of precisely *how* the recent plethora of such partnerships will bring about improvements in the health and well-being of the most vulnerable are far less common than the exhortations to form them.'

Conclusion

In this chapter we have reviewed partnership working and developed an understanding of policies and processes involved in developing and sustaining partnerships. The last twenty-five years have seen a rapid growth of interest in partnership working at local, national, international and global levels, and partnership working is now a key theme in all UK government policy. National policy documents acknowledge that partnerships are crucial since health needs to be tackled on a much broader front than the health sector could offer alone. However, some commentators have come to feel that partnership is an overused and sometimes abused term (Stewart, 2003, p. 190).

Partnership working has formed the basis for WHO's Health for All strategy since its launch during the WHO Conference on Primary Health Care in Alma Ata in 1978 (WHO, 1978). The organisation's emphasis on the development of partnerships for health has continued since then and underlies its most recent strategy *Health 21: Health for All in the 21st Century* (WHO, 1999), in which Target 20 specifically encourages the mobilisation of partnerships for health: 'by the year 2000 implementation of policies for health for all should engage individuals, groups and organizations throughout the public and private sectors and civil society, in alliances and partnerships for health' (WHO, 1999, p. 200).

Partnerships for health have been integral to the WHO's health promotion programme since its inception in the early 1980s, and they provide a consistent theme in its global health promotion conference declarations of Adelaide (WHO, 1988), Sundsvall (WHO, 1991), Jakarta (WHO, 1997) and Mexico City (WHO, 2000). Partnerships bring together skills and knowledge and, as Naidoo and Wills (2005) suggest, lead to 'the sharing of common concerns and information, the ability to influence decision making, avoiding the duplication of, or gaps in, a service response so making better use of resources, a more comprehensive and holistic approach to problems, synergy – the effect of collaboration being greater than that achieved alone' (Naidoo and Wills, 2005, p. 133).

In essence, a partnership can be greater than the sum of its parts. Yet partnership working remains a contested concept and can include many different types of partnerships, including interagency, interprofessional, collaborative, joined-up working, and community coalitions. There is a need to critically review the concept of partnerships and relate this to one's own practice and experience. Participation must be distinguished from partnership working, which involves community development and community empowerment, and people need to be given time and space to move from consultation to participation to partnership, and perhaps beyond. A key factor is the necessary commitment to a common cause, already stressed in this chapter. And, as highlighted earlier, it is crucial for partnerships to be flexible (Peckham, 2003, citing Glendinning, 2002).

Part II of the book explores notions of community development. The next chapter examines a case study of poverty and health which brings together some of the concepts explored in the last few chapters, including global, national and local policies for public health, healthy public policy, making and changing policy, the settings for health, and partnership working for health.

References

Atkinson, D. (1999) *Advocacy: A Review*, Brighton, Pavilion.

Audit Commission (1998) *A Fruitful Partnership: Effective Partnership Working*, London, Audit Commission.

Baggot, R. (2000) *Public Health: Policy and Politics*, Basingstoke, Macmillan.

Barnes, M. and Prior, D. (2000) *Private Lives as Public Policy*, Birmingham, Venture.

Barnes, M., Benzeval, M., Judge, K., Mackenzie, M. and Sullivan, H. (2005) *Health Action Zones: Partnerships for Health Equality*, Abingdon, Routledge.

Bauer, G., Davies, J.K. and Pelikan, J. (2006) 'The EUPHID Health Development Model for the classification of public health indicators', *Health Promotion International*, vol. 21, no. 2, pp. 153–8.

Bush, R.D. and Mutch, A. (2002) *A Community Capacity Index*, Brisbane, University of Queensland, Brisbane Centre for Health Care.

Byrne, D. (2004) *Enabling Good Health for All: A Reflection Process for a New EU Health Strategy*, Brussels, European Union.

Davies, J.K., Hill, C. and Linwood, E. (2004) *The Development of a European Health Promotion Monitoring System: The EUHPID Project Final Report to the European Commission*, Brighton, University of Brighton, International Health Development Research Centre.

de Leeuw, E. and Skovgaard, T. (2005) 'Utility-driven evidence for healthy cities: problems with evidence generation and application', *Social Science and Medicine*, vol. 61, no. 6, pp. 1331–41.

Delaney, F. (1994) 'Muddling through the middle ground: theoretical concerns in intersectoral collaboration and health promotion', *Health Promotion International*, vol. 9, no. 3, pp. 217–25.

Department of Health (DoH) (1998) *Our Healthier Nation*, London, The Stationery Office.

Department of Health (DoH) (1999) *Saving Lives: Our Healthier Nation*, London, The Stationery Office.

Department of Health (DoH) (2001a) *National Service Framework for Older People*, London, The Stationery Office.

Department of Health (DoH) (2001b) *Shifting the Balance of Power within the NHS*, London, The Stationery Office.

Department of Health (DoH) (2001c) *Valuing People: A New Strategy for Learning Disability for the 21st Century*, London, The Stationery Office.

Department of Health (DoH) (2006) [online], http://www.dh.gov.uk/PolicyAndGuidance/HealthAndSocialCareTopics/PrisonHealth/fs/en (Accessed 4 September 2006).

Duggan, M. (2001) *Growing Closer: A Guide to New Partnerships for Health*, London, NHS Confederation.

Earle, S., Lloyd, C.E., Sidell, M. and Spurr, S. (eds) (2007) *Theory and Research in Promoting Public Health*, London, Sage/Milton Keynes, The Open University.

EuroHealthNet (2004) *Promoting Social Exclusion and Tackling Health Inequalities in Europe: An Overview of Good Practice from the Health Field*, Brussels, EuroHealthNet.

Exworthy, M. and Powell, M. (2000) 'Variations on a theme: New Labour, health inequalities and policy failure' in Hann, A. (ed.) *Analysing Health Policy*, Aldershot, Ashgate.

Fawcett, S., Paine-Andrews, A., Franisco, J., Schultz, J., Lewis, R., Williams, E., Harris, K., Berkley, J., Lopez, C., Fisher, J. and Richter, K. (1995) 'Using empowerment theory in collaborative partnerships for community health and development', *American Journal of Community Psychology*, vol. 23, no. 5, pp. 677–97.

Funnell, R., Oldfield, K. and Speller, V. (1995) *Towards Healthier Alliances: A Tool for Planning, Evaluating and Developing Healthy Alliances*, London, Health Education Authority.

Geddes, M. (1997) *Partnerships Against Poverty and Exclusion? Local Regeneration Strategies and Excluded Communities in the UK*, Bristol, Policy.

Gillies, P. (1998) 'Effectiveness of alliances and partnerships for health promotion', *Health Promotion International*, vol. 3, no. 2, pp. 99–120.

Glendinning, C. (2002) 'Partnerships between health and social services: developing a framework for evaluation', *Policy and Politics*, vol. 30, no. 1, pp. 115–27.

Glendinning, C. and Clarke, J. (2000) 'Old wine, new bottles? Prospects for NHS/local authority partnerships under "New Labour"', paper presented to ESRC seminar on 'The third way in public services', York, April.

Global Alliance for Vaccines and Immunization (GAVI) (2006) [online], http://www.gavialliance.org/ (Accessed 4 September 2006).

Goumans, M. (1998) *Innovations in a Fuzzy Domain: Healthy Cities and (Health) Policy Development in the Netherlands and the United Kingdom*, Maastricht, University of Maastricht.

Gray, B. (1985) 'Conditions facilitating interorganizational collaboration', *Human Relations*, vol. 38, no. 10, pp. 911–36.

Gray, B. (1989) *Collaboration: Finding Common Ground for Multi-Party Problems*, San Francisco, Jossey-Bass.

Harding, A. (1998) 'Public–private partnerships in the UK' in Price, J. (ed.) *Partnerships in Urban Governance*, Basingstoke, Macmillan.

Hastings, A., McArthur, A. and McGregor, A. (1996) *Less than Equal: Community Organizations and Estate Regeneration*, Bristol, Policy.

Health Education Board for Scotland (HEBS) (2000) *Partnerships for Health: A Review*, HEBS Working Paper No. 3, Edinburgh, Health Education Board for Scotland.

Heenan, D. (2004) 'A partnership approach to health promotion: a case study from Northern Ireland', *Health Promotion International*, vol. 19, no. 1, pp. 105–13.

HP-Source.net (2003) [online], http://www.hp-source.net/ (Accessed 5 March 2007).

Hudson, B. (1987) 'Collaboration in social welfare: a framework for analysis', *Policy and Politics*, vol. 15, no. 3, pp. 175–82.

Hudson, B., Hardy, B., Henwood, M. and Wistow, G. (1999) 'In pursuit of inter-agency collaboration in the public sector: what is the contribution of theory and research?', *Public Management*, vol. 1, no. 2, pp. 235–60.

Hughes, J.K., Knox, C., Murray, M. and Greer, J. (1998) *Partnerships in Northern Ireland: The Path to Peace*, Dublin, Oak Tree Press.

Hunter, D. (2003) *Public Health Policy*, Cambridge, Polity.

Huxham, C. (1996) *Creating Collaborative Advantage*, London, Sage.

Japhet, G. and Hulme, A. (2004) 'Partnerships to promote health' in Moodie, R. and Hulme, A. (eds) *Hands On Health Promotion*, Melbourne, IP Communications.

Judge, K. and Bauld, L. (2006) 'Learning from policy failure? Health Action Zones in England', *European Journal of Public Health*, vol. 16, no. 4, pp. 341–3.

Lowndes, V. and Skelcher, C. (1998) 'The dynamics of multi-organizational partnership: an analysis of changing modes of governance', *Public Administration*, vol. 76, no. 2, pp. 313–33.

Lucas, K. and Lloyd, B. (2005) *Health Promotion: Evidence and Effectiveness*, London, Sage.

Mackintosh, M. (1992) 'Partnerships: issues of policy and negotiation', *Local Economy*, vol. 7, no. 3, pp. 210–24.

Markwell, S. (2003) *Partnership Working: A Consumer's Guide to Resources*, London, Health Development Agency.

Marmott, M. and Wilkinson, R. (2005) *Social Determinants of Health* (2nd edn), Oxford, Oxford University Press.

Mayo, M. (1997) Partnerships for regeneration and community development, *Critical Social Policy*, vol. 17, no. 52, pp. 3–26.

Naidoo, J. and Wills, J. (2005) *Public Health and Health Promotion: Developing Practice* (2nd edn), London, Baillière Tindall.

Nutbeam, D. and Harris, E. (2004) *Theory in a Nutshell*, Sydney, McGraw-Hill.

Orme, J., Powell, J., Taylor, P., Harrison, T. and Grey, M. (eds) (2003) *Public Health for the 21st Century: New Perspectives on Policy, Participation and Practice*, Maidenhead, Open University Press.

Peckham, S. (2003) 'Who are the planners in public health?' in Orme et al. (eds) (2003).

Powell, M. and Glendinning, C. (2002) 'Partnerships, quasi-networks and social policy' in Glendinning, C., Powell, M. and Rummery, K. (eds) *Partnerships, New Labour and the Governance of Welfare*, Bristol, Policy.

renewal.net (2006) *The Terrance Higgins Trust, SWISH Project* [online], http://www.coventrypartnership.com/upload/documents/document708.doc (Accessed 3 January 2007).

Roberts, V., Russell, H. and Harding, A. (1995) *Public–Private Voluntary Partnerships in Local Government*, Luton, Local Government Management Board.

Rummery, K. and Glendinning, C. (1997) 'Working together: primary care involvement in commissioning social care services' in *Debates in Primary Care No. 2*, Manchester, Manchester University, National Primary Care Research and Development Centre.

Savas, E. (2000) *Privatisation and Public–Private Partnerships*, New York, Seven Bridges.

Snape, S. and Taylor, P. (eds) (2004) *Partnership Working between Health and Local Government*, London, Frank Cass.

Statutory Instrument (2005) *The Children and Young People's Plan (England) Regulations 2005*, Statutory Instrument 2005 No. 2149, London, The Stationery Office; also available online at http://www.opsi.gov.uk/si/si2005/20052149.htm (Accessed 6 March 2007).

Stewart, M. (2003) 'Neighbourhood renewal and regeneration' in Orme et al. (eds) (2003).

Stewart, M. and Purdue, D. (2002) *Co-operation and Co-ordination in Area-based Regeneration Initiatives*, London, Department for Environment, Transport and the Regions.

Sullivan, H. and Skelcher, C. (2002) *Working across Boundaries: Collaboration in Public Services*, Basingstoke, Palgrave Macmillan.

Taket, A. and White, L. (2000) *Partnership and Participation: Decision-making in the Multi-Agency Setting*, New York, Wiley.

Tsouros, A. and Draper, R.A. (1993) 'The Healthy Cities project: new developments and research needs' in Davies, J.K. and Kelly, M.P. (eds) *Healthy Cities: Research and Practice*, New York, Routledge.

UNDESA (2006) [online], http://www.un.org/esa/sustdev/mgroups/about_mgroups.htm (Accessed 4 September 2006).

World Federation for Medical Education (WFME) (2006) *WHO/WFME Strategic Partnership to Improve Medical Education* [online], http://www.wfme.org/ (Accessed 1 September 2006).

World Health Organization (WHO) (1978) *Alma Ata Declaration*, Geneva, World Health Organization

World Health Organization (WHO) (1988) *Adelaide Recommendations on Healthy Public Policy*, Geneva, World Health Organization.

World Health Organization (WHO) (1991) *Sundsvall Statement on Supportive Environments for Health*, Geneva, World Health Organization.

World Health Organization (WHO) (1997) *The Jakarta Declaration on Leading Health Promotion into the 21st Century*, Geneva, World Health Organization.

World Health Organization (WHO) (1998) *Health Promotion Glossary*, Geneva, World Health Organization

World Health Organization (WHO) (1999) *Health 21: Health for All in the 21st Century. The Health for All Policy Framework for the European Region*, Copenhagen, World Health Organization Regional Office for Europe.

World Health Organization (WHO) (2000) *Mexico Ministerial Statement for the Promotion of Health: From Ideas to Action*, Geneva, World Health Organization.

World Health Organization (WHO) (2005) *The Bangkok Charter for Health Promotion in a Globalized World*, Geneva, World Health Organization.

World Heath Organization (WHO) (2006) *Healthy Cities and Urban Governance* [online], http://www.euro.who.int/healthy-cities (Accessed 8 January 2007).

World Heath Organization (WHO) (2007) *DOTS: The Internationally-Recommended TB Control Strategy* [online], http://www.who.int/tb/dots/en/ (Accessed 19 March 2007).

Chapter 6

Addressing poverty and health

Tom Heller, Kythé Beaumont, Sarah Earle and Jenny Douglas, incorporating previously published material from Linda Jones (2002)

Introduction

So far, this book has focused on promoting public health through public policy, examining policy making at national and international levels. It has also examined the importance of working in partnerships within and across different settings and organisations. Addressing inequalities in health and the impact of poverty on health, in particular, is one of the main concerns of public health policy in the twenty-first century. This chapter focuses on poverty, and explores how healthy public policy seeks to combat the effects of poverty on health and wellbeing.

The chapter uses the study of poverty to explore how healthy public policy at the global, national and local levels can impact on health. It starts by considering, in Section 6.1, different definitions of poverty, reflecting on which groups in society are most likely to experience and be in poverty. Section 6.2 then moves on to consider ways of measuring poverty, taking into account the differences between developed and developing countries. Section 6.3 examines the health consequences of living in poverty and compares the relative health risks between the richest and poorest groups in society. Finally, Section 6.4 examines some of the national and international policies that address inequalities in health and critically considers some of the evidence demonstrating the links between poverty and illhealth.

Your study of this chapter will help you consider the effects of poverty-related policy at global and national levels and should act as a way of revisiting some of the themes that have been explored in the previous five chapters of Part I.

6.1 Defining and experiencing poverty

Defining poverty is an important and necessary part of reducing inequalities in health. This section considers competing definitions of poverty and examines who in society is most likely to be defined as poor.

6.1.1 Definitions of poverty

The term poverty is commonly used and although it is an almost universal concept there are many definitions of poverty. The term has come to mean many different things to different people and there is considerable debate about how poverty is defined and measured (see Figure 6.1).

Figure 6.1   Items regarded as necessary by at least two-thirds of British adults (Source: adapted from McKay, 2004, pp. 220–1)

	Omnibus survey: percentage of respondents considering the item necessary
Beds and bedding for everyone	95
Heating to warm living areas of the home	94
Damp-free home	93
Visiting friends or family in hospital	92
Two meals a day	91
Medicines prescribed by doctor	90
Refrigerator	89
Fresh fruit and vegetables daily	86
Warm, waterproof coat	85
Replace or repair broken electrical goods	85
Visits to friends or family	84
Celebrations on special occasions such as Christmas	83
Money to keep home in a decent state of decoration	82
Visits to school: for example, sports day	81
Attending weddings, funerals	80
Meat, fish or vegetarian equivalent every other day	79
Insurance of contents of dwelling	79
Hobby or leisure activity	78
Washing machine	76
Collect children from school	75
Telephone	71
Appropriate clothes for job interviews	69
Deep freezer/fridge-freezer	68
Carpets in living rooms and bedrooms	67
Regular savings (of £10 per month) for rainy days or retirement	66

Laderchi et al. (2003) claim to have identified four approaches – monetary, capability, social exclusion and participatory ways of defining the concept of poverty. However, these academic approaches might seem fairly irrelevant to the millions of people throughout the world – such as those quoted in Box 6.1 – for whom the experience of insufficient resources to meet their daily needs has become a daily reality.

Box 6.1 Voices of the poor

The World Bank has conducted a project called 'Voices of the poor'. These are some of the gathered responses from poor people all over the world.

'He's lying to the people. There's no roads, no money for food, yet he'll build a huge villa. When was the last time any improvements were made here?' – said by a Roma from Bulgaria of the local mayor.

'There is much bitterness, especially in the thought that any opportunities that may come will be taken by the rich ...' – Dahshour Village, Egypt.

'Poverty is lack of freedom, enslaved by crushing daily burden, by depression and fear of what the future will bring.' – Georgia.

'If you want to do something and have no power to do it, it is talauchi (poverty).' – Nigeria.

'Lack of work worries me. My children were hungry and I told them the rice is cooking, until they fell asleep from hunger.' – an older man from Bedsa, Egypt.

'When one is poor, she has no say in public, she feels inferior. She has no food, so there is famine in her house; no clothing, and no progress in her family.' – a woman from Uganda.

(Adapted from World Bank, 2006a)

The United Nations Millennium Declaration, adopted in 2000, resolved to 'spare no effort to free our fellow men, women and children from the abject and dehumanising conditions of extreme poverty' and to halve it by 2015 (UN, 2000a). Various official organisations have attempted to produce their own definitions of poverty. The United Nations uses a rather wide definition of poverty that includes many features that take poverty away from simple measures of income: 'Poverty: a human condition characterized by the sustained or chronic deprivation of the resources, capabilities, choices, security and power necessary for the enjoyment of an adequate standard of living and other civil, cultural, economic, political and social rights' (OHCHR, 2006).

The World Bank has also attempted to add wider and more human dimensions to their definitions of poverty:

> Poverty is hunger. Poverty is a lack of shelter. Poverty is being sick and not being able to see a doctor. Poverty is not having access to school and not knowing how to read. Poverty is not having a job, is fear for the future, living one day at a time. Poverty is losing a child to illness brought about by unclean water. Poverty is powerlessness, lack of representation and freedom.
>
> (World Bank, 2006b)

In the UK there are diverse ways of defining poverty. The most commonly accepted measure of poverty has become a statistically based indicator of 'income poverty'. Households below the 'poverty line' are those deemed to have less than 'one-half of mean equivalised disposable income' (Piachaud and Sutherland, 2000, p. 5). Examples of the current income levels that would be considered below the poverty line are shown in Box 6.2.

Box 6.2 The poverty line

In 2004/05 the poverty line – the amount of money below which, after adjusting for size and composition of household and after housing costs, a family was categorised as poor – was as follows:

- £186 per week, (£9,672 per year) for a lone parent with two children aged 5 and 11.

- £268 per week (£13,936 per year) for a couple with two children aged 5 and 11.

(CPAG, 2006, p. 4)

Different definitions of poverty can pose challenges to policy makers, academics and practitioners who are interested in anti-poverty policy and practice. However, there are two commonly used concepts that relate to poverty – 'absolute poverty' and 'relative poverty'.

Thinking point: what is the difference between absolute poverty and relative poverty?

In most industrial countries, poverty is perceived as a 'relative' concept, measured in terms of people's ability to sustain a basic lifestyle in accordance with the norms and standards of their own society. Absolute poverty can be considered in terms of life and death, of not having enough nourishment, warmth or shelter to survive. In the rich countries of the world comparatively few people are in this state of absolute poverty, whereas in the poorest countries many people live under its threat. However, some groups in society are more likely to experience poverty than others; the next section focuses on this.

6.1.2 Who experiences poverty?

The groups in the population of industrialised countries most likely to find themselves in poverty are households with no paid workers, lone parents with children, disabled or long-term sick people (Gordon et al., 2000). Figure 6.2 shows the groups considered to be at greatest risk of poverty in the UK. Large families are also more at risk of poverty, as are women and people from black and minority ethnic groups (Cook and Watt, 1987; Glendinning and Millar, 1987; Madood et al., 1997). People from black and minority ethnic groups are also more likely to find themselves living in poverty because of the effects of racism and racial discrimination (Nazroo and Karlsen, 2001). Discrimination in employment may lead to people from black and minority ethnic communities being placed in low-paid jobs or becoming unemployed. Similarly, discrimination in housing policies of local authorities, private landlords, and in lending policies of banks and building societies may lead to disproportionately more people from black and minority ethnic communities living in poorer housing and areas of deprivation.

Figure 6.2   Groups at greatest risk of poverty in the UK (Source: CPAG, 2006, p. 5)

	Risk (%)
In receipt of Incapacity Benefit	46
In receipt of Tax Credits	22
In receipt of Income Support	71
Mother under 25	41
Lone parent	48
Lone parent not working	72
Couple both not in work	72
Workless households	75
Four or more children in family	50
One or more disabled adults in household	40
Pakistani/Bangladeshi ethnicity	57
Black or Black British ethnicity	43
Local Authority tenure	56
No savings	45

Certain groups within every society are more likely than others to experience poverty. The British Government has often focused its attention on child poverty and its attempts to reduce the numbers and proportion of children living in poverty have met with varying degrees of success

(CPAG, 2006). However, there has been a dearth of information about the nature of poverty experienced by older people (Howarth et al., 1999), which has led to less attention being paid to people in the later stages of the lifecourse.

'Social exclusion' is a term linked to relative poverty which has been defined by the Prime Minister as 'broadly covering those people who do not have the means, material and otherwise, to participate in social, economic, political and cultural life' (quoted in Scottish Office, 1998). The term 'social exclusion' started to gain currency in the 1980s. Initially it was used in the social policy of the French Socialist Government to refer to people without access to the system of social insurance who were living on the margins of society (Burchardt et al., 1999). When later used in the context of the European Union, it referred much more to the objective of achieving social and economic cohesion (Percy-Smith, 2000).

Demi Patsios (2006) argues that older people are more likely to be at risk of poverty because of their low income. Older pensioners, particularly those living in single-pension households and older women, are at greatest risk. Older people living in poverty are also more likely to suffer social exclusion and isolation. Box 6.3 gives some statistics relating to older people living in Northern Ireland during 2004/05.

Box 6.3 Older people in Northern Ireland 2004/05: statistical background

Ageing population:

- 16 per cent of the population is of pensionable age.
- By 2013, it is estimated that this figure will reach 24 per cent.

Poverty:

- 22.2 per cent of pensioners are living in poverty.
- 50 per cent of householders experiencing fuel poverty are aged sixty plus.
- In 2004/05, 1,280 individuals (many of whom were older people) suffered cold-associated deaths.

Isolation:

- Over 80,000 older people live on their own.
- Loneliness has been identified as a problem by 53 per cent of older people.

(Adapted from Help the Aged, 2006)

6.2 Measuring poverty

Many official measures of poverty in the developed world use the notion of 'subsistence', which is conceived as the level at which an individual or household has just enough income or resources to meet a minimum number of basic needs (for food, clothing and shelter). The official benefits system in the UK uses a similar calculation to determine benefits that will top up household income to this basic Income Support level.

Measuring the numbers of people below average income can show the relationship between the poorest groups and the rest of society. Studies between the late 1970s and early 1990s indicated that the gap between households on high incomes and those on low incomes was widening. More recently the number and percentage of children in poverty has been falling, as shown in Figure 6.3.

Figure 6.3   Number and percentage of children in poverty after housing costs (Source: CPAG, 2006, p. 2, Table 1)

Year	Millions	% of children
96/97	4.2	33
97/98	4.1	32
98/99	4.1	33
99/00	4.1	32
00/01	3.8	30
01/02	3.7	30
02/03	3.6	28
03/04	3.5	28
04/05	3.4	27

During the 1970s, only 6 per cent of the population of the UK had incomes below half of mean income. This proportion increased sharply to 21 per cent in 1991–92 and stabilised at 18–19 per cent by the late 1990s (Hills, 2004). Other analysts have used questionnaire-based research to identify the types of goods and services people need to maintain health (Townsend, 1979; Bradshaw, 1993).

Thinking point: how do you think that poverty should be measured?

One popular method of determining poverty relies on a 'basic needs basket'. Using this approach it is possible to determine the cost of providing certain basic needs for an individual or for their household. Thus, if a minimum nutritional requirement is set at approximately 2,200 calories per day, the local cost of determining that level of nutritional intake can be determined. A multiplier may be added to include non-food necessities. Traditional recommendations on how to set the poverty line within the USA have included the cost of food, clothing, shelter and a small multiplier to account for those expenses that may differ from person to person (Citro, 1995).

However, there is considerable variation between people and between cultures regarding the items that they consider to be essential. For example, Figure 6.1 summarised the results of a national survey of poverty and exclusion conducted in 1999 in Britain by Gordon et al. (2000). This survey found a high level of consensus about items regarded as necessities. Respondents went considerably beyond a subsistence approach in their view of poverty. They considered as necessities a reasonably comfortable home with modern amenities, and sufficient income to ensure participation in key social events. In any event, it is apparent that the concept of poverty is highly dependent on wider social values and norms and is relative to the prevailing culture.

Many measurements of poverty use the unit of a family or a household to consider the line below which the people in that unit could be considered to be living in poverty. Although this makes some sense, because most societies are organised around family or household units, this level of aggregation may miss significant problems with regard to the distribution of assets within the household or family unit. It remains possible for non-poor households to contain poor individuals. For example, some studies have exposed gender inequities within some households where discrimination of power and resources leave women more vulnerable to the health effects of poverty (Quisumbing, 2001).

6.2.1 Measuring poverty within a global perspective

So far this chapter has focused on poverty and income largely within the UK. Taking a more global perspective is also important and throws light on the extremes of income distribution throughout the world. Statistics can hardly start to help to make sense of the enormous disparities between rich and poor, and the enormous numbers of people living in poverty throughout the developing world. Many of the 'necessities' listed in Figure 6.1 will seem as hopelessly out of reach to the millions of people living on less than one or two dollars each day. Figure 6.4 shows a world map with the percentages of people living on incomes of less than one dollar per day.

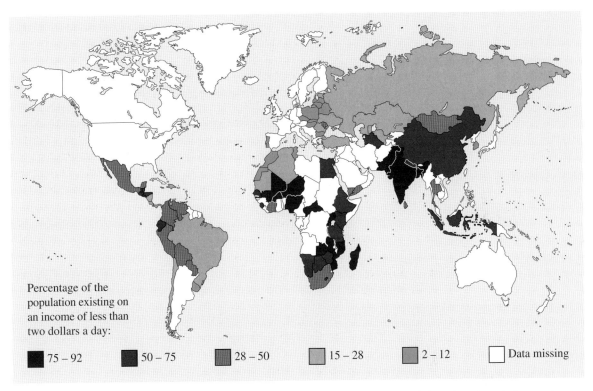

Percentage of the population existing on an income of less than two dollars a day:

| ■ 75 – 92 | ■ 50 – 75 | ■ 28 – 50 | ■ 15 – 28 | ■ 2 – 12 | □ Data missing |

Figure 6.4   The poverty lines: population living with less than two dollars a day (Source: Poverty Mapping, 2006)

Of course, the interrelationship between health and poverty runs in both directions. At an individual level, illness can put people at risk of becoming poor. In addition, the economic effect of large numbers of ill people in a community will tend to have a debilitating effect on the whole of that society. Many governments within developing countries have recognised that having a large portion of their population living in poverty and experiencing illness is unsound economically (Leon et al., 2001). A healthy population, especially good health among those who would otherwise be able to join the workforce, is essential for economic recovery. Investment in improving the health of the population becomes an economic necessity as well as a humanitarian imperative.

Even within the expanding European Union there remain considerable health inequalities. In general terms, the people living in central and eastern European countries have poorer health and reduced life expectancy compared with people living in western Europe, where levels of poverty and income differentials are considerably less extreme (Koupil, 2005).

Even in comparatively rich, developed countries, there is a variable risk of poverty and associated illness. Figure 6.5 shows the percentage of children living in relative poverty in a variety of rich nations.

Mackenbach and Bakker (2003) analysed policy developments relating to health inequalities in nine different European countries and noted that those countries are all in very different phases of awareness of, and willingness to take action on, inequalities in health: 'European trends in inequalities in mortality during the last decades of the 20th century have generally shown a widening of the gap in relative terms, and at best a stable situation in absolute terms' (Mackenbach and Bakker, 2003, p. 1413). Whether the focus is on local, regional, national or global policies, living in

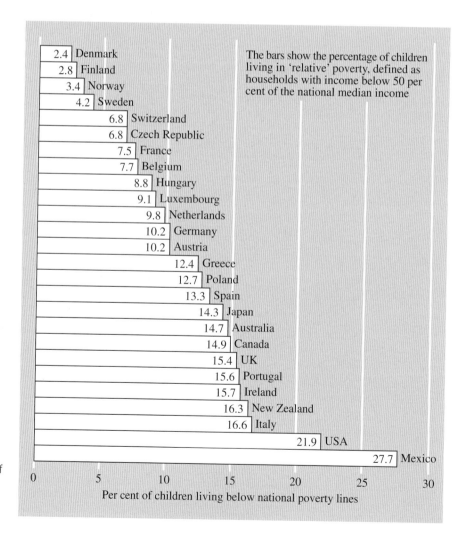

Figure 6.5   The child poverty league: percentage of children living below the national poverty lines in a range of rich nations (Source: UNICEF, 2005, p. 4, Figure 1)

poverty is an important issue for policy makers, researchers and public health practitioners – among others – because being poor can lead to poor health. The next section focuses on the health consequences of poverty.

6.3 The health consequences of poverty

There is an abundance of evidence linking poverty and disadvantage to poor health (see Graham, 2007). Obviously some of the links between poverty and illness are related to very specific factors. For example, if poverty for a family or for individual people means that they don't have access to enough food or clean water, then this will certainly lead to an immediate and severe detrimental effect on their health. Similarly, if access to health services is dependant on the ability to pay, then some people will suffer poor health because they simply are not able to afford medical fees or other healthcare costs. More subtle factors, however, might also be linked to the amount of disposable wealth and in many countries there is a very obvious gradient of health, with people at the top of the income scale performing better on almost all health parameters. For example, a study of 300,000 men in the USA showed that mortality declined progressively across twelve categories of household income from less than $7,500 to more than $32,499 per annum (Smith et al., 1996).

Some commentators have suggested that the degree of inequality between income groups is a cause of poor health in itself. Richard Wilkinson (1996) highlighted the health effects of widening income differences within a range of countries with different levels of inequality. Beyond a certain level, he concluded, it was not the absolute but the relative living standard that influenced health. In his opinion, the scale of relative deprivation, as measured by income differences between people in the same society, continues to be a powerful determinant of health and illness. His evidence compared a range of data in which the statistical associations were striking, although it is less clear that a causal relationship exists. For example, in England and Wales the proportion of children living in households below half of the national average income (the current European relative poverty measure) had grown from 10 per cent in 1979 to 31 per cent in 1990. Infant mortality in England and Wales was strikingly higher than in Sweden, where income differentials were not as great and only 2 per cent of children in one-parent families were in relative poverty. Having mapped income differentials against national standards of health, Wilkinson argued that the best way of improving health in developed countries would almost certainly be by reducing income differences. However, Gibson (2007) found little evidence to support Wilkinson's theory during his research in a working-class area of northern England. He found that there were anxieties and stress connected with living in a deprived area, but argued that most of the actual adverse health effects were understandable in terms of the material conditions in which poor people lived and worked.

Recent official government reports (e.g. DoH, 2005) seem to indicate that in England there appears to have been a widening gap in health inequalities between those in the lowest and highest social classes, and this is reflected in their health experiences. This apparently widening gap is shown in Figure 6.6 as differences in life expectancy at birth for various social classes (i.e. Social classes I to V).

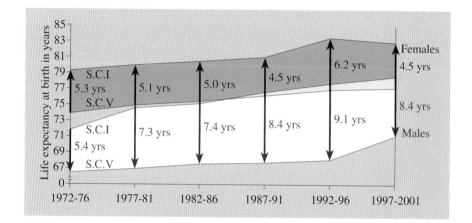

Figure 6.6   Life expectancy at birth in years, by social class and gender, 1972–2001 (Source: DoH, 2005, p. 15, Figure 1)

Thinking point: can you think of reasons other than living standards why there might appear to be an increasing health gap between social classes?

Figure 6.6 appears to show that although overall mortality fell in all social classes, there was a greater reduction in mortality in the highest social classes (social classes I and II) than in the lowest (social classes IV and V). However, in recent years, the health of all groups has improved and a general social improvement has changed the demographic pattern of society, with many people moving into higher social groupings. Those left behind have worse health than those who ascend the social scale and many ill people, especially those with mental health issues, tend to fall down the social gradients. So unless some adjustment is made for the fact that, over time, those in social classes IV and V represent a different proportion of the population and a proportion expected to have poor health, just comparing trends between social classes over time will give a misleading picture of apparently widening divisions in health between the social extremes (Heller, 2005).

6.3.1 Links between social circumstances and poor health

David Gordon, Professor in Social Justice at Bristol University, has commented extensively on the links between poverty, inequality and illness. Box 6.4 sets out some of the features of contemporary society that he feels are behind the illness experienced by the poorest people in society.

Box 6.4 The contemporary poverty and illhealth experience in Britain

- Roughly 9.5 million people in Britain cannot afford adequate housing. That is, they are unable to afford to keep their homes adequately heated, free from damp or in a decent state of decoration. The majority of the population believe that people ought to be able to afford to do this.

- 8 million people cannot afford one or more essential household goods such as refrigerator, telephone, or to repair electrical goods or furniture when they break.

- 7.5 million people cannot afford to participate in common social activities, they cannot afford to visit their friends or families, they cannot afford to attend weddings or funerals or have special celebrations like birthdays or Christmas.

- Over a third of British children go without social or material necessities. These are the things the majority of the population think they ought to be able to have, such as three meals a day, toys, out-of-school activities and adequate clothing. Nearly one fifth of children go without two or more of what the majority think are necessities of life.

- About 6.5 million adults go without essential clothing, such as a warm waterproof coat, because they don't have the money to buy it.

- 4 million people are not properly fed by today's standards in Britain.

- Over 10.5 million are financially insecure.

(Gordon, 2004, based on Gordon et al., 2000, pp. 68–9)

People on low or very low incomes suffer more illness and die earlier than those in higher income groups, as successive official and unofficial health reports have demonstrated.

Thinking point: what do you think are likely to be the specific health risks for groups of people living in poverty?

Lone mothers with children are more likely to live in sub-standard housing in a poor environment. People who are unemployed have a much higher rate of suicide (Platt, 1984). Older people are more at risk of hypothermia and malnutrition. People in social classes IV and V have a higher incidence of a whole range of diseases, including coronary heart disease, stroke, most cancers, respiratory and infectious diseases. There are about 500 deaths from hypothermia recorded each year in the UK, the vast majority of them of older people, and added to this is the much bigger problem of what is termed 'cold-associated disease' (Wilkinson et al., 2004). Older people are the most vulnerable, and in severe winters suffer up to 50 per cent excess mortality from respiratory disease and heart disease. Being in poverty or at the margins of poverty – with the fear of not being able to pay the heating bill and getting into debt – is the position in which many elderly people find themselves, and it has a direct impact on their health.

There are competing arguments about the relationship between the social environment, income inequality and health. Graham (2007) argues that poverty is linked to poor health as part of a social gradient whereby people living in poverty experience worse health than those in middle-income groups. Similarly, people in middle-income groups experience worse health than people higher up the socio-economic gradient. Lynch et al. (2000) propose that health inequalities are the result of the cumulative negative effect of lack of resources across the lifecourse.

Although social exclusion has been defined in various ways, one of the key elements of social exclusion is its extension across several different domains. Disadvantage in relation to one aspect of life is linked to disadvantage in other areas: for example, households where there are problems with housing may also be disadvantaged in terms of household income, low educational attainment and other features, which cumulatively create a situation that can be recognised under the umbrella term 'poverty'. This will reflect on policy, for while some initiatives may focus specifically on poverty and health, most public health initiatives recognise that people living in poverty experience a range of social, cultural and economic disadvantage. Action aimed at countering social disadvantage should always be prepared to focus on the wider range of factors that influence health, recognising the need to work in partnership across different organisations and settings.

6.4 Policies relating to poverty and health

So far in this chapter, evidence relating to the relationship between poverty, poor health and reduced life expectancy has been presented, along with some of the debates concerning the ways in which poverty might impact on health. We now turn to consider how healthy public policy, at the global as well as the national level, has been developed in an attempt to meet the needs of people from the poorest sectors of society.

6.4.1 National and international policies addressing poverty and inequality

Policy making is inherently a political process. Governments will usually only act if there is a political imperative that they are able to use to their advantage. This can make public health promotion particularly challenging for public health practitioners and others working at grassroots level. It particularly applies to the introduction of unpopular policies that might potentially be effective in public health terms, but disastrous at the time of the next election. For example, one could imagine that the health of the population would be improved through enormously strict controls on motoring speeds, bans on the sale and consumption of 'unhealthy foods', and the linking of certain welfare benefits to specific health behaviours, but such measures cannot be envisaged in a democratic system where consensus applies and where draconian or punitive measures are inappropriate. Targeting policies to help 'the poor' and their health status will only be popular electorally to a certain extent.

Thinking point: do you think that policies to help the poor are developed according to a pluralist/consensus or conflict model of policy making?

As discussed in Chapter 3, most governments have to negotiate in such a way that the benefits of their policies do not significantly disadvantage the rich and powerful groups within their societies. In addition, some 'healthy' policies aimed at disadvantaged members of society will be actively opposed by other interest groups concerned to protect their own position. For example, you saw in Chapter 3 that tobacco companies resist policies that restrict their ability to market and sell their products to poor people. There remains a tension between the introduction of specific poverty-related policies and the political will to implement those policies in a meaningful way. Both pluralist/consensus and conflict models of policy making are useful ways of thinking about policies relating to poverty and health.

What is the best strategy for improving public health in any given population, particularly in the context of developing nations? This subject has been a matter of intense argument and debate for many years (Leon and

Walt, 2001). On the one hand, certain political groupings insist that promoting economic growth should be given priority. In this way sufficient wealth is created so that increased expenditure can be invested in health services and programmes designed to improve the health of people at the bottom of the social gradient. The converse argument advocates a support-led series of policies designed to improve the health of people living in poverty, so that they can participate in economic activities (get a job, pay taxes, etc.) which are necessary to help the development of their society.

In addition, there are increasing calls for any policies and projects to be 'evidence-based' (Nutbeam, 2004). The rationale is difficult to fault because if policies and public health actions have not been shown to be effective, there can be no reason to invest in them. However, the research needed to demonstrate whether specific polices have led to health improvements can be notoriously difficult to undertake (see Douglas et al., 2007, for a discussion of evaluating public health interventions). Furthermore, health outcomes may take many years, if not decades, to reach significant or measurable proportions: 'there is little research funded or conducted to assess the effectiveness of interventions to tackle some of the wider social, economic and environmental determinants of health. There is very little evidence of any kind to examine the relative costs and benefits of different policy options' (Nutbeam, 2004, pp. 137–8).

The necessary public health research is difficult to undertake because of methodological, practical and ethical issues. For example, only comparatively simple public health interventions can be evaluated within classic study designs such as the RCT (randomised control trial) or even CIT (community intervention trial) (Stronks and Mackenbach, 2005). Research that may be able to determine the effectiveness of more complex 'upstream' intervention strategies, such as broader policy interventions that may influence the health of the poorer sections of society, remain elusive. In the UK, a review of public health intervention research (Milward et al., 2001) found that only 4 per cent of public health research dealt with interventions rather than descriptions of problems, and of this proportion only 10 per cent (0.4 per cent of the total) focused on the outcomes of the interventions.

In the absence of robust research evidence it is possible for governments to do nothing, or undertake high-profile activities that really do not have a research base but fulfil a political need to be seen to be 'doing something' about a visible public health problem.

6.4.2 Policy, poverty and reducing inequalities in health

Stronks and Mackenbach (2005) have identified four possible strategies that could be used by policy makers to reduce inequalities in health. These are set out in Box 6.5.

Box 6.5 Possible strategies to reduce inequalities in health

- targeting socio-economic disadvantage, such as anti-poverty policies and social benefit schemes

- reducing the effect of health on socio-economic disadvantage including benefit levels for long-term inability to work and adaptation of working conditions for chronically ill people:

- targeting factors mediating the effect of socio-economic disadvantage on health, including the promotion of healthy behaviour and healthy working conditions

- improving the accessibility and quality of health care provided to the lower socio-economic groups, including maintaining good financial accessibility of health care.

(Stronks and Mackenbach, 2005, pp. 346–7)

Each of these broad categories of health policy will have their advocates who relate to the political persuasion of the government of the time. In general terms, more left-wing, socially aware governments will tend to favour policies that are targeted at population-level policies designed to redistribute the goods of society. More right-wing governments will always be tempted to promote those policies that draw attention to the individual behaviours of people in the lowest social groups. In practice, however, most western democratic governments will attempt a mix and match policy with a variable proportion of each of these different strategies.

At a more strategic level, the World Health Organization, has continued to worry less about the precise policies that governments should follow, but suggests that they focus on health-related outcomes. Thus, the original World Health Organization 'Health For All' prerequisites (adopted at the World Health Assembly in 1977) called for 'satisfaction of basic needs', among which are listed 'adequate food and income', 'decent housing', 'secure work' and 'a satisfying role in society' (WHO, 1977). Among the thirty-eight targets for health in the European region were ones that called for all people to 'have the basic opportunity to develop and use their health potential to live socially and economically useful lives' and to 'have a better opportunity of living in houses ... which provide a healthy and safe environment' (Targets 2, 24, WHO, 1985, pp. 27, 89). The Second International Conference on Health Promotion, Adelaide, was more explicit about the need for 'ensuring an equitable distribution of resources even in adverse economic circumstances' (WHO, 1998, p. 5).

From time to time these general exhortations are reinforced by the introduction of health and social welfare targets and aspirations. For instance, in 1998 the WHO was pleading with its member states that: 'By the year 2000, the actual differences in health status between countries and between groups within countries should be reduced by at least 25% by improving the level of health of disadvantaged nations and groups' (WHO, 1998, p. 2).

Thinking point: in what ways do you think the policy directives from WHO have influenced the debate on poverty and illhealth?

The concerns expressed in the WHO prerequisites are very much about meeting basic needs and in this sense are most closely linked to a 'subsistence' or 'social coping' view of poverty. Since the WHO statements have to be acceptable to all signatory countries, it is not surprising that the view of poverty as relative deprivation does not feature, although it is implicit. 'Adequate', 'decent' and even 'basic' are bound to relate to the society to which the terms are applied and will have very different meanings in rich and poor countries.

Throughout this chapter – as also seen in Chapter 1 – it is increasingly apparent that, although it is important to develop local and national strategies to tackle poverty, global poverty will persist without an international focus on fair trade and a political commitment to eradicating it. In an attempt to sharpen up their focus on the underlying causes of illhealth, the WHO has established its own Commission on Social Determinants of Health (CSDH). The Commission's main goals are:

- To support health policy change in countries by assembling and promoting effective evidence-based models and practices that address the social determinants of health.

- To support countries in placing health equity as a shared goal to which many government departments and sectors of society contribute.

- To help build a sustainable global movement for action on health equity and social determinants, linking governments, international organizations, research institutions, civil society and communities.

(WHO, 2006, p. 5)

The last main goal listed above highlights the current drive in healthy public policy to promote public health through partnerships, within and across settings and organisations both nationally and globally. However, although many post-industrial countries now have policies designed to tackle disparities and inequalities in health, the content and context of such policies varies enormously. Exworthy et al. (2006) consider that the implementation of these policies reflects the differing political ideologies as well as the historical, social and political legacies specific to each country. Even where policies are enacted and resources are earmarked for implementation, there remain enormous challenges in measuring whether any useful progress towards the desired health-related outcomes has been achieved. Box 6.6 gives some of the health statistics that show that there is still a long way to go before inequalities in health between various social groups in the UK and the USA can be said to have been tackled.

Box 6.6 Disparities in health statistics between the UK and the USA

In the UK, access to health care is universal, but the life expectancy of a boy born into the lowest social class is more than 9 years less than that of a boy born into the most affluent class. Infant mortality rates for social class V, that of unskilled manual workers, are twice that for a boy born into the professional and management classes, social class I.

In the USA, race and ethnicity are major factors. The life expectancy of an African–American man is 69.0 years, whereas that of a white man is 75.3. Infant mortality is 5.75 per 1000 live births for white infants, 14.01 for African–American infants.

(*Lancet*, 2006, p. 1876)

Throughout all developed countries there is a substantial difference in the success rates of tackling poverty. Figure 6.7 shows the changes in child poverty rates during the 1990s. While some countries have successfully started to reduce their child poverty rates, the trend in other countries continues to rise.

This section has examined some of the broad strategies that policy makers can adopt to reduce inequalities in health. Section 6.4.3 now considers some of the strategies adopted by UK governments.

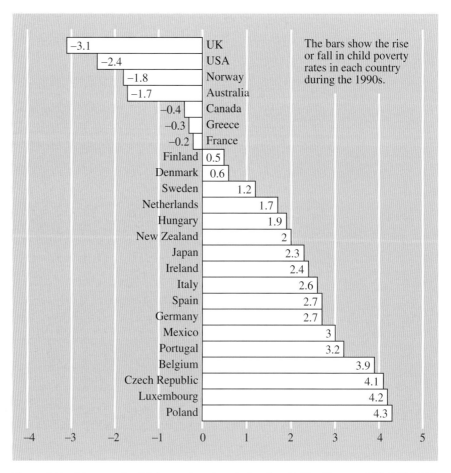

Figure 6.7   Changes in child poverty rates during the 1990s (Source: UNICEF, 2005, p. 5, Figure 2)

6.4.3 The history of inequalities on the UK health agenda

By the end of the twentieth century, issues of poverty and health were very firmly on the political and health activist agenda. The New Labour Government, elected in May 1997, pledged to address and take action on health inequality, setting up an independent inquiry (Acheson, 1998) in order to examine inequalities in health. The inquiry was chaired by Donald Acheson and backed by the then Secretary of State for Health, Frank Dobson: 'Inequality in health is the worst inequality of all. There is no more serious inequality than knowing that you'll die sooner because you're badly off' (Frank Dobson speaking in 1997, quoted in Shaw et al., 2005, p. 1017).

At the same time, the Social Exclusion Unit was set up in 1997 as an interdepartmental policy unit for England to develop integrated and sustainable approaches to the problems of the worst housing estates, including crime, drugs, unemployment, community breakdown, and bad schools (Social Exclusion Unit, 1998). In Northern Ireland, Scotland and

Wales similar aspirations were announced (Northern Ireland Office, 1999; Scottish Office, 1998; Welsh Office, 1999).

The report of the Acheson inquiry was published in November 1998 and contained thirty-nine recommendations which did not hold back from addressing the wider socio-economic determinants of health. The Acheson Report (Acheson, 1998), reinforced the bulk of the recommendations from the Black Report (DHSS, 1980), published almost twenty years previously, and concluded that the range of factors influencing inequalities in health extends far beyond the remit of the Department of Health. The report acknowledged that a response by the government as a whole would be needed to deal with the issues raised by the report. Key recommendations from Acheson included an exhortation to reduce income inequalities through the redistribution of wealth, and a commitment to tackle structural sources of inequalities, including those apparent in unemployment, incomes, education and transport.

The report recognised that improving health would mean tackling the causes of poor health. These were defined as a complex interaction between personal, social, economic and environmental factors. The report also acknowledged that, to be successful, the policies would need to attack the breeding-ground of poor health – poverty and social exclusion.

Thinking point: to what extent do you think the Acheson Report has been effective in bringing about improved health for poorer people in the UK?

Critics of the Acheson Report (Davey Smith et al., 1998), argued that the thirty-nine recommendations were not adequately prioritised or costed, and that the recommendations were too wide ranging (from water fluoridation to traffic curbing), so that the effects of poverty and income differentials were lost.

The Labour Government responded to the Acheson Report with a series of health-related White Papers, including *Our Healthier Nation: A Contract for Health* (DoH, 1998) and *Saving Lives: Our Healthier Nation* (DoH, 1999). However, these official documents gave little attention to growing income and health inequalities, and instead set rather individualised reduction targets for cancer, heart disease, accidents and mental health.

It was not until the publication of the Public Service Agreements (PSA) (DoH, 2004) that official targets addressing inequalities in health were introduced. Two of the main health targets were:

- Starting with children under one year, by 2010 to reduce the gap in mortality by at least 10 per cent between 'routine and manual' groups and the population as a whole.

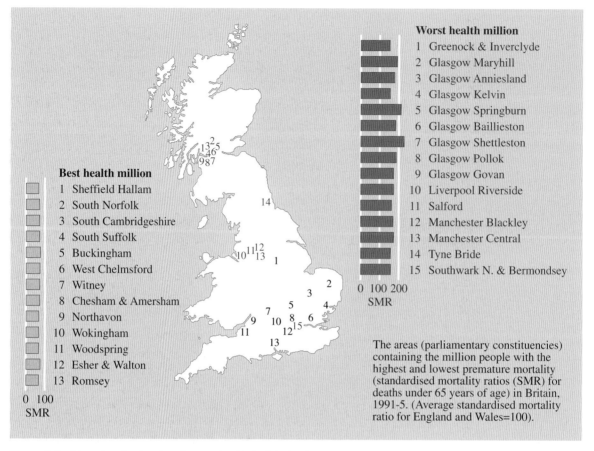

Figure 6.8   Mapping the best and worst health in Britain: the areas (parliamentary constituencies) containing the million people with the highest and lowest premature mortality (standardised mortality ratios, or SMRs, for deaths under 65 years of age) in Britain, 1991–95. (Average SMR for England and Wales = 100) (Source: Shaw et al., 2005, p. 1017, Figure 1)

•   Starting with local authorities, by 2010 to reduce the gap by at least 10 per cent between the fifth of areas with the lowest life expectancy at birth and the population as a whole.

Thinking point: what policies do you think may be the key to reducing health inequalities?

At the time of writing (2007), the Department of Health in England has established a series of initiatives designed specifically to tackle the issues associated with health inequalities. In response to their policy initiative entitled *Tackling Health Inequalities: A Programme for Action* (DoH, 2003), the Department has supported a dedicated Health Inequalities Unit (HIU), which will use Public Service Agreements (PSAs) in an attempt to reach the target of reducing inequalities in health outcomes by 10 per cent by 2010. Although there has been limited progress towards some of the targets, Figure 6.8 shows that there are still considerable differences between people's health in the north of the UK compared with the more affluent south.

The most recent figures which cover data for 2001–03 (DoH, 2005) show that the relative gap in life expectancy has increased by nearly 2 per cent for males and by 5 per cent for females in the years between 1997–99 and 2001–03. The infant mortality rate also seems resistant to the initiatives introduced to date, and the rate has gone from 13 per cent higher for the lowest social classes compared with the total population, to 19 per cent higher in 2001–03.

If the problems of poverty and illhealth seem intractable within the wealthy countries of the UK, then how much greater are the problems seen from a global perspective? Section 6.4.4 now focuses on global issues.

6.4.4 Global issues

Almost half the world's population – nearly three billion people – live on less than two dollars each day (see Figure 6.4). Approximately 790 million people in the developing world remain chronically undernourished, and Black et al. note that: 'More than 10 million children die each year, most from preventable causes and almost all in poor countries' (Black et al., 2003, p. 2226).

At a global level, the Millennium Development Goals (MDGs) (UN, 2000b) (see Figure 1.2 in Chapter 1, Section 1.2.2 in this volume), which were the product of the United Nations Millennium Summit in the year 2000, are considered the current overarching development framework and have enormous significance for health (Dodd and Cassels, 2006). The first of the UN MDGs is a commitment to 'eradicate extreme poverty and hunger' with the specific goals to 'reduce by half the proportion of people living on less than a dollar a day' and to 'reduce by half the proportion of people who suffer from hunger'.

Sachs and McArthur (2005) have outlined some of the imaginative and wide-reaching global initiatives that the Millennium Project – developed and supported by the UN Development Programme to identify practical steps to achieve the MDGs in every country – has proposed in order to reach its targets in the health sphere. Box 6.7 lists some of the 'quick wins' that are proposed by the Millennium Project to bring about speedy health benefits for people living in the developing world.

Box 6.7 Examples of 'quick wins' towards meeting the Millennium Project health goals

- The training of large numbers of village workers in health, farming and infrastructure (in one-year programmes) to ensure basic expertise and services in rural communities

- Distribution of free, long-lasting, insecticide-treated bednets to all children in malaria-endemic zones to decisively cut the burden of malaria

- Elimination of user fees for basic health services in all developing countries, financed by increased domestic and donor resources for health

- Expansion of access to sexual and reproductive health, including family planning and contraceptive information and services, by closing existing funding gaps on contraceptive supplies, family planning, and logistics

- Expansion of the use of proven effective drug combinations for AIDS, tuberculosis, and malaria, especially in places where infrastructure already exists but finance is lacking.

(Sachs and McArthur, 2005, p. 349)

However, many development activists and even some politicians remain sceptical about the progress that is being made towards the MDGs. Gordon Brown, speaking at the Labour Party Conference in 2004 pronounced that:

In 2000 the whole world came together to make a solemn promise for 2015, the Millennium Development Goals:

- the promise of primary education for every child

- the promise of an end to avoidable infant and maternal deaths and

- the promise of a halving of poverty

[...]

... at the current rates of progress in Sub-Saharan Africa:

- the promise of primary education for all will be delivered not in 2015 but 2230 (115 years too late)

- the promise for the halving of poverty not by 2015 but by 2150 (135 years too late)

- and the promise for cutting infant deaths not by 2015 but by 2165 (150 years too late)

(Gordon Brown, quoted in Gordon, 2004)

Faced with the continuing vista of official policies that may be well-meaning, but appear ineffective or inordinately slow, many development activists, including representatives from the public health movement, have been responsible for building up popular movements to combat poverty. These new organisations have devised various activities, including the use of imaginative publicity events, in order to gain public support and apply political pressure on world leaders. As you read in Chapter 1, in 2005 the leaders of the eight most powerful economic nations (G8) came together in a summit meeting at Gleneagles in Scotland. There was enormous popular pressure applied on this meeting and many hundreds of thousands of people demonstrated in the Scottish capital, Edinburgh, to ensure that the politicians understood the strength of feeling that ordinary people experience regarding the issue of world poverty. These events were replicated around the world and OXFAM (2006) estimated that 36 million people in over seventy countries united through these diverse events in their desire to express their frustration at the lack of official action on poverty and health.

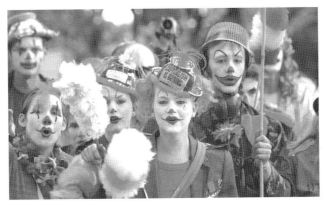

Figure 6.9   Imaginative protest is sometimes necessary to make the point about the elimination of poverty

Thinking point: do you think that mass events and demonstrations are able to influence policy makers?

In addition to the popular demonstrations, various celebrities, organised by Sir Bob Geldof, staged a series of high-profile concerts in ten large venues around the world. Although these concerts were criticised for the lack of African performers on stage, the presence of celebrities such as Paul McCartney, Bono, Robbie Williams and Madonna did increase the volume of publicity for the events. Through this mechanism knowledge of the issues and debates surrounding serious policy issues was disseminated to a very wide audience who might not otherwise have been exposed to the demands of the movement.

Partially at least because of the public pressure, the G8 leaders did agree on various measures designed to reduce the amount of poverty throughout the world, particularly those relating to Africa. The G8 agreed to cancel 100 per cent of the debts owed to the International Monetary Fund, The World Bank and the African Development Bank by some of the poorest, most indebted countries. In addition, they committed their governments to striking trade deals which would improve the ability of African nations in particular to compete in world markets. Finally, they agreed to increase the amount of help for people with HIV/AIDS and multiply the development aid targeted towards the world's poorest people.

As part of the continuing political and popular pressure following on from Make Poverty History and the Live 8 initiatives, a monitoring and campaigning organisation DATA (Debt Aids Trade Africa) has been established (DATA, 2006). This organisation, along with other development agencies and pressure groups, continues to monitor the progress made since the policy decisions that were made at the Gleneagles G8 summit meeting. They report a mixed picture, with some areas of success and other areas where no progress at all has been made, despite the promises made by the leaders of the most powerful nations of the world.

Conclusion

Combating poverty would appear to be a fundamental activity for those with an interest in promoting public health. There is now widespread acceptance of the damage done to the health of people and communities by the effects of inadequate income and the wide range of harmful material problems associated with poverty. Excess mortality and morbidity from a wide range of diseases has been demonstrated to be strongly associated with low income levels. There are still significant differences in the health status between the rich and poor people within developed countries. When a global picture is explored, the health disparities become enormous.

The health sector has been generally cautious about adopting specific anti-poverty strategies. This is not surprising, since adopting such a strategy is overtly political in nature. However, as Rose (1992, p. 129), commented, 'medicine and politics cannot and should not be kept apart', and there is a rich tradition of health workers and public health activists who are not prepared to settle for the damaging status quo. However, while there is increasing rhetoric in national and international strategies about addressing poverty, there is still evidence of an enormous gap in the health experience between rich and poor people. Global- and national-level policy change will be required to overcome poverty and, more importantly, will need to be followed by implementation of those policies. Public health practitioners can help to create pressure for change as professional workers or join in as part of the mass movements of concerned citizens.

At the same time, it is important for individuals involved in promoting public health to have a real commitment to reducing inequalities in their own practice, and to have an informed understanding of the nature and extent of poverty in their own locality. Building on such an understanding, public health workers will be better able to create 'helping relationships' that do not blame the victims of poverty, but assist individuals, households and communities in a realistic way to break out of a cycle of poverty. One of the difficulties in developing anti-poverty, work is to gain access to reliable evidence that the proposed strategies and interventions are effective. Petticrew et al. (2004) concluded that there was still a lack of information about the effectiveness and cost-effectiveness of strategies aimed at tackling inequalities in health.

Public health practitioners, whether they are professional or lay, and whether they work in or outside the health and social care sector, can have considerable influence on policy-making processes; in particular, on implementation, evaluation and policy review. Across the UK there have been a plethora of short-term initiatives, allegedly designed to reduce poverty or ameliorate some of its harmful effects. Often these initiatives are introduced in a blaze of glory as successive governments need to be seen to be active. However, after a period of time the fashionable initiative becomes starved of finance and eventually lies dormant with little evidence that it has changed the life experiences of anyone in the target group. This chapter has attempted to emphasise that long-term approaches, which seek to address the root causes of poverty, are needed. This will require redistributive policies in addition to local anti-poverty initiatives.

References

Acheson, D. (1998) *Independent Inquiry into Inequalities in Health*, London, The Stationery Office.

Black, R., Morris, S. and Bryce, J. (2003) 'Where and why are 10 million children dying every year?', *The Lancet*, vol. 361, pp. 2226–34.

Bradshaw, J. (1993) *Household Budgets and Living Standards – Findings*, York, Joseph Rowntree Foundation.

Burchardt, T., Le Grand, J. and Piachaud, D. (1999) 'Social exclusion in Britain 1991–1995', *Social Policy and Administration*, vol. 33, pp. 227–44.

Child Poverty Action Group (CPAG) (2006) *Media Briefing: The Government's Child Poverty Target*, London, CPAG; also available online at http://www.cpag.org.uk/campaigns/media/CPAG_HBAI_2006_Media_Briefing.pdf#search=%22cpag%20definition%20of%20poverty%22 (Accessed 14 September 2006).

Citro, C. (1995) *Measuring Poverty: A New Approach*, Washington, DC, National Academy Press.

Cook, J. and Watt, S. (1987) 'Racism, women and poverty' in Glendinning and Millar (eds) (1987).

Davey Smith, G., Morris, J.N. and Shaw, M. (1998) 'The Independent Inquiry into Inequalities in Health', *British Medical Journal*, vol. 17, pp. 1465–6.

Debt Aids Trade Africa (DATA) (2006) *The Data Report 2006: Executive Summary* [online], http://www.thedatareport.org/pdf/DATA_ESenglish.pdf (Accessed 12 March 2007).

Department of Health (DoH) (1998) *Our Healthier Nation: A Contract for Health*, London, The Stationery Office.

Department of Health (DoH) (1999) *Saving Lives: Our Healthier Nation*, London, The Stationery Office.

Department of Health (DoH) (2003) *Tackling Health Inequalities: A Programme for Action*, London, The Stationery Office.

Department of Health (DoH) (2004) *PSA Target* [online], http://www.dh.gov.uk/PolicyAndGuidance/HealthAndSocialCareTopics/HealthInequalities/HealthInequalitiesGeneralInformation/HealthInequalitiesGeneralArticle/fs/en?CONTENT_ID=4131685&chk=z4zsTt (Accessed 12 December 2006).

Department of Health (DoH) (2005) *Tackling Health Inequalities: Status Report on the Programme for Action* [online], http://www.dh.gov.uk/PolicyAndGuidance/HealthAndSocialCareTopics/HealthInequalities/fs/en (Accessed 21 September 2006).

Department of Health and Social Security (DHSS) (1980) *Inequalities in Health: Report of a Research Working Group* (the Black Report), London, Department of Health and Social Security.

Dodd, R. and Cassels, A. (2006) 'Health, development and the Millennium Development Goals', *Annals of Tropical Medicine and Parasitology*, vol. 100, pp. 379–87.

Douglas, J., Sidell, M., Lloyd, C. and Earle, S. (2007) 'Evaluating public health interventions' in Earle, S., Lloyd, C.E., Sidell, M. and Spurr, S. (eds) *Theory and Research in Promoting Public Health*, London, Sage/Milton Keynes, The Open University.

Exworthy, M., Bindman, A., Davies, H. and Washington, A. (2006) 'Evidence into policy and practice? Measuring the progress of US and UK policies to tackle disparities and inequalities in US and UK health and health care', *The Milbank Quarterly* vol. 84, pp. 75–109.

Gibson, A. (forthcoming) *Is Social Capital a Useful Concept in Understanding Health Inequalities?*, PhD thesis, Milton Keynes, The Open University.

Glendinning, C. and Millar, J. (eds) (1987) *Women and Poverty in Britain: The 1990s*, Hemel Hempstead, Harvester Wheatsheaf.

Gordon, D. (2004) *Eradicating Poverty in the 21st Century: When Will Social Justice be Done?*, Inaugural Lecture, Bristol, Bristol University, [online], http://www.bris.ac.uk/poverty/news_files/Inaugural%20Lecture%20Transcript%2018.10.041.doc (Accessed 30 August 2006).

Gordon, D., Adelman, A., Asworth, K., Bradshaw, J., Levitas, R., Middleton, S., Pantazis, C., Patsios, D., Payne. S., Townsend, P. and Williams, J. (2000) *Poverty and Social Exclusion in Britain*, York, Joseph Rowntree Foundation.

Graham, H. (2007) 'Poverty and health: global and national patterns' in Douglas, J., Earle, S., Handsley, S., Lloyd, C.E. and Spurr, S. (eds) *A Reader in Promoting Public Health: Challenge and Controversy*, London, Sage/Milton Keynes, The Open University.

Heller, R. (2005) *Evidence for Population Health*, Oxford, Oxford University Press.

Help the Aged (2006) *Our Work in Northern Ireland* [online] http://www.helptheaged.org.uk/en-ni/WhatWeDo/AboutUs/AcrossTheUK/ (Accessed 21 September 2006).

Hills, J. (2004) *Inequality and the State*, Oxford, Oxford University Press.

Howarth, C., Kenway, P., Palmer, G. and Miorelli, R. (1999) *Monitoring Poverty and Social Exclusion*, York, Joseph Rowntree Foundation.

Jones, L. (2002) 'The social policy contribution to health promotion' in Jones, L., Sidell, M. and Douglas, J. (eds) *The Challenge of Promoting Health: Exploration and Action* (2nd edn), Basingstoke, Palgrave Macmillan/Milton Keynes, The Open University.

Koupil, I. (2005) 'Tackling health inequalities in the enlarged European Union', *British Medical Journal*, vol. 331, pp. 855–6.

Laderchi, C., Saith, R. and Stewart, F. (2003) 'Does it matter that we don't agree on the definition of poverty? A comparison of four approaches', Queen Elizabeth House (QEH) Working Paper Series 74, Oxford, Queen Elizabeth House.

Lancet (2006) Editorial, 'Measuring progress on health disparities', *The Lancet*, vol. 367, p. 1876.

Leon, D. and Walt, G. (eds) (2001) *Poverty, Inequality and Health*: *An International Perspective*, Oxford, Oxford University Press.

Leon, D., Walt, G. and Gilson, L. (2001) 'International perspectives on health inequalities and policy', *British Medical Journal*, vol. 322, pp. 591–4.

Lynch, J.W., Smith, G.D., Kaplan, G.A. and House, J.S. (2000) 'Income inequality and mortality: importance to health of individual income, psychosocial environment, or material conditions', *British Medical Journal*, vol. 320, pp. 1200–4.

Mackenbach, J. and Bakker, M. (2003) 'Tackling socioeconomic inequalities in health: analysis of European experiences', *The Lancet*, vol. 362, pp. 1409–14.

Madood, T., Berthoud, R., Lakey, J., Nazroo, J., Smith, P., Virdee, S. and Beishon, S. (1997) *Ethnic Minorities in Britain: Diversity and Disadvantage*, London, Policy Studies Institute.

McKay, S. (2004) 'Poverty or preference: what do "consensual deprivation indicators" really measure?', *Fiscal Studies*, vol. 25, pp. 201–23.

Milward, L., Kelly, M. and Nutbeam, D. (2001) *Public Health Intervention Research: The Evidence*, London, Health Development Agency.

Nazroo, J. and Karlsen, S. (2001) 'Ethnic inequalities in health: social class, racism and identity', *Research Findings: 10*, ESRC Health Variations Programme, Lancaster, Lancaster University, [online], http://www.lancs.ac.uk/fss/apsocsci/hvp/pdf/fd10.pdf#search=%22nazroo%202001%22 (Accessed 21 September 2006).

Northern Ireland Office (1999) *New TSN: An Agenda for Targeting Health and Social Need in Northern Ireland*, Belfast, The Stationery Office.

Nutbeam, D. (2004) 'Getting evidence into policy and practice to address health inequalities', *Health Promotion International*, vol. 19, pp. 137–40.

Office of the United Nations High Commissioner for Human Rights (OHCHR) (2006) *What Is Poverty?* [online], http://www.unhchr.ch/development/poverty-02.html (Accessed 11 December 2006).

OXFAM (2006) *The View from the Summit – Gleneagles G8 One Year On*, Oxfam Briefing Note, London, OXFAM, [online], http://www.oxfam.org.uk/what_we_do/issues/debt_aid/downloads/g8_gleneagles_oneyear.pdf (Accessed 21 September 2006).

Patsios, D. (2006) 'Pensioners, poverty and social exclusion' in Pantazis, C., Gordon, D. and Levitas, R. (eds) *Poverty and Social Exclusion in Britain*, Bristol, Policy.

Percy-Smith, J. (2000) *Policy Responses to Social Exclusion: Towards Inclusion*, Buckingham, Open University Press.

Petticrew, M., Whitehead, M., Macintyre, S.J., Graham, H. and Egan, M. (2004) 'Evidence for public health policy on inequalities: 1: The reality according to policymakers', *Journal of Epidemiology and Community Health*, vol. 58, pp. 811–16.

Piachaud, D. and Sutherland, H. (2000) 'How effective is the British Government's attempt to reduce child poverty?', Case paper 38, Centre for Analysis of Social Exclusion, London, London School of Economics, [online], http://sticerd.lse.ac.uk/dps/case/cp/CASEpaper38.pdf#search=%22british%20government%20definition%20of%20poverty%22 (Accessed 14 September 2006).

Platt, M. (1984) 'Recent research on the impact of unemployment on psychological wellbeing and parasuicide' in Berryman, J.C. (ed.) *The Psychological Effects of Unemployment*, Leicester, Leicester University Press.

Poverty Mapping (2006) *The Poverty Lines: Population Living with Less than 2 Dollars and Less than 1 Dollar a Day* [online], http://www.povertymap.net/mapsgraphics/index.cfm?data_id=23417&theme (Accessed 14 September 2006).

Quisumbing, A. (2001) 'Are women overrepresented among the poor? An analysis of poverty in 10 developing countries', *Journal of Development Studies*, vol. 6, pp. 225–69.

Rose, G. (1992) *The Strategy of Preventive Medicine*, Oxford, Oxford University Press.

Sachs, J. and McArthur, J. (2005) 'The Millennium Project: a plan for meeting the Millennium Development Goals', *The Lancet*, vol. 365, pp. 347–53.

Scottish Office (1998) *Social Exclusion in Scotland: A Consultation Paper*, London, The Stationery Office; also available online at http://www.scotland.gov.uk/library/documents1/socexcl.htm (Accessed 19 March 2007).

Scottish Office (1999) *Towards a Healthier Scotland*, Edinburgh, The Stationery Office.

Shaw, M., Davey Smith, G. and Dorling, D. (2005) 'Health inequalities and New Labour: how the promises compare with real progress', *British Medical Journal*, vol. 330, pp. 1016–21.

Smith, G., Neaton, J., Wentworth, D., Stamler, R. and Stamler, J. (1996) 'Socioeconomic differentials in mortality risk among men screened for multiple risk factor intervention trial', *American Journal of Public Health*, vol. 86, pp. 486–96.

Social Exclusion Unit (1998) *Bringing Britain Together: A National Strategy for Neighbourhood Renewal*, London, The Stationery Office.

Stronks, K. and Mackenbach, J. (2005) 'Evaluating the effect of policies and interventions to address inequalities in health: lessons from a Dutch programme', *European Journal of Public Health*, vol. 16, pp. 346–53.

Townsend, P. (1979) *Poverty in the United Kingdom*, London, Penguin.

United Nations (UN) (2000a) *United Nations Millennium Declaration* [online], http://www.ohchr.org/english/law/millennium.htm (Accessed 11 December 2006).

United Nations (UN) (2000b) *Millennium Development Goals* [online], http://www.un.org/millenniumgoals/ (Accessed 21 September 2006).

United Nations Children's Fund (UNICEF) (2005) 'Child poverty in rich countries 2005: the proportion of children living in poverty has risen in a majority of the world's developed economies', Innocenti Report Card No. 6, Florence, UNICEF Innocenti Research Centre; also available online at http://www.unicef.org/sowc06/pdfs/repcard6e.pdf (Accessed 19 September 2006).

Welsh Office (1999) *Building an Inclusive Wales: Tackling the Social Exclusion Agenda*, Cardiff, Welsh Office.

Wilkinson, P., Pattenden, S., Armstrong, B., Fletcher, A., Kovats, R.S., Mangtani, P. and McMichael, A.J. (2004) 'Vulnerability to winter mortality in elderly people in Britain: population based study', *British Medical Journal*, vol. 329, pp. 647–53.

Wilkinson, R.G. (1996) *Unhealthy Societies: The Afflictions of Inequality*, London, Routledge.

World Bank (2006a) *Voices of the Poor* [online], http://www1.worldbank.org/prem/poverty/voices/index.htm (Accessed 12 September 2006).

World Bank (2006b) *Understanding Poverty* [online], http://web.worldbank.org/WBSITE/EXTERNAL/TOPICS/EXTPOVERTY/0,,contentMDK:20153855 menuPK:373757~pagePK:148956~piPK:216618~theSitePK:336992,00.html (Accessed 12 September 2006).

World Health Organization (WHO) (1977) *Health for All by the Year 2000*, Geneva, World Health Organization.

World Health Organization (WHO) (1985) *Targets for Health for All*, Copenhagen, World Health Organization Regional Office for Europe.

World Health Organization (WHO) (1998) *Second International Conference on Health Promotion, Adelaide* [online], http://www.who.int/hpr/NPH/docs/adelaide_recommendations.pdf (Accessed 12 March 2007).

World Health Organization (WHO) (2006) *Commission on Social Determinant of Health*, Geneva, World Health Organization; also available online at http://www.who.int/social_determinants/resources/csdh_brochure.pdf (Accessed 12 March 2007).

Part II
Promoting public health at a local level

The participatory and community action approach to promoting public health at a local level aims to use collaboration, collectivism and consultation to develop healthy interventions that will bring about healthy solutions and outcomes. It attempts to avoid the pitfalls of both 'victim blaming' and the paternalistic and top – down approach of much health service provision. By focusing on communities at a micro level, and on the role they play in fostering and forging healthy relationships, it is possible to explore the links between settings and to develop integrated strategies and programmes that enhance the physical, mental, social, economic and environmental wellbeing of those who live in such environments.

In the UK, commitment to community involvement has, since the mid-1980s, become both a reality and a major part of the political rhetoric, and regeneration and urban renewal of one kind or another are now the main vehicles for government's community involvement intentions. Indeed, there has long been an agenda for local government to be tuned in to communities' needs. Fresh interest in the potential of communities – clearly signalled as central in the New Deal for Communities, and in urban renaissance, reform of the planning and health systems, community strategies, local strategic partnerships and neighbourhood renewal – has come from both national and international politicians and policy makers.

Part II of this book begins with Chapter 7, 'The potential for promoting public health at a local level: community strategies and health improvement', which explores the possibilities and promise of promoting public health at a local level. Here, many of the key terms, concepts, ideas and approaches used in subsequent chapters are introduced and discussed. The chapter also explores the rationale for promoting public health at a community level, before turning to consider some of the strategies and initiatives which have led to general improvements in the health and wellbeing of local communities. This includes a brief examination of the different sectors that are responsible for promoting public health at a local level.

Chapter 8, 'Community involvement and civic engagement in multidisciplinary public health', follows on from this by investigating just how effective the mobilisation of communities in promoting the public's health has been, and how this is central to successfully addressing social injustice and health inequalities at a local level. The chapter examines the notion of community development and considers the way in which it is intended to democratise the approach to multidisciplinary public health. This chapter also explores the impact of the much-lauded patient/public involvement in the improvement of the public's health and wellbeing.

Chapter 9, 'Developing local alliance partnerships through community collaboration and participation', considers critically the role played by health alliances and local partnerships within communities in the drive to promote public health at a local level. The chapter also considers the way in which health alliances and local partnerships are central to a range of other public health-related policies and strategies, reflecting on some of the opportunities and challenges posed by local alliance partnerships. The focus here is on the importance of establishing responsibilities and structures, the need to behave properly and the significance of difference. This chapter concludes by reflecting on the concept of empowerment and ways of achieving community empowerment.

Chapter 10, 'Working with communities to promote public health', builds on previous chapters by looking at the role played by the multidisciplinary public health workforce in promoting public health at a local level. The chapter focuses on the need for many multidisciplinary public health practitioners to adopt community development approaches, and to acquire the skills needed to enable them to work effectively with communities.

The penultimate chapter – Chapter 11, 'Gauging the effectiveness of community-based public health projects' – focuses on evaluation and Health Impact Assessment as ways of establishing the effectiveness of community-based public health projects or programmes and whether or not they are making a difference. In each case, the results are used to influence policy and the decision-making process. The chapter also considers the values underpinning the evaluation of community action for health and, similarly, those of Health Impact Assessment.

Chapter 12, 'Promoting mental health and social inclusion', the final chapter of the book, introduces the key topic of mental health promotion, an area of public health which is sometimes missed off the radar of multidisciplinary public health. This chapter begins by examining what is meant by mental health and mental health promotion, before summarising some of the risks and protective factors for mental health problems. It then puts mental health promotion into context by discussing how the respective public health promotion practices and policies of each of the four nations of the UK grapple with the burning issue of mental health, and outlines the strategies that are in place to foster a climate that facilitates positive mental health and emotional wellbeing. The final section of the chapter draws together this part of the book by looking towards the future for multidisciplinary public health and mental health promotion at a local level.

Chapter 7

The potential for promoting public health at a local level: community strategies and health improvement

Stephen Handsley

Introduction

One of the key lessons learned in the last few decades of public health research is the importance of understanding the subtle, unique characteristics of the communities in which people live and work. Prevention and intervention strategies that function well in one community may fail in another simply because they fall short of addressing the specific needs of that particular population. Whatever the intervention, although changing habits and values may begin at the individual or family level, maintaining change often relies on reinforcement and approval at the community level. Public health programme efforts, therefore, need to focus on the whole community so that it becomes positive and enabling. To succeed in this endeavour, the community and its leadership must be mobilised to provide community-based public health programmes in a collaborative, consultative and participative environment. However, such action must be set within the context of the political will of politicians and policy makers.

The purpose of this chapter is to explore the potential for promoting public health at a local level, thus introducing some of the key terms, concepts, ideas and approaches which you will come across in subsequent chapters. The chapter begins by exploring the rationale for promoting public health at a community level, before turning to consider some of the strategies and initiatives that have led to general improvements in the health and wellbeing of local communities. This includes a brief examination of the different sectors that are responsible for promoting public health at a local level. The chapter ends with a brief look at the way in which locally based public health strategies and initiatives relate to practice.

7.1 Why promote public health at a local level?

Ever since the publication of the White Paper *Saving Lives: Our Healthier Nation* (DoH, 1999), a social dimension has been added to the repertoire of public health and its practice, moving from individual to collective responsibility and incorporating a social model of health. This White Paper also called for policies and services which are sensitive to the needs of local people, particularly those policies and services that target health inequalities and social injustice.

Thinking point: why promote public health at a local level? What are the benefits of such policies and practices?

According to Earle (2007), it is widely accepted that promoting public health is fundamentally a good thing. While this may, indeed, be true, it does not fully explain the rationale for promoting public health at a local level. For example, is it simply about improving the overall health of communities? Or are there more strategic, possibly political purposes, for promoting public health at a community-wide or neighbourhood level? Perhaps, like both Plant (1998) and Earle (2007), you feel that, as citizens, people have a right to benefit from locally based resources that provide health.

For some commentators, utilising local health information can be a powerful vehicle for improving the health of a community. It can highlight the existence of both problems and opportunities for improvement. It can also guide local action in support of policy changes and improve the effectiveness of programmes (Luck et al., 2006). Perhaps the most obvious reason for promoting public health at a local level is a recognition of the wider range of factors, such as income, education, employment, housing and the environment, that influence health and health inequalities, as well as the effect of these on lifestyle (Wanless, 2004). All these factors represent part of the everyday reality and priority of neighbourhoods and communities. So how might the potential for promoting public health be realised?

7.2 The potential for promoting public health at a local level

The history of public health is peppered with attempts by international bodies, successive governments, local authorities and primary care trusts (PCTs) to develop and implement strategies and interventions that address health inequalities at a local level. Many of these, although achieving some success, have been concentrated on primary care, albeit with a much broader focus. The Alma Ata declaration of 1978 (WHO, 1978), for example, placed primary care at the centre of public health. This involved universal, community-based preventative and curative services, with substantial community involvement.

As Earle (2007) has discussed, this commitment to community-based health initiatives and interventions was reinforced by the WHO Health For All strategy (WHO, 1985). This was subsequently revised in the document *Health 21: Health for All in the 21st Century* (WHO, 1999), so-called not only because it dealt with health in the twenty-first century, but also because it laid out twenty-one principles and objectives for improving the health of Europeans.

In the UK, primary care and its interface with community has traditionally been subsumed under the banner of the National Health Service (NHS). Thus, when the words 'health' and 'local' are considered together, historically many people have accepted that the face of public health at a local level is represented by the general practitioner (GP) or the primary healthcare team (PHCT). Indeed, across the UK, many of the policy publications on modernising and improving the NHS, which have been produced since the 1990s, and each country's strategy for public health and for reducing health inequalities, have placed great emphasis on primary care. Such policies positioned the issue of improving health firmly on the public health agenda and on the agendas of health authorities and primary care organisations.

The role of health authorities has been to assess the health needs of the local population, and to draw up local strategies to address those needs through the allocation of resources as determined by the development of a health improvement programme (HIMP), which involved a range of organisations from the statutory and voluntary sectors. The development of HIMPs was to be guided by a set of national standards: the national service frameworks (NSFs). For example, the National Service Framework for Older People is one of several NSFs which were introduced as part of the government's NHS Plan to invest in, and reform, the health service for the twenty-first century (DoH, 2000). One of the aims of the NSF for Older People was that local HIMPs would have to include plans to promote healthy ageing by 2003.

Health authorities were also responsible for determining the structure and functioning of local health services, setting local standards and ensuring that services met national standards; and for supporting the initial development of primary care groups (PCGs), allocating resources to them and holding them to account (depending on local circumstances, a PCG serves a population of between 50,000 and 250,000 and is a subcommittee of the local health authority). They also retained overall responsibility for promoting and protecting public health (NHSE, 1999) by developing partnerships with local authorities, PCGs, PCTs and other relevant organisations.

Other central government policies, including *Saving Lives: Our Healthier Nation* (DoH, 1999), outlined a number of initiatives aimed at addressing urban and rural deprivation, including Health Action Zones (HAZs) and Health Living Centres. These were introduced with the intention of reducing inequalities in health by working across a range of agencies, and of achieving this by involving local people. Such strategies arguably paved the way for a more community-orientated and participatory approach to public health and were part of a wider programme aimed at tackling broader social exclusion issues – through such initiatives as the New Deal for Communities (£800 million over three years). This was a key programme in the English Government's strategy to tackle multiple deprivation in the most deprived neighbourhoods in the country. The Single Regeneration Budget (£2.4 billion over three years) was another government strategy which provided resources to support regeneration initiatives in England, carried out by local regeneration partnerships.

The inception of the NHS Plan in July 2000 (DoH, 2000) seemed to reinforce the British Government's stated aims that tackling the wider determinants of health would result in healthier neighbourhoods and communities. In April 2002, the old health authorities, which were the main organisational units of the NHS for administrative and managerial purposes, were replaced by strategic health authorities (SHAs). Designed to support PCTs and NHS trusts in delivering the NHS Plan in their areas, these SHAs were seen as a key link between the Department of Health and the NHS, responsible for developing strategies for the local health services and ensuring high quality care.

This reorganisation of primary care within the NHS would, many argued, bring about fundamental changes in the way in which public health was delivered (Woodhead et al., 2002). Measures announced in *Shifting the Balance of Power within the NHS: Securing Delivery* (DoH, 2001) envisaged a situation in which PCTs would be the main vehicle for the delivery of public health locally, working with new, managed public health networks operating across SHA areas. This shift would, for example, see power and responsibility for managing the NHS locally moving to PCTs. The rationale for this was that these trusts, together with local partners, would take the lead in local communities on public health issues, mainly through the development of HIMPS and local strategic partnerships (LSPs). The three principal functions of this collaborative venture were to:

- improve the health of the communities they serve

- commission healthcare services to meet local health needs (involving local communities and frontline staff)

- provide community and primary healthcare services

(Adapted from DoH, 2001)

With the advent of the English White Paper *Choosing Health: Making Healthy Choices Easier* (DoH, 2004), the potential of communities in aiding the promotion of public health continued to be high on the political and public health agenda. The central thrust of this document was that: 'Action by local authorities working with local communities, business and voluntary groups to tackle local health issues makes a difference to the opportunities for both adults and children to choose healthier lifestyles' (DoH, 2004, p. 10). Documents which have appeared subsequently – for example, *Our Health, Our Care, Our Say: A New Direction for Community Services* (DOH, 2006) – have reinforced the view that local people in the twenty-first century should be given a 'voice' in the way in which health services are delivered.

The almost continuous reform and restructuring since the mid-1980s, which has seen the NHS shift from one locally based public health initiative to another, appears to show no sign of abating. The reorganisation of SHAs during 2006 was designed as a blueprint for citizens to reclaim the agenda on health. With the publication of *Creating a Patient-Led NHS: Delivering the NHS Improvement Plan* (DoH 2005a), PCTs were charged with changing the way the NHS works by making sure that they offered choices to patients. Part of this perpetual process of reform was that a patient-led NHS would offer a deeper insight into local communities, a process which would be locally driven and would improve the effectiveness of services by operating to a national framework and national standards (DoH, 2005a).

This, like previous health strategies, is based largely on the assumption that, at a local level, primary care services – for example, general practice or NHS supported-health centres – are natural and particularly suitable settings for promoting health. Indeed, both GPs and locally based primary care centres continue to provide valuable advice to people at a local level on promoting public health (Carlisle et al., 2002). However, since the late 1990s there has been a shift towards public health projects that are facilitated and led by local authorities, education and the voluntary sector. In many cases, such projects tend to adopt a more participatory and community-involvement approach. Both these and the continuing role of the NHS within public health will be explored below. However, given the centrality and increased emphasis on community collaboration, you are first asked to consider definitions of community within public health. The next section unpacks many of the key terms associated with the community-orientated approach, beginning with what is meant by 'community'.

7.3 Making sense of community concepts in public health

Despite the growth of community participation and public involvement in the public sector since the 1990s, there remains a certain amount of confusion and contestation around what these terms mean. For example, for some, community participation and public involvement are related to concepts such as community development, empowerment and social capital, particularly in the context of health promotion and improvement (Green, 1999). For others, community discourses tend to include references to such concepts as collaboration, consultation and collectivism (Yoo et al., 2004). Beginning with the concept of community, you are introduced to the terminology which underpins community-orientated approaches to public health.

7.3.1 Just what is meant by 'community'?

Traditional notions of communities (of interest and geography) are, it is argued, being broken down and redefined in terms of users, customers or consumers of public services, constituting an ethic of individualism (MacDonald and Smith, 2001). However, others would argue that the notion of engaging with communities – and, increasingly, the word 'community' – is used as a spray-on solution to solve complex social problems (Mowbray, 2005). For example, since coming to power in 1997, one defining characteristic of Tony Blair's Labour policy agenda has been its stated commitment to the value of community: 'Community is the governing idea of modern social democracy ... a key task for our second term is to develop greater coherence around our commitment to community' (Blair, 2002, p. 28).

Given that the word 'community' is becoming more widely used, it is important to consider some of the difficulties in attempting to define this thorny concept, and how one's understanding and knowledge of the term may affect the way in which one 'sees the world'. Hawtin et al. concur with this, arguing that: 'In reality, communities are not always comfortable homogenous entities. They are cross-cut by a variety of divisions – race, gender, and class – and contain a multitude of groups whose interests may conflict with each other' (Hawtin et al., 1999, p. 34).

Thinking point: which communities do you consider you belong to?

You could have identified a number of communities to which you belong. Perhaps you identified the area in which you live: if so, did you identify your road or street, or your estate or neighbourhood in general? Or perhaps you identified a school catchment area or a political ward, a parish or a village, a district or a county, or a nation – or even a group of nations. If you live in a large town or city, you may not feel part of any geographical community: you may not even know your neighbours, or want to know them.

The word 'community' also suggests a common bond between individuals, groups or sections of the population. A community can be an officially defined geographical area or locality, varying in size from a single street to a neighbourhood, for example, or it can be an administratively defined area, as in the case of PCTs. There are, however, other characteristics that may define a community. The people who live in a particular neighbourhood or locality, for instance, may define a community in terms of its social or emotional ties. These characteristics may include a sense of inclusiveness and belonging. Indeed, critical to the concept of 'community' is the notion of shared consciousness. Labonte (1997), for example, notes that communities are organised systems of people in relation to one another.

Conversely, a 'community' may be defined by the way in which it stigmatises, marginalises or excludes certain individuals or groups: for example, people with mental health problems, as discussed in Chapter 12. In this way, the definition of 'community' may be based on such characteristics as ethnicity, age, gender, religion, sexuality, disability, or a shared issue or problem, each of which might be used as the basis for exclusion. For instance, if you belong to a particular ethnic community, this may or may not coincide with a particular locality. If you belong to a religious group, this may provide a geographical community based on a church, temple, mosque or synagogue. Your gender or sexuality may mean that you belong to a political community such as a women's group or the gay rights movement. From this brief discussion, it can be seen that both the concept and the reality of 'community', as understood by professional and lay people, or by policy makers and recipients, can be vastly different.

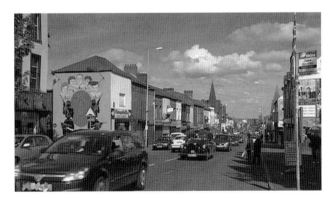

Figure 7.1   An image of a community in Belfast

Historically, community has tended to have quite a positive image. It evokes a sense of closeness and warmth: 'It is like a roof under which we shelter in heavy rain, like a fireplace at which we warm our hands on a frosty day' (Bauman, 2001, p. 1). However, as Brent (1997) argues, such sentimentalism fails to overcome the problems inherent in the operationalisation of approaches to community development; in short, any type of community activity often creates conflict and division. Despite this, 'community', 'community involvement' and 'community action' have, over recent years, as Jewkes and Murcott (1996) have argued, become part of the daily discourse of those engaged in public health. Indeed, such attention to 'community' and 'community participation' has been deliberately introduced as an integral part of their roles. This can be seen in Figure 7.2, which lists ways that public health professionals might identify the characteristics of a community.

Figure 7.2   Definitions of 'community' that may be generated by health professionals (Source: adapted from Emmel and Conn, 2004, p. 9)

Definition of community	Examples
Geographically	A particular and clearly demarcated population
Shared characteristics	Young employed men, lone mothers
Communities of interest	People from minority ethnic groups
A numerically defined community	A census aggregate
An administrative area	The population within a PCT
An at-risk group	Men who smoke and have high cholesterol
A GP's list	A practice's population

There are both advantages and disadvantages to such definitions. The advantage of the range of definitions given in Figure 7.2 is that it allows public health professionals to define clearly the boundaries of particular groups with whom they work. Geographical communities, for instance, are clearly recognisable. This, in turn, means that it is easier to plan and account for resource allocation. Similarly, it is possible to measure changes in attitudes, practices and health status among communities with clearly defined characteristics. The disadvantages of such models are that they have a tendency to become prescriptive, leading to a lack of innovation in the way community concepts are applied. As Emmel and Conn argue:

> Disadvantaged groups of the marginalised and powerless are more likely to be missed when definitions of community defined by an *outsider observer* are applied (Jewkes and Murcott, 1996). Communities defined by members may either assert their difference and exclude themselves, or be excluded because they are powerless and do not have an adequate voice to make themselves heard in decision making.
>
> (Emmel and Conn, 2004, p. 10)

Thus, it can be seen that the term 'community' may be defined in many ways to mean different things to different people. The terminology that forms a central part of community-orientated approaches to public health involves a similar range of definitions, and this is explored below.

7.3.2 Understanding the language of community concepts and participatory approaches

According to a number of scholars, community involvement can improve health and social wellbeing through the development of healthier public policy and better services (Yoo et al., 2004). However, differences remain in the way in which 'community involvement' is both defined and practised (ODPM, 2003). For example, the term 'community involvement' is applied loosely to activities which involve lay people with little or no powers of achievement. This has important implications for practice since defining or labelling a programme as community involvement, where another term – for example, community consultation – would be more appropriate, leads to disillusionment among professionals and communities because expectations are not met. Both communities and professionals should have a clear sense of purpose in developing community involvement strategies (Emmel and Conn, 2004). In short, community-orientated approaches include a wide and diverse range of activities. Although many of these concepts surrounding community activity are revisited in later chapters, Figure 7.3 offers some useful definitions of the key terms used in the field.

Thinking point: can you discern any similarities or differences between these terms?

Figure 7.3   Community activity in multidisciplinary public health: some useful concepts and definitions

Concept	Definition
Community action	Collective action by local communities, with the aim of increasing people's control over the area in which they live. Community action often involves campaigning activities in response to specific local problems, such as housing conditions, crime and vandalism, or the availability and quality of play facilities
Community development in health	A process whereby people, both individually and in groups, exercise their right to play an active and direct role in the development of appropriate health services, in ensuring the conditions for sustained better health, and in supporting the empowerment of communities for health development
Community involvement	Entails both consultation and participation, with local people participating in the development of policies to improve the health of their community, as well as having a say in the prioritising, planning and delivery of services

Communitarianism	Based on the application of reciprocity in care and compassion, the idea that individuals should play a key role in furnishing the needs of their neighbours. Once they have met their personal responsibilities, they have an obligation to promote the wellbeing of relatives, friends and others in the various communities to which they belong. These include all types of social groups, such as schools, organisations, families, neighbourhoods and interest groups
Community participation	Refers to a group of people who share an interest, a neighbourhood, or a common set of circumstances. They may or may not acknowledge membership of a particular community. Community participation is the process of involving community members in decision making about the issues that affect them, including service planning, policy development, setting priorities and addressing quality issues in the delivery of services. It includes developing formal partnerships; inviting public comment through public meetings, forums and documents for consultation; conducting focus groups, surveys, interviews and workshops; forming community councils, and advisory and consultative committees; developing networks of consumers, carers and community representatives; and appointing representatives to health committees
Capacity building	Developmental work and activities (e.g. the provision of financial or computer training) which increase the abilities of an organisation or a community to take action or provide services. Capacity building is used to support the process of helping local groups to take part in the social and economic regeneration of their area by encouraging and developing people's skills and confidence, building up an infrastructure by setting up and strengthening networks, and improving organisation and procedures
Civic engagement	Active participation in the institutions of civil society. Civic engagement includes activities such as signing a petition, contacting a local councillor or public official working for a local council, attending a public meeting or rally, or contacting a member of parliament
Consultation	Allows for a higher level of involvement than does the giving of information. People may be asked for their views of and comments on problems and be offered options, which are then taken into account and perhaps proceeded with after negotiation. In other words, consultation takes place when people are offered choices on what might be done, but not the opportunity to develop their own ideas or to participate in putting plans into action
Empowerment	A social process that promotes the participation of individuals, organisations and communities in actions with the goal of increased individual and community control, political efficacy, improved quality of life and social justice
Social capital	The features of social life, such as networks, norms and social trust, that facilitate co-ordination and co-operation for mutual benefit. Represents the degree of social cohesion that exists in communities

The concept of community participation is not new. It has been utilised in many different ways for many years, not only within health but more broadly within social practice and development, regeneration and neighbourhood renewal (WHO, 2002). For Zakus and Lysack (1998, p. 1), however, it is at 'the local level where day-to-day realities of incorporating community participation into health service delivery are confronted'.

To avoid confusion, it is important to be clear about the distinctions between such terms as 'consultation', 'participation' and 'empowerment'. Although these concepts are covered in greater depth in Chapter 9, an early appreciation and understanding of them is essential both to the implementation and application of community-based healthy interventions and to your grasp of community-orientated approaches. The differences are outlined in Figure 7.4.

Figure 7.4   Distinctions between 'consultation', 'participation' and 'empowerment' (Source: adapted from HDA, 2005, p. 50)

Consultation	Seeking local people's opinions on a particular issue or issues: for example, by setting up a focus group
Participation	Encouraging local people to become involved in initiatives and structures to improve communities by, for example, being community representatives on partnership boards or becoming involved in area forums. Unlike consultation, participation is about mobilising people to do something, but it is not always clear that participation empowers people
Empowerment	Strengthening communities by achieving measurable outcomes and providing education and training

Empowerment has become something of a key theme in much political rhetoric in recent years (Laverack and Wallerstein, 2001). It conveys a sense of personal psychological control and actual influence in social, political and economic spheres (Rapoport, 1987). Figure 7.5 reinforces the links between community involvement, empowerment and health, suggesting a virtuous cycle between these.

Empowerment applies equally to communities and professionals. For example, empowered communities have control over the process of defining their health needs and identifying how these might be addressed: professionals then help to direct the flow of service delivery and the application of targets to be achieved. As Earle (2007) and others have shown, the concept of empowerment emerged from the work of Paulo Freire (1970), a Brazilian philosopher and educator who was concerned with the powerlessness of the lowest social classes and the relationship between power and knowledge. However, empowerment is not just a

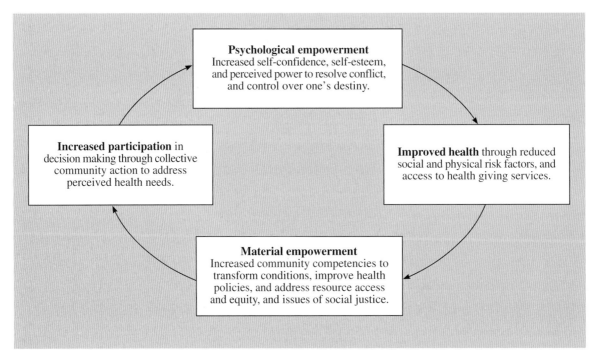

Figure 7.5   A virtuous cycle of empowerment, health and community involvement (Source: Emmel and Conn, 2004, p. 15, Figure 3)

process, but can be a goal, in that it has also been defined as the possession of power (Tones, 1994). Nutbeam (1998) makes the distinction between individual and community empowerment. Individual empowerment (or self-empowerment) refers to the ability of the individual to have power over his or her own life. Community empowerment has been defined as 'a social action process in which people and communities gain mastery and control over their lives' (Wallerstein, 1999, p. 40). It refers to the way in which individuals can act collectively to influence the determinants of health and the quality of life in their community. Although the concept of empowerment is not without criticism, it has become the cornerstone of practice for many individuals and groups engaged in public health action.

Like community involvement, civic engagement is both a community and an individual quality. Individuals differ in the degree to which they are civically minded, but the capacity of a community to work together to solve problems is a resource that people within the community can access. Although there is no single, widely agreed meaning for the term 'civic engagement', the following definition is a useful one: 'Civic engagement is the degree to which citizens participate in activities that affect the political decision-making process at all levels. Voting is one such activity, but so is membership in special-interest lobbying groups' (Temkin and Rohe, 1998, p. 63). For some, such a definition places a limit on civic engagement, with its reference to more formal activities. For example, for Robert Putnam (2000), civic engagement also takes in informal aspects of community life, such as club meetings, visits with friends, committee service, church attendance, philanthropic generosity and card games.

Whereas community involvement might be considered the informal end of the community participation spectrum, 'civic engagement is thought to take a more formal approach and describes how an active citizen participates in the life of a community in order to improve conditions for others or to help shape the communities' future' (Adler and Goggin, 2005, p. 241). So what form might this definition take in practice? Box 7.1 shows how one local resident is engaging with a locally based mental health project.

Box 7.1 Be Active, Stay Active (BASA)

Janice, an ordinary member of the local community in Alloa, Scotland, has, during the last few years, become engaged as a volunteer at BASA, a mental health project based in the local community. Janice is an active participant in the project, giving her time freely and helping those with mental health problems to become self-sufficient. As Janice points out:

> It's important for members of the community like myself to be involved in volunteering and especially so for this group because, hopefully, I can give them a wee bit of what it can be like to be really healthy ... you know, peace of mind. It's been sort of a learning experience for me because I was never aware of all the aspects of mental illness. I've been really fortunate because no one in my family or round about me has ever had a problem with mental illness so you get this thing about mental, you know, barriers come up and this has been a great experience for me. It's quite a humbling experience too because they're all so supportive and just before Christmas time I had a family bereavement and they were really supportive to me so I'm getting a two-way thing, you know, I'm giving them something but I'm getting things back.

(Open University, 2007)

7.4 Recognising the public health potential of communities

Once equipped with an appreciation and understanding of the language and discourses of community-orientated approaches, entry into the community by the public health practitioner should be much smoother. However, realising the potential of communities to promote public health is also about recognising the different groups and agencies that are involved in the health promotion process.

7.4.1 Community participation and public health

Since the mid-1970s, the focus on the potential of communities as centres of action and activity for promoting public health has been enthusiastically embraced by each of the four nations of the UK. Indeed, there is widespread agreement among all four nations that communities are often centres of social innovation in the way they create opportunities for action to address inequalities in health (NAW, 2001b).

Although this philosophy must be applauded, such community participation often comes at a price. Indeed, for many, utilising communities as part of the process of promoting public health is often closely tied to a political agenda. For example, a key thread of the Department of Health's public service agreement (PSA) (DoH, 2005b), is the need to meet a range of political objectives and targets. Despite this, the underlying philosophy of community participation is, as Dockery et al. (2001) suggest, a sound one, which has produced significant health gains since the mid-1970s. In fact, as Marilyn Taylor (2003) has argued, effecting change in communities in the 1960s and 1970s involved confrontation with local government as the centralised provider of local services. This is in contrast to the 1990s and the early twenty-first century, since when local government has been increasingly disempowered by shifts in power and decision making as it recognises that effective policy delivery is more likely if local stakeholders are fully engaged.

Thinking point: how might people be encouraged to engage in the process of participation?

Engaging stakeholders in the process of participation requires certain steps to be taken. Zakus and Lysack (1998) have identified several factors which, they argue, successfully lead to effective community participation in public health-related interventions. These include:

- recognition of the right and duty of people to participate in public and community affairs, including personal health

- the inability of institutionalised health systems to provide for all health-related needs

- recognition that planned social changes in health can only be achieved by focusing on the community as the major locus of participation

- raising standards of living and increasing education levels, and an awareness of this among those on low incomes, leading to raised health expectations

- diminished confidence in policies made solely by health experts, professionals and programme managers

- concerns about the costs associated with health services and the best use of limited resources

- an increasingly older population with chronic and disabling conditions, while preventable communicable diseases continue to threaten large populations

- a perceived untapped resource of voluntary public input to improve health services, and the belief that such an input can make a positive difference.

(Adapted from Zakus and Lysack, 1998, p. 2)

Community participation can be both an outcome of empowerment and an effective empowerment strategy. The actual process of participation can inherently empower individuals and communities to understand their own situations and to gain increased control over the factors that affect their lives. In turn, this can enhance their sense of wellbeing and quality of life. How far this has been effective in empowering people has, however, been disputed (Zakus and Lysack, 1998). For example, many of the barriers to participation are embedded in the traditional and institutionalised structures of the formal health system which, as Zakus and Lysack (1998, p. 8) note, 'often present major obstacles to meaningful involvement in health promotion and community empowerment activities'.

Barriers to participation are increasingly acknowledged and it has been argued that, in certain cases, participation may be little more than an exercise in top–down legitimation and incorporation (Skelcher et al., 2004). Thus, the coercive capacity of governments or local authorities to influence community participation must not be ignored.

As a result, activists believe that community participation has been used as an all-purpose panacea for health and development problems, and that real collaboration and consultation has been jettisoned in favour of a moderate, watered-down form of continuing education for health professionals: one that fosters an 'outsider knows best' approach. For activists, community participation involves a more proactive approach: one that responds to challenges, generates new ideas, and values new experiences and opportunities to tackle problems and difficult tasks. Activists tend to act first and consider the consequences afterwards. So, for example, in the case of the Indian city of Mumbai, regular spraying in the slums in order to eliminate the insect vector, the anopheles mosquito, which is responsible for malaria, was initiated by community activists (Emmel, 2004). However, in one slum investigated, a respondent explained how a women's group, under the guidance of a community health worker, had first written to the health officer. After receiving no response, they organised a demonstration to the ward office, demanding that insect control measures be taken. This visit had been effective: the health officer promised that insect control would be carried out every three months. The control team visited twice, but failed to arrive in the ninth month. The women returned to the health officer and demanded that the service be continued: 'Every so often we have to go and remind the Health Officer', the respondent noted, 'that is the way it is here.' At the time of writing, and after several more trips by this women's group, to 'remind' the health officer, insect control is now carried out regularly in the slum neighbourhood (Emmel, 1998, cited in Emmel, 2004, p. 24).

Pragmatists, by contrast, favour a utilitarian approach of 'respectful collaboration' among stakeholders, community representatives and local health authorities to achieve mutual goals. For pragmatists, it is all about finding a balance between zeal and caution; often they act as 'conduits' between communities and policy or decision makers. Less strident than activists, for them local communities must compromise in the drive for total empowerment by acknowledging and accepting that policy makers, managers and planners, as experts in understanding community, know best and are, therefore, more productive and effective in identifying healthy interventions and initiatives (Morgan, 2001). As a result, pragmatists often perform the function of managing the momentum for new initiatives. Thus, using the Mumbai example above, pragmatists would be guided by the words and actions of the health officer.

Whichever philosophy you choose to accept, in order for community-based health interventions to be successful, not only do they need to be located within communities, but the communities themselves need to be involved in their implementation. For example, locally based food initiatives, located in such settings as community cafes and school breakfast clubs, are at the vanguard of promoting healthy eating. Many such projects fall under the auspices of local authorities, a great many of which champion the type of democratic public health interventions that empower individuals as citizens and thereby contribute to their overall heath and wellbeing. The next section takes up this theme.

7.4.2 Local authorities and public health

In helping to realise the potential for promoting public health at a local level, local authorities have, since the early 2000s, been at the forefront of efforts to improve the health of neighbourhoods and communities. Often working in partnership to improve both the health and life chances of the most disadvantaged groups, by focusing on the wider determinants of health, local authorities lie at the heart of many current public health activities. For example, social services are just one of several local authority functions which may directly, or indirectly, influence local population health and wellbeing (Glendinning et al., 2001). In many cases, such local authority interests are represented by local strategic partnerships. These are discussed further in Chapter 9 in terms of their partnership capabilities, but it is important here to establish the full potential of LSPs in promoting public health at a local level.

Introduced into the eighty-eight neighbourhood renewal areas in England in 2001 as a means of drawing local agencies and local communities together to tackle deprivation, LSPs have contributed to improved health and health promotion, and to the overall quality of life at a local level, and continue to offer great potential. Now established in all areas, their role – which goes beyond the remit of any one partner – is to jointly set out the vision of an area and co-ordinate and drive the delivery of local services. The overall objective is the improvement of mainstream services, such as public health, in the most deprived areas, which in turn contributes to sustainable development (see Box 7.2).

Box 7.2 What are local strategic partnerships?

A local strategic partnership is a single body that:

- brings together at a local level the different parts of the public sector, as well as the private, business, community and voluntary sectors, in order that different initiatives and services are able to support each other and work together

- is a non-statutory, non-executive organisation

- operates at a level that enables strategic decisions to be taken, and is close enough to individual neighbourhoods to allow actions to be determined at community level

- should be aligned with local authority boundaries.

(Adapted from ODPM, 2005b)

In addition, LSPs often include local counsellors, GPs or other health professionals, members of the local police constabulary or fire service, educators and community representatives.

Linked to LSPs are local area agreements (LAAs) and local public service agreements (LPSAs). Created by the Office of the Deputy Prime Minister (ODPM), LPSAs were established in 2001 and LAAs in 2004. They formed part of the developing agenda for local government and were designed to provide a real opportunity to bring public health into the forefront of local community planning.

An example of a LAA is provided in Box 7.3, set out beneath headings that are standard to all LAAs. These headings relate to broad-themed categories, or 'functional blocks', under which specific agreements can be placed. The functional blocks are:

- healthy communities and older people

- children and young people

- stronger and safer communities.

Box 7.3 The health content of an existing local area agreement

Local authority: Barnsley Metropolitan Council LAA, agreed March 2005.

Healthy communities and older people
- 3 per cent reduction in prevalence of smoking by 2008
- all NHS premises and schools to be smoke free by April 2006
- 10 per cent reduction in prevalence of smoking in people with chronic disease
- decrease in the number of people dependent on incapacity benefit
- decrease to 1.9 per cent the number of older people requiring hospital admissions as a result of a fall
- 10 per cent reduction in the number of people aged 75 or over who have a fall resulting in a fracture of the femur
- 10 per cent reduction in the number of admissions to residential or nursing care as a result of a fall.

Children and young people
- increase take-up of school meals by children who are entitled to free school meals
- local prevalence of obesity not to exceed 15.5 per cent for children aged between two and ten years
- meet the national targets for sport and fitness-related activity for young people
- promote parental and child emotional wellbeing and self-esteem through co-ordination of children's centres, Sure Start, family centres and family support
- learning centre to cover drugs, smoking and sexual health.

Safer and stronger communities
- increase people's satisfaction with the quality of cleanliness and public open space in their neighbourhoods.

(Adapted from DoH, 2005b)

Although setting such targets shows a commitment by local authorities to tackle health inequalities, how does this appear in practice? A real-life example of both the scope and the success of a community-orientated public health project supported by a local authority is given in Box 7.4.

Box 7.4 Coventry City Council Keeping Active Programme

Context: Coventry established a Keeping Active Programme, after it became apparent older members of the community, including ethnic minorities and disabled persons did not have access to mainstream sports centres.

Response: The Keeping Active Programme was established to target these groups including a teaching programme to allow members to lead groups.

EHP Action: The council's health development unit leads the Keeping Active Programme, including the establishment of a multi-agency steering group.

Outcomes: Around 200 people used the voucher [for a free exercise session] and one in five of these used it to access their chosen activity for the first time, while over 250 people have benefited from keeping active classes.

(Chartered Institute of Environmental Health, 2006, p. 1)

Another body committed to locally based, democratic health provision is the Local Government Association (LGA). Formed in 1997, this is a voluntary lobbying organisation whose aim is to realise a shared vision of local government – that is, between national governments and communities – in both England and Wales: in short, a vision that will enable local people to shape a distinctive and better future for their community. A cornerstone of the LGA's ambitious plans for 2006 was the prospect of greater freedom for councils if they, in turn, devolved more power to communities and neighbourhoods (LGA, 2006). One such scheme is the Healthier Communities Shared Priority Project – a joint endeavour between the LGA and the Department of Health – designed to promote healthier communities and to narrow health inequalities by engaging with communities. According to a recent evaluation report, this project achieved a considerable level of success (HDA, 2005).

Local involvement and community action for health has, moreover, become embedded in the Comprehensive Performance Assessment (CPA) and Beacon Council Scheme (ODPM, 2005a). Carried out by the Audit Commission, the CPA looks at how well a council is run (often described as its corporate capability) in order to help it plan for improvement in the future. The CPA also looks at how well a council currently delivers services, such as education, social care, housing and planning. The council is then placed in a category based on this information. The categories are: poor, weak, fair, good and excellent.

The Beacon Scheme aims to raise standards in all councils by spreading best practice. Each year about twelve direct service and cross-cutting service areas are chosen for the award of Beacon status. Authorities awarded Beacon status are given funding to enable them to share best practice with others over a three-year period following the award.

Thus, local authorities apparently appear to be realising the full potential of communities in helping to promote public health. Might the same be said of the voluntary sector? This question is addressed in following section.

7.4.3 Voluntary sector public health

Local authorities are not alone in responding to the potential of locally orientated public health projects. A growing reliance on the voluntary sector by communities has seen many successful public health interventions and initiatives mushroom since the mid-1990s. However, as Alcock et al. (2004) have pointed out, the voluntary sector has a long history in the delivery of public policy in the UK, with voluntary organisations leading the way in the development of welfare services for a wide range of British citizens, particularly in the fields of health and social care.

Thinking point: how might the voluntary sector be involved in public health?

Voluntary organisations are often commissioned to provide outreach services to communities and to deliver locally based projects, having established strong local networks with their client groups. They include many charities and organisations that provide accessible services for vulnerable groups. Such bodies are able to advocate on behalf of local people and are important partners in much community development work. Efforts to maximise the impact of the voluntary sector in public health have resulted in some truly innovative projects. For example, Share and Repair England is a charity that provides help and support with housing modifications so that older and disabled people can live independently in their own homes for as long as possible.

The expansion of voluntary sector involvement in the delivery of mainstream public services has continued to grow as the modernisation of service provision has led to an increase in the 'contract culture' of funding for voluntary organisations providing public services. This, together with the wider role of the voluntary sector in the civil renewal agenda, has certainly shifted the nature of relations between the voluntary and statutory sectors. For example, the Welsh Assembly Government is committed to working closely with the voluntary sector under the Voluntary Sector Scheme, which is required by the Government of Wales Act 1998. As part of this commitment, grants are available to support multidisciplinary public health work by the voluntary sector at a national level in Wales.

The increased involvement of the voluntary sector in multidisciplinary public health has, however, meant that sources of funding have had to be found to meet the cost of such projects. For many, this has come in the form of the Big Lottery Fund, which has been responsible for giving out half the money for good causes raised by the National Lottery. Many of the beneficiaries have been those organisations working in public health (see Box 7.5).

Box 7.5 Sandwell Healthy Living Network

The Big Lottery has funded The Sandwell Healthy Living Network (SHLN) for a period of four years. The award from the lottery amounted to £1.7 million and was match funded by the PCT, the local authority and voluntary sector organisations by another £2.1 million. The funding was for both revenue and capital costs.

The SHLN consists of twenty projects with three strands:

1   public information

2   healthy eating

3   physical activity.

The aim of the network is to improve the health of Sandwell residents by promoting and supporting healthier lifestyles, taking an integrated approach to tackling the causes of illhealth, creating an environment in which people can make healthy choices within their lives, and encouraging organisations involved in the projects to collaborate and make best use of limited resources and appropriateness of their services.

The main objectives of the SHLN are to develop the infrastructure for a high-quality information network covering housing; legal, debt, benefits and social services; training; education; employment; health services; health promotion; and specialist information (e.g. mental health and cancer).

(Adapted from Sandwell Primary Care Trusts, 2002)

7.4.4 The role of the private sector in public health

The role of the private sector in health has, since the early 2000s, caused much concern to those who simply see its involvement as part of the creeping privatisation of the NHS. Such providers can, however, 'contribute to public health improvement by enabling customers to have fuller information about health related issues and supporting health promoting behaviours' (Newbould and Taylor, 2006, p. 1). Many well-known, high street brands, including B&Q, McDonalds, Boots, Sainsbury and Tesco, are keen supporters of activities related to public health promotion (Newbould and Taylor, 2006). Box 7.6, for example, shows how Boots, the pharmaceutical company, has become a major player in the business of public health promotion.

Box 7.6 Individual membership, collective benefits

Boots launched in April 2006 the Boots Health Club. This enables individuals who elect to join to identify areas of health of special interest to them. They can choose to receive mailings and emails on topics like heart health, stopping smoking, children's health, weight loss, vitamins and diet supplements, women's health and pain relief and allergies. Customers are encouraged to ask health experts for additional advice as and when it is needed. In addition, the Boots Health Club has its own website (www.boots.com/checkitout) and links with Boots' prescription collection service. There are monthly 'in store' healthcare events for Health Club members (and other customers). Illustrative topics include asthma and hayfever management. To date, over a million people have joined the Boots Health Club.

(Newbould and Taylor, 2006, p. 3)

In many cases, the LSPs mentioned earlier include private-sector representatives. For example, Coventry Strategic Partnership has representatives from local businesses such as Jaguar Cars, PSA Peugeot-Citroën, along with EON Energy (Coventry Partnership, 2003). Other options include representation through local chambers of commerce, a business forum and key local employers.

While many applaud such involvement, for others a further concern about the role of the private sector in public health relates to potential barriers to achieving a healthy lifestyle, which certain aspects of private sector activity create. For example, there are particular problems of access to large 'out-of-town' supermarkets, but the range of foodstuffs available in disadvantaged areas is limited, often lacking in freshness and quality, and sometimes expensive. People in these areas are less likely to have their own transport, and this impedes ready access to supermarkets and stores in other localities, which stock quality products at competitive prices. However, economic considerations militate against major retailers locating their stores in deprived areas.

Nonetheless, there is some evidence that supermarkets are potential sites for collaboration between the health sector, the food industry and the sales business in public health promotion work. In Finland, for example, Närhinen et al. (1999) showed how one supermarket was at the forefront of a community-based initiative to reduce the intake of salt and saturated fat in a small town with a population of 33,000 people. As an example of partnership working, the project also made it possible for the voluntary heart health organisation to start working in co-operation with the supermarket.

Although the private, voluntary and local authority sectors remain pivotal in efforts to demonstrate the potential for the promotion of public health at a local level, it is the primary care sector that still occupies a central role in the process.

7.5 Primary care and multidisciplinary public health

Attempts to strengthen the public health function of primary care organisations in the UK have a long history. Ever since the NHS reorganisation in 1974, when responsibility for public health came under the auspices of local health authorities, primary care has played a major part in helping to promote the public's health and wellbeing, because primary care teams have regular contact with their local communities.

An individual's first contact with healthcare and advice is often at a local level, usually through their own GP or another member of the primary care team. Thus, primary care has a long tradition of authority and trust built up between the primary care team and the community, such that GPs, for example, are authoritative figures to deliver public health messages. In fact, as well as commissioning and service provision roles, primary care organisations have come to hold a significant public health role, expected, as they are, to take the lead in improving the health of their local populations (DoH, 2000).

However, it has been suggested that primary care – in the shape of the macro, monolithic and unwieldy NHS – is not sufficiently capable of campaigning on public health issues, particularly those at a micro level (Crowley and Hunter, 2005). Indeed, the thrust of the Department of Health's 2002 report *Shifting the Balance of Power: The Next Steps* was that the centralised and institutionalised shackles of the NHS would stifle community-based interventions (DoH, 2002). Despite this, the same report concluded that primary care staff were 'uniquely placed to have an overview of services in the community and in hospitals, of public health and health services and of local authorities and the NHS' (DoH, 2002, p. 8). Furthermore, it was argued that PCTs gave them 'the opportunity to take the lead in developing and redesigning systems in primary and secondary care as well as tackling public health issues locally' (DoH, 2002, p. 8).

In Wales, local health boards are the link between primary care and the community. These twenty-two organisations are care trusts, which have been set up to be coterminous with local authorities, and report directly to the Welsh Assembly Government, providing a real link between the public and government. Community health councils across Wales monitor the quality of services and ensure that the views and needs of communities influence the policies and plans put in place by health providers. The emphasis of these and other local health groups in Wales is on developing partnerships between primary care, the secondary sector (also known as the acute sector), other health and social care providers and local communities.

In Scotland, too, the funding of primary care under PCTs reflects the move away from the individual practice model towards a collective arrangement managed through the local health care co-operatives. One of the objectives of these co-operatives is to: 'work with the support of public health medicine to develop plans which reflect the clinical priorities for the area, whilst taking into account specific health needs of the registered patient population covered by the Co-operative' (Scottish Executive, 2005). Similarly, since the scrapping of Scotland's NHS trusts in 2004, regionally based health boards, together with community health partnerships, oversee health improvement (Trueland and Sloman, 2006).

In Northern Ireland, a strategic framework for primary care (which already included both health and social aspects of care) was published in 2005, which emphasised engaging with communities about service design and delivery. Greater accessibility of services and more effective partnership working are two of the envisaged outcomes.

In England, at the time of writing, rapid changes are taking place in the way in which primary care is delivered. For example, since the early 2000s, PCTs have been at the centre of primary care development in the UK. Despite not being given enough time to demonstrate their effectiveness, by the end of 2006 these were reduced significantly in number, becoming primary care groups, in order to achieve 15 per cent efficiency savings. Simultaneously, their commissioning function was strengthened by the devolvement of more commissioning to GP practices and the contracting out of the provision of NHS services (House of Commons, 2006).

Although, at the time of writing, it is difficult to measure the implications of PCGs for locally based multidisciplinary public health, reactions are mixed. For some, these changes represent a worrying shift in the ways in which public health and health promotion are delivered (House of Commons, 2006). Others have expressed concern that, despite being seen as a way of ensuring that commissioning is based on local needs, PCGs are not geared towards user involvement (MacDonald and Smith, 2001). However, many point to good practice in terms of community development projects in primary care, although they argue that 'the commitment of professionals significantly influences both the development and the overall success of community involvement initiatives' (Fawcett and South, 2005, p. 196). Indeed, it could be argued that such changes may provide fresh and exciting possibilities that can only benefit local communities.

Many of the changes in primary care can be traced back to the 1990s when the then UK Conservative Government started to develop an explicit policy on health promotion in general practice. Of course, many activities in general practice, which might be defined as health promotion, had gone on before this time, and health promotion in general practice continues to be much more than that framed by official policy. Nevertheless, the organisational arrangements have been highly significant in defining the approach to health promotion in general practice and, some would argue, in preventing other approaches from flourishing (GLACHC, 1995).

In 1990, for the first time health promotion became part of a GP's terms of service. The new GP contract defined the basic role of health promotion within the relationship between the patient and the GP (DoH, 1990). In 1996, new arrangements were introduced whereby GPs were paid on the basis of locally agreed health promotion initiatives. Health authorities only had limited influence over health promotion activities and were not involved in detailed monitoring activities, which were focused mainly on disease prevention. In a national evaluation study commissioned by the Department of Health to assess the extent of health promotion activity under the new arrangements (Adams et al., 2001), researchers concluded that the most common focus of health promotion activity related to coronary heart disease and stroke. They also concluded that the regulatory role of health promotion committees – set up in 1996 in each health authority locality to regulate health promotion activities – was diminishing and being overshadowed by health improvement programmes and primary care groups.

There has been widespread lack of agreement on what constitutes appropriate and effective health promotion within general practice. Health promotion policy in general practice was seen by some as the site of tensions between government and doctors over the control of general practice. For example, Taylor and Bloor suggest that many doctors believed that the main purpose of the 1990 contract was ultimately to weaken the authority of the profession, and that health promotion policy in general practice has 'come to symbolise the entire issue of professional judgement and commitment versus government/management "interference"' (Taylor and Bloor, 1994, p. 85).

As we move towards the next decade, the question of GP contracts is, once again, in the news, with some suggesting that, despite the unprecedented bonanza of substantial pay rises, the performance of many GPs in preventative health is far from impressive. For example, recent research found that during visits to their GP, half of all patients with high blood pressure were not diagnosed, half of those diagnosed were not treated, and half of those treated received inadequate treatment (*Guardian*, 19 April 2006). In fact, according to some, GPs are often untrained as health educators, and have a narrow view of health promotion and limited experience of community development activities (Gillam and Florin, 2002). On the other hand, for the Faculty of Public Health, despite recognising their shortcomings, GPs would seem to be a main plank of the public health function (Faculty of Public Health, 2007).

Thus, although many primary care providers are politically antipathetic to social intervention in the guise of health promotion, particularly if the opportunity costs of such activities compromise their traditional caring role, the overall impact of the aforementioned restructuring and reformulation has yet to be fully felt.

For some GPs, however, the new opportunities created by the general medical services contract are already having an impact in providing public health programmes locally for patients:

> Increasingly, [GPs] ... are providing public health programmes locally for patients, sometimes by developing the skills of their staff or by offering more broad-based 'lifestyle' services for patients, such as smoking cessation clinics, weight management or blood pressure checks.
>
> [...]
>
> The quality and outcomes framework introduced under the new GP contract ... means practices now send information on the prevalence of diseases to registers of public health data.
>
> (Laurent, 2005, p. 12)

An example of a GP practice in the north of England, which has embedded a public health ethos into the surgery by adopting 'a new model of practice based on health promotion' (Thorp, 2005, p. 12), is given in Box 7.7.

Box 7.7 Innovation and regeneration in public health

[At Seaforth village GP practice in Liverpool, instead of simply treating illnesses they have] adopted an approach whereby every interaction with a patient becomes an opportunity to improve their long-term health.

[...]

Patient consultations are viewed as an opportunity for GPs to consider the wider health of the patient, rather than just treating an ailment. 'We see the contact with the patient as an opportunity to discuss health in the holistic sense rather than just treating their illness,' says Dr Steve Fraser, one of the two GPs at the practice. Newly registered patients receive a health promotion pack full of leaflets on local services and advice on healthy living. The GPs, practice nurse and receptionists talk patients through the contents, so they understand what is being offered and are, hopefully, encouraged to tap into community facilities and resources.

A health promoting approach has been embedded into ongoing patient–clinician consultations through a technique known as motivational interviewing. This is a style of consulting that aims to elicit the patients' readiness to change their lifestyle in ways that could improve their health ...

(Thorp, 2005, p. 12)

Establishing the last of the core functions vested in PCTs – to improve population health and address inequalities – is challenging. Nonetheless, in response to this challenge the White Paper *Our Health, Our Care, Our Say: A New Direction for Community Services* (DoH, 2006) signals the English Government's intention to shift the emphasis of health and social care from acute and intensive interventions, to community and preventative services. For example, the ability of GP practices to hold commissioning budgets will provide an opportunity for an expansion of community-based services. Similarly, reforms ongoing at the time of writing imply new roles for both practice-based commissioners (PBCs) and PCTs. A similar shift has occurred in Wales since the late 1990s, where new approaches, in which agencies work together to identify and meet unmet needs in the community, have been developed (NAW, 2001a). A key element of this strategy has been the responsibility of primary care to play its full part in the prevention and early detection of disease and illhealth.

Conclusion

The focus of this chapter has been the potential or otherwise for promoting public health at a local level. You have read about how multidisciplinary public health is delivered in a variety of ways and settings, many of which are located or embedded at the very heart of communities. While this democratisation in the delivery of public health at a local level is in contrast to the 'I plan, you participate' philosophy of the past – a move that must be welcomed – this is not to suggest that 'everything in the garden is rosy'.

On the contrary, despite claims that there has been a shift in the balance of power, critics point to both the structural and institutional barriers – embedded structures that have a disempowering effect and which are designed to subvert community action and activity – erected by gatekeepers and politicians as they strive to maintain the powerful status quo (Taylor, 2003).

What is apparent is that bridging the gap between health professionals and communities not only requires political will, but also the need to recognise the informal and everyday as important sites for governance and decision making (Van der Platt and Barrett, 2006). Effective governance and community participation require an informed, engaged citizenry which participates in decision making and works with service providers in designing, delivering and monitoring services. To create this requires public bodies to go beyond the now routine provision of opportunities for consultation and participation. It means embarking on a process – as many have already shown with the changing discourses around involvement and participation – in which local authorities, PCTs and other organisations responsible for health truly commit themselves to a cultural change in the way in which public health promotion is delivered. This includes more community action, local ward committees, advisory panels and the like. Those organisations that are not prepared to face up to such a commitment need to recognise that limited consultation – which is presented as an opportunity for active participation – is likely to lead to consultation fatigue and disillusionment in their local communities.

References

Adams, C.J., Baeza, J.I. and Calnan, M. (2001) 'The new health promotion arrangements in general medical practice in England: results from a national evaluation', *Health Education Journal*, vol. 6, no.1, pp. 45–58.

Adler, R.P. and Goggin, J. (2005) 'What do we mean by "civic engagement"?', *Journal of Transformative Education*, vol. 3, no. 3, pp. 236–53.

Alcock, P., Brannelly, T. and Ross, L. (2004) *Formality or Flexibility? Voluntary Sector Contracting in Social Care and Health*, London, The National Council for Voluntary Organisations.

Bauman, Z. (2001) *The Individualised Society*, Cambridge, Polity.

Blair, T. (2002) 'My vision for Britain, *Observer*, 10 November, p. 28.

Brent, J. (1997) 'Community without unity' in Hoggett, P. (ed.) *Contested Communities: Experiences, Struggles, Policies*, Bristol, Policy.

Carlisle, R., Avery, A.J. and Marsh, P. (2002) 'Primary care teams working harder in deprived areas', *Journal of Public Health Medicine*, vol. 24, no. 1, pp. 43–8.

Chartered Institute of Environmental Health (2006) *Case Study: Coventry City Council Keeping Active Programme* [online], http://www.cieh.org (Accessed 17 June 2006).

Coventry Partnership (2003) *Community Plan 2003–2010: Raising our Game, Closing the Gap – Partnership for Inclusion, Equality and Excellence*, Coventry, The Coventry Partnership.

Crowley, P. and Hunter, D.J. (2005) 'Putting the public back into public health', *Journal of Epidemiology and Community Health*, vol. 59, no. 4, pp. 265–7.

Department of Health (DoH) (1990) *General Practice in the NHS: The 1990 Contract*, London, HMSO.

Department of Health (DoH) (1999) *Saving Lives: Our Healthier Nation*, London, The Stationery Office.

Department of Health (DoH) (2000) *The NHS Plan: A Plan for Investment, A Plan for Reform*, London, The Stationery Office.

Department of Health (DoH) (2001) *Shifting the Balance of Power within the NHS: Securing Delivery*, London, The Stationery Office.

Department of Health (DoH) (2002) *Shifting the Balance of Power within the NHS: The Next Steps*, London, The Stationery Office.

Department of Health (DoH) (2004) *Choosing Health: Making Healthy Choices Easier*, London, The Stationery Office.

Department of Health (DoH) (2005a) *Creating a Patient-Led NHS: Delivering the NHS Improvement Plan*, London, The Stationery Office.

Department of Health (DoH) (2005b) *Local Area Agreements and Local Public Service Agreements*, London, The Stationery Office.

Department of Health (DoH) (2006) *Our Health, Our Care, Our Say: A New Direction for Community Services*, London, The Stationery Office.

Dockery, G., Barry, L. and Heley, E. (2001) 'Community participation in health: how does it work?' in Martineau, T., Price, J. and Cole, R. (2001) *Health by the People: A Celebration of the Life of Ken Newell*, proceedings of a colloquium held on 23 and 24 March 2000, Liverpool, Liverpool School of Tropical Medicine.

Earle, S. (2007) 'Promoting public health: exploring the issues' in Earle, S., Lloyd, C.E., Sidell, M. and Spurr, S. (eds) *Theory and Research in Promoting Public Health*, London, Sage/Milton Keynes, The Open University.

Emmel, N.D. (1998) *Perceptions of Health and the Value Placed on Health Care Deliverers in the Slums of Bombay*, PhD Thesis (unpublished), Leeds, University of Leeds.

Emmel, N. (2004) *Towards Community Involvement: Strategies for Health and Social Care Providers. Guide 21A The Complexity of Communities and Lessons for Community Involvement*, Leeds, University of Leeds, Nuffield Institute for Health.

Emmel, N. and Conn, C. (2004) *Towards Community Involvement: Strategies for Health and Social Care Providers. Guide 1 Identifying the Goal and Objectives of Community Involvement*, Leeds, University of Leeds, Nuffield Institute for Health.

Faculty of Public Health (2007) *Public Health Training Curriculum 2007* [online], http://www.fphm.org.uk/training/downloads/curriculum_2007.pdf (Accessed 1 March 2007).

Fawcett, B. and South, J. (2005) 'Community involvement and primary care trusts: the case for social entrepreneurship', *Critical Public Health*, vol. 15, no. 2, pp. 191–204.

Freire, P. (1970) *Pedagogy of the Oppressed*, New York, Continuum.

Gillam, S. and Florin, D. (2002) *Reducing Health Inequalities: Primary Care Organisations and Public Health*, London, King's Fund.

Glendinning, C., Abbott, S. and Coleman, A. (2001) '"Bridging the gap": new relationships between primary care groups and local authorities', *Social Policy and Administration*, vol. 35, no. 4, pp. 411–25.

Greater London Association of Community Health Councils (GLACHC) (1995) *A Review of Health Promotion in Primary Care: From GP Health Promotion Contract to Promoting Health with Local Communities*, London, Greater London Association of Community Health Councils.

Green, J. (1999) *Community Action on Health: Summary Report*, Newcastle, University of Northumbria at Newcastle, Social Welfare Research Unit.

Guardian (2006) Editorial, 'NHS reforms. Right goals, too many wrong results', *Guardian*, 19 April.

Hawtin, M., Hughes, G., Percy-Smith, J. and Foreman, A. (1999) *Community Profiling: Auditing Social Needs*, Maidenhead, Open University Press.

Health Development Agency (HDA) (2005) *The Healthier Communities Shared Priority Project*, London, Health Development Agency.

House of Commons (2006) *Changes to Primary Care Trusts: Second Report of Session 2005–06*, HC 646, London, The Stationery Office.

Jewkes, R. and Murcott, A. (1996) 'Meanings of community', *Social Science and Medicine*, vol. 43, no. 4, pp. 555–63.

Labonte, R. (1997) 'Community organizing and "partnerships for health"' in Minkler, M. (ed.) *Community Organising and Health*, New Brunswick, NJ, Rutgers University Press.

Laurent, C. (2005) 'Doctor knows best', *Public Health News*, vol. 27, pp. 12–13.

Laverack, G. and Wallerstein, N. (2001) 'Measuring community empowerment: a fresh look at organizational domains', *Health Promotion International*, vol. 16, no. 2, pp. 179–85.

Local Government Association (LGA) (2006) *Closer to People and Places: A New Vision for Local Government*, London, Local Government Association.

Luck, J., Chang, C., Brown, E.R. and Lumpkin, J. (2006) 'Using local health information to promote public health: issues, barriers, and proposed solutions to improve information flow', *Health Affairs*, vol. 25, no. 4, pp. 979–91.

MacDonald, G. and Smith, P. (2001) 'Collaborative working in primary care groups: a case of incommensurable paradigms?', *Critical Public Health*, vol. 11, no. 3, pp. 253–66.

Morgan, L.M. (2001) 'Community participation in health: perpetual allure, persistent challenge', *Health Policy and Planning*, vol. 16, no. 3, pp. 221–30.

Mowbray, M. (2005) 'How to make social capital: *Bowling Alone's* sequel, *Better Together*', *Community Development Journal*, vol. 40, no. 4, pp. 459–74.

Närhinen, M., Nissinen, A. and Puska, P. (1999) 'Healthier choices in a supermarket: the municipal food control can promote health', *British Food Journal*, vol. 101, no. 2, pp. 99–107.

National Assembly for Wales (NAW) (2001a) *Improving Health in Wales: A Plan for the NHS with its Partners*, Cardiff, National Assembly for Wales.

National Assembly for Wales (NAW) (2001b) *Improving Health in Wales: The Future of Primary Care*, Cardiff, National Assembly for Wales.

National Health Service Executive (NHSE) (1999) *Leadership for Health: The Heath Authority Role*, London, Department of Health.

Newbould, J. and Taylor, D. (2006) *Action for Better Public Health*, London, University of London, School of Pharmacy/Boots.

Nutbeam, D. (1998) 'Evaluating health promotion – progress, problems and solutions', *Health Promotion International*, vol. 13, no. 1, pp. 27–44.

Office of the Deputy Prime Minister (ODPM) (2003) *Searching for Solid Foundations: Community Involvement and Urban Policy*, London, Office of the Deputy Prime Minister.

Office of the Deputy Prime Minister (ODPM) (2005a) *Government Response to the Review of the Beacon Council Scheme*, London, Office of the Deputy Prime Minister.

Office of the Deputy Prime Minister (ODPM) (2005b) *Local Strategic Partnerships: Shaping their Future*, London, Office of the Deputy Prime Minister.

Open University (2007) K311 *Promoting Public Health: Skills, Perspectives and Practice*, DVD, Milton Keynes, The Open University.

Plant, R. (1998) 'Citizenship, rights, welfare' in Franklin, J. (ed.) *Social Policy and Social Justice: The IPPR Reader*, Cambridge, Polity.

Putnam, R. (2000) *Bowling Alone: The Collapse and Revival of American Community*, New York, Simon & Schuster.

Rapoport, J. (1987) 'Terms of empowerment/exemplars of prevention: towards a theory of community psychology', *American Journal of Community Psychology*, vol. 15, no. 2, pp. 121–48.

Sandwell Primary Care Trusts (2002) *What Works for Health in Sandwell?*, West Bromwich, Sandwell Primary Care Trusts.

Scottish Executive (2005) *Designed to Care: Renewing the National Health Service in Scotland*, Edinburgh, Scottish Executive; also available online at http://www.scotland.gov.uk/library/documents1/care_05.htm (Accessed 1 March 2007).

Skelcher, C., Mathur, N. and Smith, M. (2004) *Effective Partnership and Good Governance: Lessons for Policy and Practice*, Birmingham, University of Birmingham.

Taylor, D. and Bloor, K. (1994) *Health Care, Health Promotion and the Future General Practice*, The Nuffield Provincial Hospitals Trust, London, Royal Society of Medicine Press.

Taylor, M. (2003) *Public Policy and the Community*, Basingstoke, Palgrave.

Temkin, K. and Rohe, W.M. (1998) 'Social capital and neighborhood stability: an empirical investigation', *Housing Policy Debate*, vol. 9, no. 1, pp. 61–88.

Thorp, S. (2005) 'Innovation and regeneration', *Public Health News*, July, pp. 12–13.

Tones, B.K. (1994) 'Health promotion, empowerment and action competence' in Jensen, B.B. and Schnack, K. (eds) *Action and Action Competence as Key Concepts in Critical Pedagogy*, Didaktiske Studier Vol. 12, Copenhagen, Royal Danish School of Educational Studies.

Trueland, J. and Sloman, L. (2006) 'Can England learn from its neighbours?', *Guardian*, 12 April.

Van der Platt, M. and Barrett, G. (2006) 'Building community capacity in governance and decision making', *Community Development Journal*, vol. 41, no. 1, pp. 25–36.

Wallerstein, N. (1999) 'Power between evaluator and community: research relationships within New Mexico's healthier communities', *Social Science and Medicine*, vol. 49, no. 1, pp. 39–53.

Wanless, D. (2004) *Securing Good Health for the Whole Population: Final Report*, London, HM Treasury.

Woodhead, D., Jochelson, K. and Tennant, R. (2002) *Public Health in the Balance: Getting it Right for London*, London, King's Fund.

World Health Organization (WHO) (1978) *Alma Ata Declaration*, Geneva, World Health Organization.

World Health Organization (WHO) (1985) *Health for All in Europe by the Year 2000: Regional Targets*, Copenhagen, World Health Organization.

World Health Organization (WHO) (1999) *Health 21: Health for All in the 21st Century*, Copenhagen, World Health Organization Regional Office for Europe.

World Health Organization (WHO) (2002) *Community Participation in Local Health and Sustainable Development: Approaches and Techniques*, European Sustainable Development and Health Series 4, Copenhagen, World Health Organization Regional Office for Europe.

Yoo, S., Weed, N.E., Lempa, M.L., Mbondo, M., Shada, R.E. and Goodman, R.M. (2004) 'Collaborative community empowerment: an illustration of a six-step process', *Health Promotion Practice*, vol. 5, no. 3, pp. 256–65.

Zakus, D.L. and Lysack, C.L. (1998) 'Revisiting community participation', *Health Policy and Planning*, vol. 13, no. 1, pp. 1–12.

Chapter 8

Community involvement and civic engagement in multidisciplinary public health

Stephen Handsley

Introduction

In Chapter 7, you were introduced to the potential for promoting public health at a local level. This chapter investigates the importance of such an approach by examining some of the practical ways in which this is successfully achieved, as well as some of the difficulties. It examines the effectiveness of the mobilisation of communities in promoting the public's health and how this is key to successfully addressing social injustice and health inequalities at a local level. It explores some of the difficulties and dilemmas faced by both public health practitioners and lay people when attempting to implement community-based and people-led healthy interventions and initiatives.

The first section builds on Chapter 7 and looks at the degree to which people participate in community life, and the extent to which they feel empowered to change their community. Section 8.2 then turns to the notion of community development and begins to lay the foundations for this approach. Having considered the way in which community development is designed to democratise the approach to multidisciplinary public health, in Section 8.3 you are asked to think about how successful this has proved in recognising and legitimating local voices. This same section then begins to explore some of the alternatives to community development. The chapter concludes by exploring the impact of the much lauded patient and public involvement in the improvement of the public's health and wellbeing.

8.1 Mobilising communities in the delivery of multidisciplinary public health

As discussed elsewhere, delivering modern multidisciplinary public health in the twenty-first century includes a wide range of activities, reflecting the diversity of its historical origins (Earle et al., 2007). Many such activities occur at a local level and entail some sort of community involvement. As earlier chapters have demonstrated, community involvement in health has become something of a buzzword as the World Health Organization (WHO), governments and local authorities pursue a participatory and collaborative solution to the ever-increasing widening of health inequalities. Community involvement is most often used, in both policy and practice, to mean the involvement of people from a given locality or a given section of the local population in public decision making. This may mean inviting local residents as individuals to join or put forward their views to, for example, a council committee, an area forum or, as pointed out in earlier chapters, local strategic partnerships (LSPs). Or, it may entail the election or nomination of people to put forward the viewpoint of a particular grouping within the population.

People are not always involved on a collective basis; they may also be involved at a more individualistic level. Others may be involved against their will. For example, as Dhesi (2000) points out, people's personal and social objectives are not necessarily commensurate in all situations, and some may feel pressured into being involved rather than face communal exclusion. Other groups or individuals may feel excluded on, for instance, the basis of their ethnicity, sexuality, gender, religion, age and social class (Campbell and McLean, 2002).

One meaning of community involvement less prominent in policy, but more fundamental and colloquial, is the participation of people in what might be thought of as 'real-life' community activities. The great majority of these activities – whether friendship groups, volunteering, sports clubs, social clubs, faith groups, carers' groups, or others – are not about representation or participation in council mechanisms. Rather, they are either about the activities themselves or simply a form of social interaction. A large proportion of community-orientated approaches, however, are about representation in the sense of campaigning for local health improvements or public causes, or representing people's interests as stakeholders. Involvement in such organisations is seen as important in creating social capital, as it facilitates interaction with others. You consider this more fully below.

8.1.1 Social capital and communities

Social capital, at its most basic, refers to the features of social life, such as networks, norms and social trust, that facilitate co-ordination and co-operation for mutual benefit, and represents the degree of social cohesion that exists in communities. Key elements of social capital include:

- Social resources – e.g. informal arrangements between neighbours or within a faith community

- Collective resources – e.g. self-help groups, credit unions, community safety schemes

- Economic resources – e.g. levels of employment; access to green, open spaces

- Cultural resources – e.g. libraries, art centres, local schools.

Communities where social capital is abundant are often characterised by:

- High levels of trust between friends and neighbours

- Shared norms and values

- Local people engaging in civic and community life.

(HDA, 2004a, p. 1)

Through such networks and norms, people can learn more about their community, develop their sense of efficacy and promote trust, both between similar types of people (bonding social capital, or exclusive) and diverse types of people (bridging social capital, or inclusive) (Putnam, 2000). Whereas the former may be more inward-looking and have a tendency to reinforce exclusive identities and homogeneous groups, the latter may be more outward-looking and encompass people across different social divides (Putnam, 2000, p. 22). Either way, by working collectively, people can, it is argued, make improvements to their communities and solve local problems. For example, in parts of Northern Ireland, community engagement is now a key part of the public health strategy. Such an approach has led successfully to the expansion of a Health Information Workers programme, in which local women act as volunteers sharing information about health and wellbeing, within local neighbourhoods in north and west Belfast led by the Women's Information Group (DHSSPS, 2004).

However, this is not necessarily as straightforward as it might sound since, as Ritchie et al. (2004) argue, there are many different levels at which the community may participate, and at one extreme this may amount to little more than tokenism. In many cases, involvement is still something of a mantra, much invoked but still neglected or confused in practice. Moreover, communities do not always have the same access as local authority organisations and government agencies to the type of resources which might enable them to define and set the agendas and participate on an equal footing.

Thus, despite the support for involvement and participation, many argue that much of it remains at a rhetorical or ideological level and that it fails to match the reality on the ground. Indeed, full participation in community-based health promotion activities often implies not only action and agency, but also control. (This is discussed further in Section 8.2.1 where the ways in which community-based models differ in scope from community development models are illustrated in Figure 8.2.) However, as with national government, many health authorities, LSPs or local councils often resist transferring authority to communities, preferring instead to retain power: a debate which is unpacked in Chapter 9.

8.1.2 The process of community involvement

To appreciate fully the reasons why communities get involved in promoting public health in the first place, it is worth repeating the claim by Earle et al. (2007) that a social model of health is based on the understanding that health chances and health choices are shaped, to a great extent, by the wider social, political and economic conditions in which people live. In short, it is those places where people live and work that influence if, how or why they promote health.

Thinking point: what does this mean for the process of community engagement?

In Chapter 7, you were introduced to certain concepts that feature widely in community-orientated approaches. For example, it was argued that community engagement and neighbourhood participation involve empowering individuals through collective action and activity to challenge and change the socio-economic environment, and to redistribute power and resources in order to enhance the health chances of hitherto disadvantaged groups. Such an approach requires the participation of local people in working together to promote public health – their own and that of others – and is based on the principles of collectivism rather than individualism. Although critics argue that such meaningful participation and democratisation eludes many groups and individuals (Higgins, 1999), the key to this approach is illustrated in Figure 8.1, which features a framework outlining the stages required in the effective mobilisation of communities.

Empowering communities to have more say in the shaping of policies influencing health represents something of a break with earlier traditions of public health associated with top–down social engineering (Petersen and Lupton, 1996). The adoption of a community development or capacity-building approach to public health promotion is underpinned by its ideological commitment to remedy inequalities and to achieve better and fairer distribution of resources for communities (Tones and Tilford, 2001). This approach is one that aims to assist communities in identifying problems, developing solutions and facilitating change and this too is

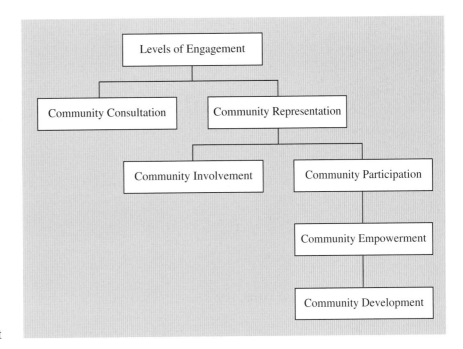

Figure 8.1   Levels of
community engagement

achieved ideally through participatory processes and bottom–up planning
(Smith et al., 2001). Within this collectivist ideology, individuals combine
and take responsibility for each other's health and wellbeing. The individual
is not submerged or lost in the collective, but is located within it rather than
existing in isolation and competition with others (Collins, 1997). A more
individualistic approach lays responsibility firmly on individuals where they
may need to compete with others to improve their own health and wellbeing.

Thinking point: what do you think collectivist and individualist approaches have to say
about promoting public health?

While both approaches have their respective supporters, the main
differences lie in the ideological principles which inform such thinking.
Community-orientated practice seeks healthful change for the whole
community's benefit. The focus is on the collective or common good
instead of individual health. Here, change is intended to affect the whole
community, including all units of service, not just the individual, family, or
specific aggregate (Goeppinger and Shuster, 1992).

With its emphasis on the common good, a communitarian approach considers
duty as the main principle of morality. It regards the individual's duty to
contribute to the welfare and survival of the group at large as paramount,
while remaining wedded to the principles of collectivism. So, using the
example of immunisation, a communitarian perspective would trust each
individual member of the community to use their moral judgment over the
dangers their actions might present to the welfare of the whole community,

rather than to them as individuals, if they chose not to have either themselves or their children protected against the dangers of infectious diseases.

This account of the concept of community often leads to the assumption that individuals are denied rights and personal choice, that their choice of way of life in these communities is constrained by the community's pursuit of shared ends, and that in the pursuit of the common good as the prime goal, people are expected to sacrifice their individuality or uniqueness.

Thinking point: how might this approach result in the individual becoming submerged within the community?

Indeed, adopting a communitarian approach may, at first sight, appear to overlook the needs of particular individuals as the community races towards its collective goal. For example, according to this model the distribution of health services or public health initiatives is not determined by the individual or his or her individual needs, but by what 'the community' considers as necessary for the common good. This is, in turn, determined by the values and standards of a given community and can be different for different communities. Such a one-sided approach, it is argued, leaves individuals disempowered and lacking choice in their public health requirements (Hoedemaekers and Dekkers, 2003).

However, Teffo and Roux's (1998) answer to this is: not at all! They argue that communal societies recognise the difference between individuals, on the one hand, and sets of individuals on the other; and accepts the uniqueness of individuals, their fates, fortunes and misfortunes. They also recognise individuals' unique talents and contributions, for instance, in terms of originality and creativity in problem solving and other activities of the community. They caution that, although to an outsider members of collectivist cultures may seem to relinquish primary control and autonomy through their socio-ethical role or commitment to the wellbeing of the community, we must not lose sight of the fact that they gain a sense of purpose, belonging and security in their families and communities.

Although there is some similarity in the ideology, this communitarian approach is not to be confused with the individualist approach to public health promotion. The latter approach fosters notions of individual responsibility and assumes that individuals can afford to choose health and buy healthcare in situations where the state does not provide or purchase this. Communitarian thinking, on the other hand, is based on the assumption that, without collective co-operation, individuals will not achieve their personal goals. Indeed, as Putnam (2000) has shown, it is known that strong, cohesive and sustainable communities provide a better environment for health outcomes and wellbeing than weak communities. Likewise, strong and sustainable social relationships and social networks are proven indicators of health and a sense of wellbeing (East, 1998). This philosophy is illustrated in Box 8.1, which relates the story of how one local community has taken control of the development of health services in its neighbourhood.

Box 8.1 Community health shop, Barlanark, Glasgow

The doctors' surgery in Barlanark, a largely local authority housing scheme in Easterhouse, Glasgow, was situated in a dilapidated portakabin within the grounds of a local primary school. In the winter the wind would blow through the spaces in the window frames and in the summer it felt like sitting in a greenhouse.

Local people signed a petition and presented it to the local councillor. At the same time, the Greater Easterhouse Partnership was looking for health inclusion projects to support and pilot through their Pathfinder scheme. A steering group composed of community representatives, the local councillor, the Pathfinder Co-ordinator, the East Glasgow Local Health Care Co-operative (LHCC) General Manager and a representative from the Health Promotion department of what is now Greater Glasgow NHS Board (GGNHSB) met regularly to develop proposals to improve health services in the South Suburb of Greater Easterhouse.

From this group the idea of a 'Community Health Shop' was developed. Two shop units were leased and internally refitted to a custom design, and in October 1999 the shop was opened by Jackie Baillie MSP, Deputy Minister for Communities.

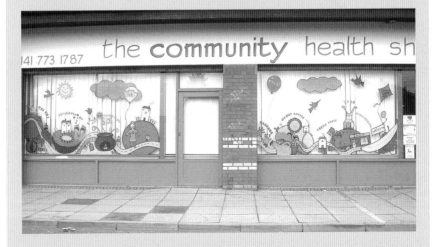

Initially, services were limited to those who made no charge, such as GP, health visitor, practice nurse, dietician, podiatrist, and other local services such as money advice.

Two posts were created: co-ordinator and administrator; and the shop became a company limited by guarantee and was granted charitable status. Community representatives made up to 75 per cent of the Board and the rest were from the main funders: Pathfinder, LHCC and GGNHSB.

To increase and improve the services, funding was sought from the National Lottery through their New Opportunities Fund for Health. In August 2001, Healthy Living Centre status was granted and over £500,000 funding over five years was awarded.

The Commmunity Health Shop now has over twenty-seven services, with new ones being added regularly. The main challenge for the Board now is to secure sustainability for the shop by fundraising for the future, beyond the five years which have already been secured.

(Adapted from Community Health Shop, 2006)

Communitarian thinking is not without risks, however. Communities are known for expecting great sacrifices from their members for the benefit of the public good. Citizens may feel coerced to do things they don't like and they experience state intervention as oppressive (Melnyk, 1985). Moreover, Muntaner et al. (2001) warn that communitarians tend to overlook issues of class, gender and ethnicity, along with the role of individual subjectivity in mediating the relation between inequality and health.

8.1.3 What does community involvement look like?

Community-orientated approaches have become integral in the push towards narrowing the health inequalities gap and are, therefore, a central plank of recent legislation in each of the four nations of the UK. To complement such policies, public and patient partnerships, leading to the empowerment of local people, have also become enshrined within health and regeneration policy initiatives since early 2000. For example, Health Improvement and Modernisation Plans (HIMPs) and Health Action Zones (HAZs) were founded on the 'bottom–up' meets 'top–down' principles of collaboration and consultation. Through these initiatives, inequalities and exclusion were to be tackled in some of the most deprived areas of the UK. This, it was envisaged, was to be achieved through partnerships between the public, private and voluntary sectors, and most significantly, communities themselves (Crawshaw et al., 2003).

As discussed in Chapter 5, Heath Action Zones were identified as one of the initiatives reflecting the 'Third Way' policies espoused by the UK New Labour Government. The Third Way has been associated with the reduced role of the state, privatisation of health and social services, non-governmental organisations, modern philanthropy and the demise of the welfare state (Muntaner and Lynch, 1999). As mentioned above, and like other area-based or zone initiatives, HAZ programmes were designed to tackle inequalities and exclusion in some of the most deprived areas of the UK. Box 8.2 illustrates some of the key principles of area-based initiatives (ABIs), using one particular HAZ.

Box 8.2 Merseyside HAZ principles of community involvement

Merseyside HAZ Implementation Plan included some basic principles of community involvement which recognised that:

- Communities could be geographic, or communities of interest.
- It is important to ensure that marginalised and excluded people have a voice.
- Inclusiveness requires addressing cultural, physical or material barriers to involvement.
- Public information is a critical prerequisite.
- Meaningful involvement requires information, support, resources and training.
- There is a continuum of involvement, from being informed to initiating and leading.
- A long-term strategic approach is more effective than one-off consultation processes.
- There is an overlap between community and staff involvement.
- Voluntary and community organisations have a valuable role to play.
- Organisational development is needed for staff in partner organisations.
- There is a variety of methods for facilitating involvement, especially of 'hard-to-reach' groups.

(Adapted from Liverpool Partnership Group Self-Assessment, 2002)

Despite the push by politicians to convince the general public that community action is, indeed, participatory, equitable and egalitarian, achieving what Tony Blair has referred to as 'modernised social democracy' (Blair, 1998, p. 1), it is debatable whether or not communities are truly involved and, moreover, how effective these strategies are in producing meaningful outcomes. Similar concerns have been voiced within the health sector (Smith et al., 2001).

Taking a capacity-building or participatory approach, on the other hand, is intended to go beyond mobilisation: that is, to foster *initiation* of action by community members (Smith et al., 2001). Capacity building is the essence of community development and is a process of working democratically with a community to determine its needs and strengths, and to develop ways of utilising its strengths to meet its needs. According to Smith et al., besides increasing social solidarity, strengthening the capacity-building approaches of social networks 'contribute[s] to the broader goal of creating a public able to engage in collective social and political life, the ideal of active citizenship' (Smith et al., 2001, p. 36). Indeed, such an approach, it is argued, serves to create a healthier community: one that is actively engaged in promoting its own health. The role of the health professional in such an approach is to facilitate this process through participation, collaboration and consultation.

8.2 Developing healthier communities: laying the foundations

As outlined in Chapter 7, how you define or understand 'community' is likely to underpin your practice or way of thinking. The task of developing healthier communities is, therefore, likely to require a fundamental awareness and appreciation of the importance of laying strong foundations; in short, in awareness that communities themselves are vital in improving health, and can play a significant role in promoting individual self-esteem and mental wellbeing and reducing social exclusion. Given the health-promoting effect of social and communal interaction, it is this collaborative ethos that underpins the community development and community action approach to health – an approach that helps to lay the foundations of a more equitable and egalitarian philosophy around multidisciplinary public health – and which is the focus of this section.

8.2.1 Contemplating community development

At its most basic, community development is about the development of 'community' – the capacity of local populations to respond collectively to events and issues that affect them. Community action for health operates within a diverse range of communities and, because they are not always harmonious, it is important to appreciate that part of such an approach may well involve attempts to reconcile various conflicts. For example, the relationship of health to these various notions of community may be strong or extremely weak, or even non-existent. On the other hand, for many, health is often the catalyst and motivating force for bringing people together. Working with communities to identify these problems, to facilitate both action and participation, and to encourage informed and powerful community partnerships, is a key function of community development in health (Amos, 2002).

Thinking point: how might a community development approach influence or impact on public health?

Community development in health (CDH) aims to enable the active involvement of people, especially those most oppressed and marginalised, in issues, decision making and organisations which affect their health and wellbeing in general. In considering such an approach as community development, it is important to recognise how it differs in scope from a community-based model. Figure 8.2 illustrates some of these differences.

Figure 8.2   Characteristics of community-based versus community development models (Source: adapted from HDA, 2004b, p. 5, Box 1.2)

Community-based models	Community development models
Problem, targets and action defined by sponsoring body	Problem, targets and action defined by community
Community seen as medium, venue or setting for intervention	Community itself the target of intervention in respect of capacity building and empowerment
Notion of 'community' relatively unproblematic	'Community' recognised as complex, changing, subject to power imbalances and conflict
Target largely individuals within either geographical area, or specific subgroup in geographical area defined by sponsoring body	Target may be community structures or services and policies that impact on the health of the community
Activities largely health oriented	Activities may be quite broad based, targeting wider factors with an impact on health, but with indirect health outcomes (empowerment, social capital)

As Figure 8.2 shows, the two approaches differ in their ideological content. A key task of community action is to address these differences and ideological divisions. Bridging the gap between public health practitioners and communities, community action for health can involve both lay people and practitioners. Rather than remaining passive, communities define their own health agendas, and inform and influence decision making with practitioners.

However, it is also important to recognise that any difference in philosophy can manifest itself in friction between lay and professional perspectives whereby 'top–down', or results-driven, approaches conflict with the more organic methods of 'bottom–up' approaches forged and fermented by grass-roots community workers. The concept and reality of 'community' between professionals and lay people, or policy makers and recipients, therefore, can be vastly different. This can only mean that different priorities for change will arise.

A community development approach embraces a set of categorical and complex principles which give it a sound practical and empirical foundation and which are embodied in the Standing Conference for Community Development (SCCD) charter. These principles are set out in Box 8.3.

Box 8.3 A statement on community development

Community development is about building active and sustainable communities based on social justice and mutual respect.

It is about changing power structures to remove the barriers that prevent people from participating in the issues that affect their lives.

Community workers support individuals, groups and organisations in this process on the basis of the following values and commitments.

Values

Social Justice – enabling people to claim their human rights, meet their needs and have greater control over the decision-making processes which affect their lives.

Participation – facilitating democratic involvement by people in the issues which affect their lives, based on full citizenship, autonomy, and shared power, skills, knowledge and experience.

Equality – challenging the attitudes of individuals, and the practices of institutions and society, which discriminate against and marginalise people.

Learning – recognising the skills, knowledge and expertise that people contribute and develop by taking action to tackle social, economic, political and environmental problems.

Co-operation – working together to identify and implement action, based on mutual respect of diverse cultures and contributions.

Commitments

Challenging discrimination and oppressive practices within organisations, institutions and communities.

Developing practice and policy that protects the environment.

Encouraging networking and connections between communities and organisations.

Ensuring access and choice for all groups and individuals within society.

Influencing policy and programmes from the perspective of communities.

Prioritising the issues of concern to people experiencing poverty and social exclusion.

Promoting social change that is long-term and sustainable.

Reversing inequality and the imbalance of power relationships in society.

Supporting community-led collective action.

(SCCD, 2001, p. 5)

Participation and involvement are recurrent themes. The charter stresses the collective and active involvement of people in issues that affect their lives. It is concerned with issues of powerlessness, disadvantage, injustice and social exclusion, and it is no accident that community development projects were not set up in affluent residential areas. The process is concerned with the empowering and enabling of those who are traditionally deprived of power and control over their common affairs. How, then, might this philosophy match what happens on the ground?

In Scotland, the Scottish Community Development Centre (SCDC) has developed a programme of training and support materials called Achieving Better Community Development (ABCD): a model they believe provides a practical framework for planning and learning from community development interventions (Barr and Hashagen, 2000). The SCDC claim that this model encourages those involved in community development to be clear about what they are trying to achieve, how they should go about it, and how they can change things in the light of experience. The 'pyramid diagram' given in Figure 8.3 shows how this is achieved.

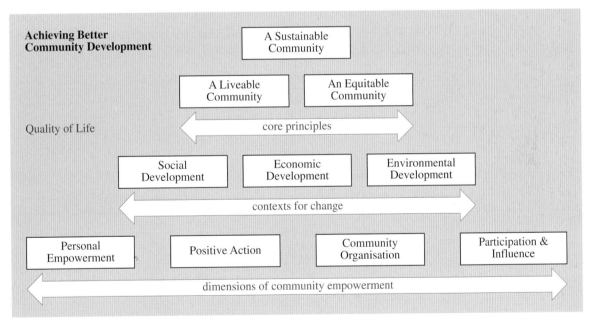

Figure 8.3   Model illustrating ways of achieving better community development (Source: adapted from HDA, 2004c, p. 22)

Similarly, in Wales, the community development approach is represented in the ethos of Community Development Cymru (CDC). CDC is an all-Wales, member-led independent organisation which aims to work across sectors to promote and facilitate community development at all levels, throughout Wales (CDC, 2006).

Achieving good practice for community development and health work calls for a series of clear guidelines, and these were set out by the Health Development Agency (HDA), now part of the National Institute for Health and Clinical Excellence (NICE). These guidelines state that there should be:

- a clear and realistic role and remit

- adequate and appropriate resources to meet the project remit

- adequate and appropriate management and evaluation to support the project

- recognition of the importance of the wider environment within which projects operate

- building in long-term sustainability.

(Adapted from HDA, 2004a, pp. 35–6)

Thinking point: how might the effectiveness of the community development in health approach be measured?

Although many of the outcomes of a community development approach are, it is argued, often intangible (Gilchrist, 2003), the aforementioned ABCD model presents a useful framework for also evaluating its effectiveness. Figure 8.4 gives the outcomes of community development as suggested by this framework.

The aim of community development for health is, in the spirit of communitarianism, a process whereby the community defines its own health needs, works out how those needs can best be met and collectively decides on a course of action to achieve the desired outcomes. Although the strength of a community development approach is that it builds community capacity, this is certainly not achieved overnight. Rather, it takes time, perhaps two or three years, to build up trust, involvement and understanding of local issues and concerns. Some projects start by setting up in a local community centre or shopping precinct. Or, the community development worker may knock on doors, visit local groups, or frequent play areas or launderettes. Undertaking a community profile or needs assessment by involving local people and groups in the process is becoming increasingly popular. This then becomes not only an information-gathering exercise, but allows people to learn new skills as well as share experiences. The project worker may become involved in setting up mutual support

Figure 8.4   Evaluation framework for achieving better community development (Source: SCCD, 2001, p. 9)

Community empowerment	
Process	Outcome
Personal empowerment	A learning community
Positive action	A fair and just community
Community organising and volunteer support	An active and organised community
Participation and involvement	An influential community
Quality of life	
Process	Outcome
Community economic development	A shared wealth
Social and service development	A caring community
Community environmental action	A safe and healthy community
Community arts and cultural development	A creative community
Governance and development	A citizens' community

groups and action groups. These may wish to influence statutory service provision, or they may become involved in setting up their own initiatives (such as food co-operatives), or they may campaign around a particular issue, such as improving the safety of children on their own estate.

Some of the tools required, using a community development approach, when working with the community to promote health include being able to:

- understand key concepts, principles and the history of community development, of health improvement and of reducing health inequalities, and be able to appraise their value

- relate practice to these key values and principles

- have an awareness of evidence that supports a community development approach to health improvement and reducing health inequalities

- understand the objectives of relevant government policies, and know how to keep abreast of policy changes, in particular via websites

- discuss different government policies in relation to community development

- compare local programmes and strategies

- make connections between national policies and local initiatives

- distinguish different approaches to community involvement and development in policies and programmes

- assess one's own practice in relation to these policies and programmes, and relate community development to one's practice.

(Adapted from HDA, 2004a, p. 58)

Although this sounds fine in theory, how might it look in practice? For Hull Developing our Communities (DOC) community workers operating on the ground, this meant initially taking time getting to know people and their communities, meeting up with people and listening to their stories and experiences, their hopes, aspirations and needs. Each community has different identities and cultures, and many factors have an impact on quality of life and on opportunities to influence decision making. This initial work builds trust, confidence and a sense of value and self-worth within communities. It includes outreach to marginalised people so that confidence and learning increase, community networks are strengthened and people feel more able to have a collective voice in decision-making processes. Examples of the type of work involved in developing communities by Hull DOC include:

- Community celebrations – bringing people together to facilitate a community event such as parties, community plays, lunches, poetry workshops.

- Carrying out a participatory appraisal – involving communities in looking at what is going on in an area and finding ways to collectively improve community life.

- Creative training – away days to local colleges, universities and community centres – helping to break down barriers.

- Community information – developing an interactive web-site with communities.

- Meeting people in their locality – office bases located in communities providing access, facilities and resources. Workers attend community group meetings.

- Creating an informal local reference group – so that residents, groups and organisations can network, raise issues and develop priorities for Hull DOC's work and influence its decision making. This includes nominating people to sit on a Community Chest panel which awards grants to community groups.

(SCCD, 2001, p. 10)

This approach led to some local residents compiling a poem to celebrate the success of Hull DOC:

> 'Don't put yourself down, they said,
> Until you've really tried it.
> We organised our tenants group
> Sat on committees too
> Then we applied for funding
> For the things we had to do.
> We took our tenants out on trips
> What a difference in the block!
> Who made all this possible?
> It was, of course, Hull DOC'

('Part of a poem from Gatwick House, supported by Hull DOC', SCCD, 2001, p. 10)

Thinking point: how might this success be achieved?

Achieving the type of success illustrated by this poem means, first, recognising the importance of different research methods when adopting a community development in health (or CDH) approach. For example, many professionals, practitioners and local people have begun to embrace a participatory action research approach (Earle et al., 2007). A similar collaborative approach to building bridges with communities is community-based participatory research. This is a collaborative partnership approach to research that equitably involves, in all aspects of the research process, those who are affected by the issue being studied – community members, organisational representatives, and researchers (Israel et al., 1998). Another approach that has several benefits is peer research, whereby volunteers from the community undertake research with others in the community. This is an excellent way of reaching those who are the most excluded, as well as developing the skills and capacity of individuals undertaking the work. The peer researchers should be closely involved in deciding the best way to undertake the research and in designing the event or survey questions. Their knowledge of how best to reach others in the community, and the types of questions to ask, will be invaluable in ensuring that the views and voices of the target audience are heard. One example of this approach can be found in the city of Leicester where local parents were trained as peer researchers (see Box 8.4).

Although those who work within CDH projects are very positive and sometimes evangelical about their work, they are not without their critics. For example, CDH has been described as 'sometimes unforgivably naive in its claim to be able to transform the lives and social prospects of deprived groups' (Beattie, 1991, p. 178). Beattie also points out that there is 'the persistent doubt whether local action can ever achieve more than marginal and token victories in the face of the larger social inequalities and social

Box 8.4 Young parents as peer researchers

Joan

My name is Joan. I'm 18 and have two children. Jameelah who is 2 and Akeem, 4 months. I found out about the project from my support worker at Sure Start St Matthews. I got involved because I'd never done anything like this before and I thought it would be good working with people of my own age group who were also young parents.

I've gained a lot of experience from doing this. I know now when people are listening and when they're not and when they're being patronising! I've got a bit wiser and learnt a lot. It's given me a good outlook on other people.

It's helped me to help other young parents and give them advice. I hope that the results of this project will improve services for young parents.

(Hall et al., 2002, p. 3)

injustices which, of course, reflect policies at national level' (Beattie, 1991, p. 178). Proponents of CDH would counter that, although they recognise the need to change policy at national and international levels, their endeavours are focused on helping deprived and oppressed groups to 'find a voice' (Rosenthal, 1983).

The challenge for many government agencies, therefore, has been to develop a system that would allow an increase in the participation of communities in the promotion of public health, while simultaneously developing community cohesion and social capital among the diverse range of people and agencies working together in the local community. CDH has gone some way to fulfilling this obligation.

Thus, a community group's 'purpose' might not be primarily to redress social inequalities. It may simply be to provide a community centre where local people can meet and organise local activities. There are many small steps on the road to achieving the CDH workers' aim to empower communities to take control over their own affairs (issues of empowerment are developed further in the next chapter). Although an ultimate aim would be to promote equity, they would identify many other categories of activity that achieve a health gain.

The role itself is not without its dilemmas, but CDH project workers' loyalties are usually firmly located in their community, and they see themselves as having a pivotal role in supporting the community and facilitating group action, as well as securing resources and access to policy makers.

Thinking point: what might be some of the challenges facing CDH workers?

Although CDH has begun to embrace the idea of citizen participation within the broad spectrum of civil society, new concepts and rights have emerged, which pose challenges and opportunities for the profession: for example, the need to continue engaging key stakeholders, to recognise the heterogeneity of communities, to champion a partnership approach, to attract resources, to link with local action and to encourage greater use of health impact assessment. Empowerment models have, in recent years, presented CDH practitioners with opportunities to not only foster action and involvement, but also to promote a philosophy that fundamentally embraces a 'people-centred' approach emphasising human and social development. Box 8.5 neatly illustrates the practical successes of such an approach.

Box 8.5 The empowering potential of community development approaches in health promotion

The Report of the Health Select Committee praised the Beacon Project on a housing estate in Falmouth, Cornwall, which was awarded a Nye Bevan award in 1999 for its remarkable contribution to health improvement. This project used community development approaches to bring about a range of social and environmental improvements in the poorest ward in Cornwall. As the report of the Health Select Committee says, '*the results of the project have been nothing short of remarkable:*

- *post natal depression is down by 80%*

- *the number of children on the child protection register is down by 60%*

- *the child accident rate is down by 50%*

- *the overall crime rate is down by 50%*

- *residents' fuel bills have been cut by £80–£360 pa*

- *boys' SATs results have improved by 100%; girls' by 25%.*'

[Second Report of the Health Select Committee (2001), paragraphs 115–16]

(Duggan et al., 2002, p. 15)

Despite the obvious successes of CDH, there are some who argue that this approach is not conducive to all aspects of multidisciplinary public health. Considering the practice of community development in heart health promotion, Robinson and Elliot (2000, p. 230) found that it is not always realistic to advocate such an approach as the goal to which all communities should strive since, they argue, 'project objectives are often limited to those that will generate measurable and numeric outcomes rather than allowing for the process in community development approaches'. Likewise, many argue that CDH raises false expectations: 'Community development projects that are devolved too early to the community; that are under-resourced (both financially and in terms of working with local social infrastructure); that inflate community expectations and then leave the community to fend for itself, are unlikely to enjoy long-term success' (Simpson et al., 2003, p. 284). Although this may indeed sometimes be the case, overall the use of CDH has proved extremely effective in promoting health and in addressing health inequalities (Fisher et al., 1999).

By now you should have a comprehensive grasp not only of the potential for communities to influence public health initiatives and interventions, but also of how this action is fostered and facilitated utilising a community development approach. However, while community development remains a source of hope in terms of social justice and equitability, not all community-orientated approaches follow this pathway, as Section 8.2.2 shows.

8.2.2 Communities and the individual

Although community development has become something of a catch-all term in public health circles, this is not the only approach when engaging with communities to promote public health. Strategies that use a more individualistic approach can still be found embedded within communities. For example, many sexual health clinics are geared towards personal, rather than communal, health promotion activity. Such examples reflect the traditional model of personal behaviour change, long associated with health education practice in Britain (Amos, 2002). This model is in contrast to the more radical, social action approach epitomised by community development, as outlined above, in which communities are encouraged to 'take on social action roles that facilitate the development of social capital as the health-related link between social structure and human agency'(Whitehead, 2004, p. 314). It is the latter, collective (as opposed to individual) approaches, however, that critics argue are popular, simply because the implications for policy are that they are cheaper than the goal of reducing costly health inequalities, thus placing responsibility on the community itself. This also encourages an element of victim blaming, implying that poor people are unhealthy because they do not devote enough energy to participation in community activities (Muntaner and Lynch, 1999).

However, some community-based interventions have begun a return to a more targeted, individual approach. This approach involves targeting people from specific groups within the community or with particular health issues, and working with them on a one-to-one basis to improve their health and wellbeing. An example is the Pals in Pregnancy programme in Coventry, which involves recruiting local women, known to have had problems in pregnancy, to help others in similar situations. The women can meet with their 'Pal' in person, talk over the telephone or attend a group session if they prefer. An evaluation of the programme found that over half of clients felt their Pal had had a positive effect on their pregnancy, simply by listening to their problems in confidence and offering a link into other helping agencies and support services (Visram and Drinkwater, 2005).

On the other hand, some public heath interventions favour a more generic individual approach. Here the intention is that health trainers, for example, will employ this approach, attempting to improve the health of their local population by promoting health behaviour change with individuals on a one-to-one basis. One example of such an approach is the public health assistants (PHAs) pilot project within Camden Primary Care Trust (PCT). The five PHAs represent the diversity of the local population and work out of various bases within the community. They have undergone extensive training, including psychology-based methods in behaviour change, and are able to signpost people to preventative and other services (Visram and Drinkwater, 2005).

Although such individualistic approaches serve to promote public health, it could be argued that they simply represent a traditional top–down model in which individuals are judged to be passive objects rather than active subjects. This theme of whether or not local people are at the heart of public health is picked up in the following section.

8.3 Legitimating local voices: putting people at the heart of public health?

The current approach to community development has its roots in the community development projects that were set up in 1969 by the UK government as 'a neighbourhood-based experiment aimed at finding new ways of meeting the needs of people living in areas of high social deprivation' (Jones et al., 2002, p. 34). As noted above, it was expected that this would be achieved by mobilising communities, placing people at the heart of public health in an effort to enforce change by addressing health inequalities and social injustice. Indeed, many key user movements and projects – for example, the women's health movement and black and minority ethnic health action groups – successfully campaigned on specific issues in their locality utilising a community development approach. While the ultimate goal of these movements was to improve health and address health inequalities, many of them were not primarily about health but helped facilitate wellbeing and healthy outcomes.

Most self-help groups are thoroughly participatory in that they are usually set up and organised by the members themselves. They are therefore genuine grass-roots organisations. But Gareth Williams has questioned the degree to which they are collectivist in the ideological sense. He claims that most self-help groups are: '"Janus headed" in that they straddle both the individualist and collectivist ideologies and that an uneasy compromise exists between different impulses ... self-care or social support, counselling or activism, personal change or political change' (Williams, 1989, p. 154).

8.3.1 Community campaign groups with a health component

Despite often coming together to campaign about a whole range of social issues, these grass-roots organisations may, however, include a health component even though the main motivation underpinning their establishment was not health. For example, the campaign may be about an environmental issue such as pollution from a local factory, which has wider implications: health being just one of them. On the other hand, the organisation may be a pensioners' group concerned about the transport needs of older people; or a parents' action group campaigning for a safe play area for their children; or a tenants' association campaigning for better housing. Whatever the reason for coming together, many of these campaign groups adopt a community activist approach. For example, although a national organisation, the Tenant Participation Advisory Service (TPAS) has made a substantial impact in helping to raise awareness of how poor housing is a contributory factor in health at a community level (TPAS, 2005).

Thinking point: can you think of any such campaigns in your locality, and can you identify a health component?

Community campaigns can be reactive or proactive, but they tend to come together for a particular purpose and do not necessarily form long-term groupings, although, as with TPAS, some do form lasting links and campaign over many years. Undoubtedly such campaigns are prime examples of collective action, but the acronym NIMBY ('not in my backyard') could well be applied to many campaigns, especially those that campaign against the siting of an undesirable object: for example, a mobile phone mast. If the fact that this object may be placed in the territory of less active or articulate communities is of no concern, then in ideological terms these groups are exhibiting many of the features of individualism. If on the other hand, a chain of community protest is set up, such as with the anti-road protesters, then the ideals of collectivism are being met. Similar contradictions can be observed within some self-help groups.

8.3.2 Obstacles to working with communities: reality meets rhetoric

Despite the positive dimension of community participation and community involvement, facilitating the process – for both practitioners and policy makers – is often filled with potential obstacles, some of which may lead to the destruction of area-based initiatives. These include:

- Local residents' lack of time or interest in the activities of the initiative. For example, emerging evidence suggests that it is easier to attract local residents to become involved in community projects that concern housing, poverty or young people's prospects than in schemes focusing solely on economic development, employment or training.

- The provision of separate channels for involvement for particular groups (e.g. those with a particular age or ethnicity) can be worthwhile, but they require a lot of support. Both targeted and universal strategies need to be adopted to promote more widespread community involvement.

- A lack of recognition of any lessons learned from earlier activities in previous area-based initiatives in the same area.

- A rigid agenda set in advance, which is not open to the influence of community involvement and consultation.

- The use of questionnaires and/or surveys alone when engaging in community consultation.

- Undue 'out-of-hours' pressures on local residents and the risk of intimidation.

- A small number of local people (sometimes disparagingly referred to as 'the usual suspects') who sometimes dominate community involvement. However, the longevity of involvement by a few community members can, under certain circumstances, be beneficial as some initiatives suffer from a problem of high turnover and consequential loss of community memory and experience.

- Lack of sufficient funding although no general agreement was found as to what constitutes sufficient funding.

- The risk of focusing the available funding on facilitating community engagement at the expense of ensuring the sustainability of the area based initiative.

(Adapted from Home Office, 2004)

When working to develop community health, both community groups and professionals working and campaigning for health, despite being committed to a bottom–up approach to community action, often have to face up to the reality that, to achieve the success they desire, an element of compromise has to be part of the process. This often means having to trade their enthusiasm and ambitions for a slightly 'watered-down' version of any intervention or initiative. Whether or not such a compromise is a political reality or simply based on rhetoric is highly debatable.

So, in the case of agency-sponsored projects, the agency has the power to define the basis of membership and to establish the formal rules of the dialogue, thereby 'marginalising the voices of the counter publics in the dialogic process' (Barnes et al., 2003, p. 396). However, there is now widespread recognition of the practical difficulties associated with establishing equitable community partnerships, many of which often result in a blame culture which leads to a chasm between rhetoric and operations (Weiss, 1981). Indeed, conflict as an enduring process has, in many cases, created considerable barriers to effecting healthy outcomes (Hudson et al., 1999). A number of ways of overcoming such obstacles has been put forward with, in some cases, conflict helping to facilitate collaboration.

Gray (1985) argues that stakeholders need to have an appreciation of their interdependence as well as their independence. Gray recognises that complex problems (such as health and social care problems) are not soluble by any one organisation and are therefore not their sole property; individuals or organisations who are directly affected by the problem also have a stake. In defining problems in this way, stakeholders are forced to recognise their interdependence, and in so doing can claim a right to influence the collaboration agenda.

Gilchrist (1998) proposes a 'twelve-step' model of conflict – one that might be used by community development workers to create consensus and develop lasting coalitions between communities and decision makers. She outlines a series of phases through which people move, from a position of mutual hostility to an agreed settlement. The key to this approach is the proactive formation of connections between people and the vitality of relationships which develop as a result.

Step One – Recognition
There is an awareness of the conflict as a problem and a shared desire to change the situation.

Step Two – Tolerance
The parties to the conflict accept and tolerate each other's existence, acknowledging that they all have some rights and responsibilities in dealing with issues arising from the conflict.

Step Three – Information exchange
Communication is established between the parties, allowing them to exchange information and develop knowledge of each other.

Step Four – Dialogue
The parties enter into discussion, learning about their different experiences and grievances in relation to the conflict. Dialogue allows analysis to develop, but not necessarily consensus.

Step Five – Empathy
At a personal level, individuals from different sides of the conflict begin to understand each other's perspectives and to empathise with one another.

Step Six – Mediation
Through further discussion, possibly mediated by an 'outsider', areas of agreement are highlighted which address common concerns and identify shared values.

Step Seven – Shared commitment
A joint vision of how the conflict could be resolved is developed, probably achieved through some compromises and re-framing of the problem.

Step Eight – Negotiation
Agreement on limited objectives emerges after negotiation, and co-operation around these is developed.

Step Nine – Trust
The experience of working together consolidates personal relationships and organisational procedures, based on mutual trust and respect.

Step Ten – Coalitions
More formal arrangements are set up to promote partnership and create mechanisms for dealing with tensions and difficulties that have arisen from conflicting interests and viewpoints.

Step Eleven – Alliances
Alliances are formed around a range of issues which cross the barriers of the original conflict. There is progressive integration and development of informal networks.

Step Twelve – Resolution and justice
Reconciliation and peaceful co-existence is achieved based on a just and equitable solution to the conflict. Antagonistic identities ('us and them') fade away and a new sense of community emerges.

(Gilchrist, 1998, pp. 105–6)

Thus, in working to promote health at a local level, it is important to recognise that there are likely to be differences between potential collaborators over the value and virtues they place on joint activities. Nonetheless, this should not prevent them from working in tandem to achieve their shared aim.
The issue of collaboration is explored further in Chapter 9.

8.4 Community patient and public involvement in action

Whereas the benefits of CDH to locally based initiatives and interventions have been well documented, less so is the way in which community development has much to offer large health service organisations and primary care groups. Although the reasons for this are many, a major factor that influenced the shift away from the provision of healthy interventions by the statutory sector to the voluntary and community sectors was the publication of the Black Report (DHSS, 1980). This argued that many of the problems of health inequalities lay outside the scope of the NHS, being related to social and economic factors, such as income, employment, environment, education, housing, transport and lifestyle.

With the advent of such initiatives as patient and public involvement (PPI) forums, the National Primary Health Care Team, practice nurses based in GP surgeries, and a shift in the NHS philosophy from cure to one of prevention, the statutory sector is, once again, seen as the key player in promoting the public's health. Indeed, a greater emphasis on the role of NHS Trusts in relation to population health was outlined in *Shifting the Balance of Power* (DoH, 2002), a major recommendation of which was that the role of public health should be confined predominantly to working within primary care.

Thus, at the time of writing (2007), the mutual improvement of health and healthcare lies with an amalgam of community projects as well as with large health service organisations and primary care groups. Indeed, PPI forums – as a mechanism for bringing together primary care and locally based health improvements – have for many years been a cornerstone of attempts to put patients at the centre of everything the NHS does.

Community development workers, who once saw themselves on the other side of the battle lines attacking statutory provision or state bureaucracy, now often find themselves acting as go-betweens. Is this a welcome development? Does it represent a new awareness on the part of the statutory services? The late Wendy Farrant was sceptical about the new rhetoric of user participation and community involvement. She wrote: 'The belated interest of the NHS in community development needs to be seen in relation to the crisis in the welfare state, and broader debates around such issues as community care, volunteerism, decentralisation and consumerism' (Farrant, 1991, p. 14). She went on to argue that this new interest is largely concerned with consumerist notions of community participation which she believed 'undermines the fundamental principles of community development' (Farrant, 1991, p. 17). Nonetheless, the involvement of patients and the public in health decision making is now a central theme of national and local policy in all four nations of the UK. Such involvement illuminates the patient experience and helps to shape a health service that is truly responsive to individual and community needs. On both a practical and a cultural level, the current government is clear that it wants to change the way in which people's needs are incorporated into the NHS: 'The importance of involving all local communities, including so-called "hard to reach" groups such as ethnic groups, children and young people, is widely recognised. Collaboration and partnership with the voluntary and community sectors is an effective route to building community relationships' (DoH, 2004, p. 3).

So, why is it so important to involve patients and the public? Edwards and Elwyn have identified some of the reasons:

People who become active in decisions about their care, experience:

- reduced anxiety and psychological distress

- symptom resolution

- reduced blood pressure

- enhanced functional and health status, and mood.

And there are obvious benefits to organisations, for example:

- helping design services that will meet people's needs

- assisting the development of alternative proposals

- helping to build accountability and trust in NHS organisations if these pay attention to what people say.

(Adapted from Edwards and Elwyn, 2004)

Although these benefits are a welcome result of PPI, how does this transfer to practice? For some, it means collaboration between other agencies. Box 8.6 offers a practical illustration of the possible benefits accrued using this approach.

Box 8.6 Collaboration with the voluntary and community sectors is an effective approach to patient and public involvement

A hospital trust paid for seven volunteers from a local cancer voluntary organisation to be trained as focus group facilitators. These facilitators ran a series of focus groups with people living with cancer and produced a report for the trust's Cancer Services Review Group.

The aim of the process was to improve the service in line with user views. Although there were some difficulties initially, the experience gained by the trust and the voluntary organisation ensured that the programme changed and evolved over time.

This model has been extended to two other trusts and is supported financially by the local cancer network.

(DoH, 2004, p. 40, Box 7.4)

Critics point out that, despite the rhetoric behind PPI, there is a political agenda geared towards decision makers rather than communities (Rowe and Shepherd, 2002). In spite of such cynicism, however, feedback from patients during 2006 suggested that they valued being able to choose where to go for their treatment, and the convenience of choosing the time and date of their appointment (DoH, 2006).

In June 2006, a further step towards making it easier for people to get involved in their local health services was announced by the then Health Minister, Rosie Winterton. A new national Patient and Public Involvement Resource Centre, to develop and support NHS staff and organisations to involve people in local health services, would open its doors. The Resource Centre, operated by a consortium made up of the University of Warwick, the Centre for Public Scrutiny and the Long-term Medical Conditions Alliance, will promote the value of involving people and will work with NHS organisations, staff and patients to build on the foundations of involvement that are already in place in many parts of the country.

The rise in lay people wishing to join PPI forums, facilitated by the Commission for Patient and Public Involvement in Health (CPPIH), also suggests that many communities are keen to be involved in influencing the way in which local health services are delivered. Indeed, given that these forums also look at wider health issues, such as social care, transport or housing, they appear to signal a move towards real community empowerment. However, there have been concerns about possible cultural constraints to local involvement (Rowe and Shepherd, 2002).

In 2006, the CPPIH suggested that the current PPI forum system would not be successful unless it changed. It must, they argued, allow community input on major issues of public health (CPPIH, 2006). Such changes would, they believed, see accountability functions delivered in the future by an independent system of 'local involvement networks' (LINs), covering a geographical primary care trust area instead of being linked to a particular organisation. The plan was that such bodies would include local people and community-led health and social care organizations, with the networks acting as a mechanism for gathering and bringing together the views and concerns from a wide variety of local patient and public interest groups across the health and social care arena.

Conclusion

Community involvement and civic engagement are now an integral part of the landscape of twenty-first century multidisciplinary public health and governments from each of the four nations of the UK appear committed to this approach. Indeed, there is increasing acceptance that communities are seeing a shift in the way multidisciplinary public health promotion is delivered, with the increased use of a community development approach acting as a key to fostering and facilitating community competence and capacity. The value of such an approach is that it is judged to be much more democratic, concentrating, as it does, on enabling and empowering local people. However, community-orientated approaches to promoting public health are not all about community development, with some taking a more individualistic approach. Whichever approach you choose, the shift in the balance of power, which, during the last decade, has seen a sea change in the way primary care is delivered in the UK, seems set to see the continuance of such community-orientated policies and practices: ones that seek to mobilise communities in the delivery of multidisciplinary public health.

References

Amos, M. (2002) 'Community development' in Adams, L., Amos, M. and Munroe, J. (eds) *Promoting Health: Politics and Practice*, London, Sage.

Barnes, M., Newman, J., Knops, A. and Sullivan, H. (2003) 'Constituting the "public" in public participation', *Public Administration*, vol. 81, no. 2, pp. 379–99.

Barr, A. and Hashagen, S. (2000) *ABCD Handbook: A Framework for Evaluating Community Development*, London, Community Development Foundation.

Beattie, A. (1991) *The Evaluation of Community Development Initiatives in Health Promotion: A Review of Current Strategies*, Health Education Unit Occasional Papers, vol. 1, no. 3, Milton Keynes, The Open University.

Blair, T. (1998) *The Third Way: New Politics for the New Century*, Fabian Pamphlet 588, London, Fabian Society.

Campbell, C. and McLean, C. (2002) 'Ethnic identities, social capital and health inequalities: factors shaping African-Caribbean participation in local community networks in the UK', *Social Science and Medicine*, vol. 55, no. 4, pp. 643–57.

Collins, W.A. (1997) 'Relationships and development during adolescence: interpersonal adaptation to individual change', *Personal Relationships*, vol. 4, no. 1, pp. 1–14.

Commission for Patient and Public Involvement in Health (CPPIH) (2006) *Patient and Public Involvement (PPI) Forums* [online], http://www.cppih.org (Accessed 12 September 2006).

Community Development Cymru (CDC) (2006) *A National Strategic Framework for Community Development in Wales* [online], http://www.cdc.cymru.org/main.php (Accessed 24 October 2006).

Community Health Shop (2006) [online],http://www.community-health-shop.org (Accessed 1 November 2006).

Crawshaw, P., Bunton, R. and Gillen, K. (2003) 'Health Action Zones and the problem of community', *Health and Social Care in the Community*, vol. 11, no. 1, pp. 36–44.

Department of Health (DoH) (2002) *Shifting the Balance of Power*, London, The Stationery Office.

Department of Health (DoH) (2004) *Patient and Public Involvement in Health: The Evidence for Policy Implementation*, London, The Stationery Office.

Department of Health (DoH) (2006) *The GP Patient Survey – Your Doctor, Your Experience, Your Say (formerly known as the National Patient Experience Survey 2006/7) – Update for Strategic Health Authorities (SHAs), Primary Care Trusts (PCTs) and Primary Care Contracting Advisors (PCCAs)*, London, The Stationery Office.

Department of Health and Social Security (DHSS) (1980) *Inequalities in Health: Report of a Research Working Group* (the Black Report), London, Department of Health and Social Security.

Department of Health, Social Services and Public Safety (DHSSPS) (2004) *A Healthier Future: A Twenty Year Vision for Health and Wellbeing in Northern Ireland 2005–2025*, Belfast, Department of Health, Social Services and Public Safety.

Dhesi, A.S. (2000) 'Social capital and community development', *Community Development Journal*, vol. 35, no. 3, pp. 199–214.

Duggan, M. with Cooper, A. and Foster, J. (2002) *Modernising the Social Model in Mental Health: A Discussion Paper*, SPN Paper 1, Social Perspectives Network/TOPSS (Training Organisation for the Personal Social Services) England.

Earle, S., Lloyd, C.E., Sidell, M. and Spurr, S. (eds) (2007) *Theory and Research in Promoting Public Health*, London, Sage/Milton Keynes, The Open University.

East, L. (1998) 'The quality of social relationships as a public health issue: exploring the relationship between health and community in a disadvantaged neighbourhood', *Health and Social Care in the Community*, vol. 6, no. 3, pp. 189–95.

Edwards, A. and Elwyn, G. (2004) 'Involving patients in decision making and communicating risk: a longitudinal evaluation of doctors' attitudes and confidence during a randomized trial', *Journal of Evaluation in Clinical Practice*, vol. 10, no. 3, pp. 431–7.

Farrant, W. (1991) 'Addressing the contradictions: health promotion and community health action in the United Kingdom', *International Journal of Health Services*, vol. 21, no. 3, pp. 423–39.

Fisher, B., Neve, H. and Heritage, Z. (1999) 'Community development, user involvement, and primary health care', *British Medical Journal*, vol. 318, pp. 749–50.

Gilchrist, A. (1998) 'A more excellent way: developing coalitions and consensus through informal networks', *Community Development Journal*, vol. 33, no. 2, pp. 100–8.

Gilchrist, A. (2003) 'Community development in the UK – possibilities and paradoxes', *Community Development Journal*, vol. 38, no. 1, pp. 16–25.

Goeppinger, J. and Shuster, G.F. (1992) 'Community as client, using the nursing process to promote health' in Stanhope, M. and Lancaster, J. (eds) *Community Health Nursing, Process and Practice for Promoting Health* (3rd edn), St Louis, MO, Mosby.

Gray, B. (1985) 'Conditions facilitating interorganizational collaboration', *Human Relations*, vol. 38, no. 10, pp. 911–36.

Hall, D., Rae, C. and Jarvis, M. (compilers) (2002) *Young Parent Peer Research Project*, Leicester, Connexions Leicestershire.

Health Development Agency (HDA) (2000b) *Evaluation of Community-Level Interventions for Health Improvement: A Review of Experience in the UK*, London, Health Development Agency.

Health Development Agency (HDA) (2004a) *Developing Healthier Communities*, London, Health Development Agency.

Health Development Agency (HDA) (2004c) *Social Capital*, London, Health Development Agency.

Higgins, J.W. (1999) 'Citizenship and empowerment: a remedy for citizen participation in health reform', *Community Development Journal*, vol. 34, no. 4, pp. 287–307.

Hoedemaekers, R. and Dekkers, W. (2003) 'Key concepts in health care priority setting', *Health Care Analysis*, vol. 11, no. 4, pp. 309–23.

Home Office (2004) *What Works in Community Involvement in Area-Based Initiatives? A Systematic Review of the Literature*, London, Home Office Research and Development Office.

Hudson, B., Hardy, B., Henwodd, M. and Wistow, G. (1999) 'In pursuit of interagency collaboration in the public sector. What is the contribution of theory and research?', *Public Management: An International Journal of Research and Theory*, vol. 1, no. 2, pp. 235–60.

Israel, B.A., Schulz, A.J., Parker, E.A. and Becker, A.B. (1998) 'Review of community-based research: assessing partnership approaches to improve public health', *Annual Review of Public Health*, vol. 19, pp. 173–202.

Jones, L., Sidell, M. and Douglas, J. (eds) (2002) *The Challenge of Promoting Health: Exploration and Action* (2nd edn), Basingstoke, Palgrave Macmillan/Milton Keynes, The Open University.

Liverpool Partnership Group Self-Assessment (2002) *Merseyside HAZ Principles of Community Involvement* [online], http://www.liverpoolfirst.org/doc/T5.doc (Accessed 12 October 2006).

Melnyk, G. (1985) *The Search for Community: From Utopia to a Co-operative Society*, Montreal and Buffalo, Black Rose Books.

Muntaner, C. and Lynch, J. (1999) 'Income inequality and social cohesion versus class relations: a critique of Wilkinson's neo-Durkheimian research program', *International Journal of Health Services*, vol. 29, no. 1, pp. 59–82.

Muntaner, C., Lynch, J. and Davey-Smith, G. (2001) 'Social capital, disorganised communities, and the Third Way: understanding the retreat from structural inequalities in epidemiology and public health', *International Journal of Health Services*, vol. 31, no. 2, pp. 213–37.

Petersen, A. and Lupton, D. (1996) *The New Public Health and Self in the Age of Risk*, St Leonards, Australia, Allen & Unwin.

Putnam, R. (2000) *Bowling Alone: The Collapse and Revival of American Community*, London, Simon & Schuster.

Ritchie, D., Parry, O., Gnich, W. and Platt, S. (2004) 'Issues of participation, ownership and empowerment in a community development programme: tackling smoking in a low income area in Scotland', *Health Promotion International*, vol. 19, no. 1, pp. 51–9.

Robinson, K.L. and Elliot, S.J. (2000) 'The practice of community development approaches in heart health promotion', *Health Education Research*, vol. 15, no. 2, pp. 219–31.

Rosenthal, H. (1983) 'Neighbourhood health projects: some new approaches to health and community work in parts of the United Kingdom', *Community Development Journal*, vol. 18, no. 2, pp. 120–31.

Rowe, R. and Shepherd, M. (2002) 'Public participation in the new NHS: no closer to citizen control?', *Social Policy and Administration*, vol. 6, no. 3, pp. 275–90.

Scottish Centre for Regeneration (2005) *Community Engagement Case Studies* [online], http://www.communitiesscotland.gov.uk/stellent/groups/public/documents/webpages/scrcs_008622.hcspwww (Accessed 15 October 2006).

Simpson, L., Wood, L. and Daws, L. (2003) 'Community capacity building: starting with people not projects', *Community Development Journal*, vol. 38, no. 4, pp. 277–86.

Smith, N., Littlejohns, L.B. and Thompson, D. (2001) 'Shaking out the cobwebs: insights into community capacity and its relation to health outcomes', *Community Development Journal*, vol. 36, no. 1, pp. 30–41.

Standing Conference for Community Development (SCCD) (2001) *Strategic Framework for Community Development*, Sheffield, Standing Conference for Community Development.

Teffo, L.J. and Roux, A.P.J. (1998) 'Metaphysical thinking in Africa' in Coetzee, P.H. and Roux, A.P.J. (eds) *The African Philosophy Reader*, London, Routledge.

Tenant Participation Advisory Service (TPAS) (2005) *Campaigning for Better Housing* [online], http://www.tpas.org.uk/sub_page.asp?id=1&cat=49 (Accessed 26 September 2006).

Tones, K. and Tilford, S. (2001) *Health Promotion: Effectiveness, Efficiency and Equity*, Cheltenham, Nelson Thornes.

Visram, S. and Drinkwater, C. (2005) *Health Trainers: A Review of the Evidence*, Primary Care Development Centre [online], http://www.pcdc.org.uk (Accessed 12 October 2006).

Weiss, J.A. (1981) 'Substance vs. symbol in administrative reform: the case of human services coordination', *Policy Analysis*, vol. 7, no. 1, pp. 21–45.

Whitehead, D. (2004) 'Health promotion and health education: advancing the concepts', *Journal of Advanced Nursing*, vol. 47, no. 3, pp. 311–20.

Williams, G. (1989) 'Hope for the humblest? The role of self-help in chronic illness: the case of ankylosing spondylitis', *Sociology of Health and Illness*, vol. 11, no. 2, pp. 135–59.

Chapter 9

Developing local alliance partnerships through community collaboration and participation

Angela Scriven

Introduction

Enabling and encouraging people to participate in defining and promoting their collective concerns in relation to health are important public health processes. If community groups operate in isolation, they will make less of an impact on the organisations and agencies that affect their health and wellbeing. How local communities and providers of services can engage effectively with each other to define their needs and plan and provide services is the subject of this chapter.

At the outset there is a discussion of terms, concepts, opportunities, challenges and roles of community-based health alliances and the way in which these partnerships are central to a range of public health-related policies and strategies. This is followed in Section 9.2 with a detailed consideration of the development of local partnerships and alliances, exploring the 'pushes' and 'pulls' that influence practice. The emphasis in Section 9.3 is on how to form local alliance partnerships and on the importance of establishing responsibilities and structures. Section 9.4 focuses on the various forms of community participation and collaboration, and the final section of the chapter reflects on the concept of empowerment and ways of achieving empowered communities.

9.1 Health alliances and partnerships at a local level

The practice of participatory approaches involving the community in active collaboration and partnership work with statutory and voluntary agencies is well established within the public health arena. As noted in previous chapters, as early as 1978 the full participation of the community in the multidimensional work of health improvement became one of the pillars of the Health for All movement, launched at the Alma Ata conference (WHO, 1978). The declaration from this conference confirmed that people have not only the right but also the duty to participate individually and collectively in the planning and implementation of their healthcare. This was developed further in 1986 when the Ottawa Charter identified strengthening community action as one of five key priorities for proactive health creation (WHO, 1986). A wide range of international policies has followed, which have adopted and reaffirmed these ideas. A recent international declaration from the World Health Organization (WHO), the Bangkok Charter, prioritises local partnerships and calls for the strengthening of the capacity of civil society and decision makers to act collectively to exert control over the factors that influence health. The Charter asserts that active participation, especially by the community, is essential for the sustainability of public health efforts. The challenge, to make a reality the commitment to engage and empower people, is clearly laid out for public health professionals. The formation of partnerships with public, private and non-governmental organisations (NGOs) is prioritised and designed to create sustainable actions across sectors to address the determinants of health (WHO, 2005).

Thinking point: what does the term 'health alliance' mean to you?

In the UK, the term 'healthy alliances' was introduced to public health professionals in the early 1990s in the first government public health strategy in England (DoH, 1992). From this first use, a healthy alliance (or health alliance) has been used to describe coalitions or partnerships among different organisations, groups and communities that share the common goal of improving health. Although the term 'health alliance' is still used to describe multisectoral public health action, it is often employed interchangeably with the term 'partnerships' to mean the same thing. The second English government strategy (DoH, 1999), for example, re-emphasised the importance of 'partnerships' between people, their communities, local government, voluntary agencies, health services, and business, in order to make health everyone's responsibility.

Working together is also an underpinning principle of *Choosing Health* (DoH, 2004a), the third public health strategy in England. This principle is based on the assertion that government and individuals alone cannot make progress on healthier choices. Real progress depends on effective partnerships across communities, including local government, the NHS, business, advertisers, retailers, the voluntary sector, communities, the media, faith organisations and many others (DoH, 2004a).

Similar ideas are expressed internationally in public health pronouncements, and are firmly embedded in the public health White Papers and strategies from Wales, Scotland and Northern Ireland. Local authorities across Wales, for example, have been active in setting up local health alliances whose role is to engage with local communities in order to identify and address health and wellbeing issues (NAW, 2001). *Improving*

Health in Wales, the health strategy of the National Assembly for Wales (NAW), seeks to enter into partnerships with the people of Wales (NAW, 2001). Participation is seen as a fundamentally important principle underpinning the improvement of public health, the assumption being that people have a right to participate in decisions that affect not only their individual health, but that of the society in which they live, and that they should be enabled to do this. Local health alliances are now well established across Wales. One of these is illustrated in Box 9.3 in Section 9.3.4 below.

The promotion of local partnership working is also at the core of a range of other public health-related policies and strategies, such as neighbourhood renewal. As outlined in Chapter 7, of particular note at a local level in England are local strategic partnerships (LSPs), which form a single non-statutory, multi-agency body, match local authority boundaries and aim to bring together at a local level the different parts of the public, private, community and voluntary sectors. LSPs have been central to the delivery of the Social Exclusion Unit's *New Commitment to Neighbourhood Renewal: National Strategy Action Plan* (SEU, 2001). (Further information relating to LSPs can be obtained from the national policy document *Local Strategic Partnerships: Government Guidelines* [DETR, 2001], and from the Neighbourhood Renewal Unit [2007]).

However, the public heath potential of LSPs has, since their inception, seen them charged with tackling deep-seated, multifaceted problems, requiring a range of responses from different bodies. For example, local public, private, community and voluntary sector partners working through LSPs (see DoT, 2003, for a breakdown of LSP membership) have been responsible for taking many of the major decisions about public health priorities for their local areas. This work was supported by a resource pack on how to create healthy communities by engaging in local partnerships (DoH, 2005).

It is clear from international and national policies and strategies, some of which are discussed above, that joint working that involves communities in collaboration and partnership has become a fundamental platform for delivering public health. Moreover, there is a general accord within the various policy documents that agencies or sectors working in isolation from the community are unlikely to make a real difference to quality of life or health gain (DoH, 2004a, 2004b, 2004c). Through joint planning, resource sharing and increased political strength, local collaboration and partnerships are presented as being able to accomplish more than groups acting alone in advocating and affecting change on the broader factors that influence health (Baldwin et al., 2005).

Much of the rhetoric around partnership working either implicitly or explicitly assumes that partnerships are beneficial. Entwistle (2006,

p. 228) goes as far as suggesting that they are: 'third only to motherhood and apple pie' in their intuitive appeal. This may or may not be the case, but what is certainly true is that 'partnership' is a favourite word in the lexicon of New Labour (Falconer and McLaughlin, 2000). It is surprising, therefore, given the popularity of alliance partnerships as a strategy in the public health agenda since the mid-1990s, that there is little hard evidence that they are as effective as policy developers and politicians would have us believe. Although reflecting the government spin on the benefits of working with the community and voluntary groups, the *Voluntary and Community Sector Review* (HM Treasury, 2004), in examining the state of local partnerships, found that their impact was variable, ranging from real change at best to tokenism or one-sided compacts at worst. Huxham and Vangen (2000) echo the findings of this review and argue that many partnerships do not get near to achieving collaborative advantage, which is one of the main rationales for their existence.

Thinking point: what obstacles do you think might detract from the success of a local alliance partnership?

Coulson (2005), in an article carrying the barbed title 'A plague on all partnerships', offers insights into why some local health alliances may not achieve their goals. He suggests a number of reasons for lack of success, including incompatibility in the aims of the different partners, or their cultures and histories being too diverse to be brought into harmony. There may also be a lack of understanding of their different organisational structures, particularly when local informal groups engage with larger statutory organisations. The problem of unequal power relations in partnership arrangements that include community representation is another factor and a point picked up later in this chapter. There may also be an imbalance in what each partner is putting into the alliance and what each is getting out of it.

Entwistle (2006) has strong views on this and claims that partnership working is second to none in the generation of frustration and disappointment. He points to local authorities in England and Wales struggling to fully appreciate the number and complexity of local partnerships operating in their patch, with new partnerships being created to address all manner of social problems. One reason suggested for this proliferation is that what used to be called committees, networks or working groups are being relabelled as partnerships (Entwistle, 2006, p. 228). There are, therefore, perhaps in some areas, too many partnerships at the local level, which overstretch the capacity of local populations to engage fully in alliance work. This may result in collaborative fatigue or even cynicism. Some of these issues will create barriers for statutory and non-statutory organisations to effective collaboration with the community. Nonetheless, because citizen-centred services and community participation are strongly embedded in current policy agendas, public health practitioners are expected to work closely with local communities to achieve public health targets. It is important, therefore, to understand how to establish and maintain alliances for health, and overcome some of the problems cited above.

9.2 Forming alliance partnerships

To a great extent the reasons for an alliance will determine who initiates the partnership and which groups are involved. Forming partnerships and collaborations and building a health alliance can involve a two-way push and pull process. The push effect occurs when the impetus for the partnership or collaboration comes from a community group that wants to widen its sphere of influence, mobilise resources or gather support from other groups or organisations. The pull effect occurs when professionals approach the community for consultation or invite them to participate in activities that affect their community, such as making the delivery of services more accountable to local needs. The push effect of a community seeking a partnership can be described as a 'bottom–up', grass-roots alliance; the pull effect of public health practitioners inviting the community to participate in decision making in relation to their health needs represents a more 'top–down', expert-led alliance. In practice this distinction may not be as clear cut. When you read the three case-studies of local alliance partnerships in Section 9.4.3, it should become apparent that in some of these alliances both a push and a pull effect are present.

9.2.1 Bottom–up local public health alliances

The following are some of the possible benefits to communities when establishing bottom–up local alliances:

- creation of a service within a community where one did not previously exist

- modification to service delivery so that it more closely meets community needs

- access to resources, and/or resource maximisation

- policy development at organisational or community levels

- system development and change through the modification of relationships between the community and statutory and non-statutory organisations

- social and community development aimed at strengthening communities.

(Adapted from Walker, 2002)

As discussed in the previous section, however, there are disadvantages and potential drawbacks to working collaboratively. In order to be effective in achieving their goals, community groups need to share with the professionals with whom they form an alliance a common vision and agenda, agreed priorities, openness about self-interests, mutual respect, trust and cultural sensitivity.

The fact that the health sector is now more responsive to meeting community-identified health needs will perhaps make bottom–up alliances easier to establish and sustain. Health and social care professionals are being encouraged to systematically engage with, and listen to, their local communities (NHSE, 1999, p. 9). Although the new needs-led, user-responsive National Health Service (NHS) is more sensitive to consumer interests, alliances that are initiated by policy makers and providers of services will have a different motivation from that of more bottom–up initiatives.

9.2.2 Top–down local public health alliances

As indicated above, top–down partnerships are often motivated by the desire to break down barriers that exist between providers and recipients of services. An example of a top–down approach is Health Connect. East Renfrewshire Health Connect (2007), for instance, has been established to provide health and lifestyle services to individuals and groups in some of the most deprived communities in the East Renfrewshire area of Scotland. The main aim is to reduce inequalities in health by promoting mental health. A wide range of voluntary and community groups are included, and local people have been involved through health needs assessment and People's Panel surveys, and were also on the steering group to develop the funding bid. The knowledge and experience of the community are valued, and local involvement is encouraged wherever possible. Local people are members of the Health Connect Task Group and take part in consultations to help design services. In return, Health Connect provides support and training when required.

One of the main difficulties faced by those, such as Health Connect, who consult with communities, is how to gain access and how to identify who is knowledgeable about a particular community. Key informants in the community can be interviewed using qualitative interview techniques in order to try to build up a number of perspectives that are representative of the community. Key informants have been described in a number of ways, but are generally regarded as those people who:

- work within a community and have a professional understanding of issues, and often interpret communities from their particular disciplinary vantage point, such as school teachers, the police, social workers and health visitors

- are recognised community leaders and are seen to represent the community or a section of it, such as councillors, faith leaders, chairs of self-help groups

- are important within informal networks and often play a central role in local communications, such as shop owners or local publicans.

Thinking point: what might be some of the main problems and benefits associated with selecting and identifying key informants?

The practice of selecting key informants may inadvertently identify people with their own strong agendas, which may or may not reflect the agendas of the local population. Other problems could include that the key informants might be:

- uninformed of the views of the whole community

- subjective or self-focused and unable to see the wider community interests

- biased or prejudiced

- emotive and incapable of rigorous or rational analysis because the issues being addressed are too personal.

Despite these potential problems, there are still benefits associated with engaging with community leaders as representatives of the community in top–down alliances. When decisions are being taken in relation to the public health needs of the community, community leaders can offer a contrasting perspective to the views of the professionals. These contrasting views can result in the generation of more creative solutions to public health problems. The application of common sense and important understanding and expertise, which laypersons representing a community perspective can bring to consultations, can act as a form of 'reality check' (Burton, 2003).

In order to ensure that consultation with and fuller participation by either key informants or the wider community are undertaken appropriately and effectively, public health practitioners need to understand what constitutes good practice in relation to participatory approaches. This is the subject of the next section.

9.3 Good practice in developing alliances

With the renewed emphasis on community participation, a number of agencies have developed good practice guidelines for forming and sustaining alliance partnerships with communities. Many of these guidelines address the different levels of power that partners hold. Earlier chapters have shown how community members can be marginalised by the larger organisations or professionals involved in partnerships. Such organisations or professionals can take over at the expense of local people, which can breed resentment and lack of trust. Renwal.net, a government website for neighbourhood renewal, offers a range of publications on partnership working with local communities. The guidelines outlined below are adapted from *Working in Partnership* (Renwal.net, undated), one of the toolkits available from Renwal.net. The toolkit focuses on three fundamental issues:

1   establishing responsibilities and structures

2   behaving properly

3   respecting difference.

9.3.1 Establishing responsibilities and structures

Local alliance partnerships may need to establish structures, which might involve, for example, sub-groups, forums and resource management teams. Not all partner organisations work in the same way and the cultures and habits of a statutory agency will be different from those of a small voluntary organisation or community group. Protocols need to be established so that everyone knows the ways in which the alliance partnership is to be conducted.

Roles and responsibilities need to be identified, and the relationship between members and the different roles that members might play need to be established at the outset. In order to ensure that the partnership is conducted in an open, consistent and clear way, and so that everyone knows what is happening, it is important to have rules about procedures: about who does what and when they do it, who has to be asked, and so on. This covers:

*   establishing a constitution (where necessary)

*   consultative, planning, operational and decision-making structures

*   roles of members (and separation of roles where necessary)

*   formal positions (leadership, chairs)

*   running successful meetings (agendas, when to speak, when to vote, time management and note taking).

9.3.2 Behaving properly

Relationships within a local alliance are influenced by the way in which people interact with each other. Setting standards for behaviour and language in order to build trust and respect is crucial. Health alliances should operate in ways that complement the philosophy of inclusion. Certain forms of language or dress, and choice of location or timing of meetings can all lead to misunderstandings and lack of trust. Trust relates to social capital and ideas about capacity building in communities. Social capital involves mutuality, sharing, joining in community organisation, and increasing cohesion within neighbourhoods. It is built when people begin to listen to each other and to behave as equals in terms of personal relations, whatever the resources or skills they bring.

To summarise, the key issues linked to behaviour in the development of health alliances through partnerships are:

- careful consideration of location, language, dress and conventions of behaviour for meetings in order to ensure inclusivity

- power relations: the need to strive for equity

- transparency: the need to ensure open lines of communication

- handling of conflict: the need to establish a protocol.

Leaders, from whatever sector, play an important function as role models. If the leaders do not behave as if they are real partners, why should anyone else do so? Leadership and how it should be exercised in alliance partnerships, and the need to build community leadership capability for partnership working, are crucial issues. In addition, since consensus and agreement is sometimes difficult to reach, there is a need for skills in handling conflicting views.

9.3.3 Respecting difference

Local alliance partnership working can bring together organisations and people who hold very different views about the community and community needs. Recognising and respecting these differences is central to successful partnerships. A range of different interests need to be engaged as a result of the differences between:

- **communities of place:** the community or communities within a particular neighbourhood

- **communities of interest:** those people who belong to different groups whose identities do not derive only from where they live, but also from their particular characteristics, histories and cultures. Communities of interest, which spread right across cities and towns, must not be forgotten. The most obvious communities of interest in relation to respecting difference include those relating to ethnicity, gender, disability, sexual orientation and age.

A key challenge is to engage minority interests and create equal partners in local health alliances. Gender may be an important explanation of different forms of behaviour. Formal partnership structures, such as LSPs, are often dominated by men, but neighbourhood-based community work is often led and supported primarily by women. Such gender imbalances reflect those at a national level, in which women are unevenly represented in the decision-making processes. Other communities of interest may also feel marginalised in partnership working, such as disabled people or people from minority ethnic groups. It is not easy to resolve many of these power issues and to facilitate the empowerment of those who are at the edge of a partnership, but it is important to try to recognise and respect the strengths that difference and variety can bring to local health alliances.

9.3.4 Steps in establishing a local health alliance partnership

Guidelines produced by the National Assembly for Wales (NAW, 1999) provide a useful checklist on setting up public health alliances. Although they refer more to establishing strategic alliances that cross more formal organisational boundaries and are top–down in ethos, they also reflect the steps that need to be taken in establishing local community bottom–up alliances. These are to:

- identify key players
- set up a steering group
- canvas other sectors (public, voluntary, private, academic and community) for support
- ensure top-level support
- bring existing partnerships into the alliance, where relevant
- train members to understand each other and the influences on health
- develop a vision of what the alliance could achieve
- undertake a review or 'audit' of health indicators and existing provision
- define respective roles and responsibilities
- draw up a strategy and plan for implementation
- set up monitoring and evaluation mechanisms.

(Adapted from NAW, 1999)

Some local health alliances may need to be formed only for a limited period, whereas others may require ongoing commitment. There are many reasons for sustaining alliances, which usually reflect the overall purpose of setting up an alliance in the first instance.

Thinking point: what might be some of the main ways of sustaining alliances?

Baldwin et al. (2005) argue that it is the perceived benefits that the representatives in an alliance receive for their efforts, both for themselves and for the community as a whole, that is crucial to sustainability. Drawing on a range of literature, Baldwin et al. identify a number of important issues related to keeping an alliance going, including the need for flexibility to allow for change and the requirement for good communication, with the use of information technology, to maintain commitment and the involvement of partners. Having an alliance co-ordinator and ensuring that there are regular reviews of ongoing work are also key factors linked to sustainability.

Despite the availability of guidelines such as those outlined above, many partnerships at a local level will prove complex to establish and difficult to sustain. What follows are three case-studies of successful local health alliances, one from Scotland, one from England and one from Wales. As you read through these, think about both the benefits and the problems encountered in each situation.

Box 9.1 Roots and Fruits: a rural project for towns and villages in East Lothian

Roots and Fruits grew out of a community conference organised by East Lothian Voluntary Organisation Network (ELVON) when local people decided there was a need to tackle food, health and poverty issues in their area. With community help, a group of volunteers bought a second-hand minibus and began delivering fruit and vegetables to rural areas, where it was sold at just above wholesale prices. In 2001, Roots and Fruits won a National Lottery Award which allowed them to purchase a £29,000 purpose-built mobile shop, specially converted to allow wheelchair access. Now a registered charity, Roots and Fruits delivers low-cost fresh fruit and vegetables and tinned foods to approximately 3,000 customers across nineteen towns and villages in East Lothian. The mobile shop is part of a wide-ranging health promotion project which also includes local food co-operatives, a community garden and deliveries to nursery schools, day centres and sheltered housing. A community development worker co-ordinates the whole project and also runs cookery classes and workshops, and regularly involves community groups in the work of the project.

The overall aim of Roots and Fruits is to promote good health among the people of East Lothian by encouraging healthier eating and providing access to good quality fruit and vegetables at an affordable price to local communities. A specific objective is to enable the community to participate in the project.

Community members can take an active part in the project by becoming volunteers or joining the management committee. The project is currently overseen by a voluntary management committee of twelve members, which includes ELVON, East Lothian NHS Board and local residents. Community involvement has helped to secure a steadily developing project. Funding comes from a range of statutory bodies and charities. However, continually tapping into short-term funding streams has proved to be time consuming and a drain on the resources. Ongoing evaluation is a further cost.

Potential continues to grow as Roots and Fruits discovers and responds to community needs. The van's weekly visits are a social occasion and, for some, the driver of the mobile shop may be the only person they see that day. The linked activities, such as the community garden, offer scope for widening the partnership to involve schools, but this potential for expansion may not be realised because it will overstretch staff capacity. Future developments are therefore reliant on a strong relationship with funders.

Roots and Fruits is perceived as a model of good local collaborative work. The NHS Board in Scotland has described it as providing 'all sorts of added value that straight contracted services would not provide, good community service, good neighbourhood stuff'. It is recognised that the project provides community education and action, and has facilitated the development of a community focus on health, food and poverty, with a growth in community-focused solutions.

(Adapted from NHS Scotland, 2004, pp. 30–1)

Roots and Fruits is an example of a bottom–up alliance that has applied community development approaches to its work, involving local residents and other partners from the beginning. This has encouraged a strong sense of community ownership and has helped the project to identify and respond to expressed needs specific to the local community. The structure involves a management committee, and the aims of the project were outlined from the start: all partners had a clear idea of what the project was set up to do, and why. However, if a community is included as an equal partner in the way illustrated here, then a degree of flexibility in the aims of the partnership is required in order to ensure that lessons are learned and any necessary changes incorporated into both the aims and ways of meeting these, so that the work continues to meet community needs.

It is clear from this case-study that flexibility is a feature of the work, with linked activities seen as a way of widening the partnership. This is particularly important for Roots and Fruits as the van's visit encourages new contact with the community, which sometimes reveals further opportunities for project development. A significant problem for sustainability of a small alliance partnership project of this type is the uncertainty of funding streams, and the need to commit resources to evaluating the work and for applying for annual funding.

Box 9.2 Grange Park Community Partnership

Grange Park is a council-built estate on the north-east side of Blackpool and sits in one of the most deprived wards in England. The estate comprises almost 1,800 dwellings, with 1940s and 1970s housing stock. The area experiences some of the worst social and economic conditions in the north-west, with high levels of multiple deprivation and social exclusion. In many ways, the community is isolated from other areas of population and employment and, as a consequence, many residents experience exclusion from labour markets and from many of the services that other communities take for granted. Car ownership is low. The key issues that characterise the community in Grange Park are:

- high levels of under-achievement and low educational attainment
- marginalisation caused by low incomes and limited access to statutory family and other support networks
- considerable barriers to employment and training
- high levels of long-term illhealth, and problems with drug and alcohol abuse
- concerns over the safety of the community.

The original local partnership was initiated from a groundswell of people who lived and worked on the estate. This grew and was picked up by the health authority and the council. A community audit was commissioned by the council, which brought together the residents' views and highlighted the long-term health issues. A community forum was established, followed by various partnerships, to address the problems identified by the audit. Health, youth and council agencies responded alongside the residents, schools, the police, and housing departments. Several consultations have taken place in the community, and the local partnership has adopted a holistic way of working. Partners want to create a safe, healthy place where people can live, work, play, shop and, above all, feel part of the community. The primary aim of all the collaborative efforts is to work to improve the quality of life of the residents and the opportunities and choices open to them.

As a result of joint working, crime rates have been considerably reduced, making the estate a safer place to live. The Fire Service offers free smoke detectors to every household, and works closely with the council's environmental action team to remove any rubbish in the streets. In May 2005, for example, ten tonnes of rubbish were removed and fires were reduced by 61 per cent.

Blocks of bedsits have been demolished and replaced by family housing. A campus has been built which consists of a health centre, a primary school, a city learning centre, a housing estate office, a family centre and a Sure Start. Home-Start and Sure Start have addressed health issues through healthy eating initiatives, including a community café, and cook-and-eat sessions. The community café was set up as a direct result of consultation with families: they wanted somewhere they could meet others. The cook-and-eat sessions were prioritised and initiated by the community, demonstrating a bottoms–up approach. Health roadshows have been run in partnership with health agencies, the Fire Service, the police, local shops, schools, and the environmental health department. Community-identified needs have resulted in the provision of a dog warden, employed to address issues concerning roaming dogs, and the setting up of a Wellbeing Centre, which includes hairdressing, beauty therapy and homeopathy.

In recognition of all the hard work carried out over the years on Grange Park, the partnership was awarded the Deputy Prime Minister's 'Sustainable Communities Award' in 2005. The Awards Panel described Grange Park as: 'An excellent example of the sustainable transformation of a deprived community. The holistic approach addresses every aspect of the estate's life, and represents a model partnership-based local authority initiative'.

(Adapted from ODPM, 2005)

Grange Park is an example of how a bottom–up approach by local people can result in their community-defined needs being linked effectively to statutory services and provision; the case-study shows both a push and a pull effect. The community-dominated objectives are being addressed alongside health and social welfare more normative, professionally driven agendas and action, demonstrating that statutory services can work in partnership with the community in ways that result in a diverse range of health needs being identified and met. Through the local alliance structures involving a community forum, local people have prioritised health-related activities that are specific to their expressed needs, such as the dog warden and the wellbeing centre. By actively engaging statutory services, the community has tapped into resources that may not otherwise have been available to them, so the problematic resource issues identified in the Roots and Fruits case-study are not as significant here. In contrast, the next case-study illustrates how statutory services can actively engage the community from a top–down standpoint in a manner that allows the community to participate in partnerships which allow local heath needs to be met effectively.

Box 9.3 Caerphilly Health Alliance

Caerphilly Borough is situated in the valleys of south-east Wales and has a population of approximately 170,000. Due to a dramatic decline in the traditional heavy industries of coal and iron, the 1980s saw a rise in unemployment to some of the highest levels in the UK. In several parts of the borough, the combination of unemployment, poor health, and environmental and social problems has led to a spiral of decline. Caerphilly Borough Health Alliance has been in existence since 1999, following the publication of *Developing Local Health Alliances* by the National Assembly for Wales (NAW, 1999). Membership, representation and structure for the Alliance were originally agreed at a multi-agency partnership conference during which it was decided to concentrate on five priority health areas in a number of key settings. These priority areas were nutrition, physical activity, tobacco control, sexual health, and injury prevention, and the original target settings were schools and workplaces. Since 1999, the work of the Health Alliance has been supported by a co-ordinator, together with a team focused on specific areas of work, such as the Healthy Schools Scheme and healthy workplaces. In 2004, the Healthy Living Centre staff within the borough also joined the team. Each of the priority areas has a working group of professionals, voluntary sector and community representatives and elected members who meet on a regular basis to take forward work to address relevant issues. Each working group has developed an action plan of work programmes, which includes target areas and timescales. These programmes can involve anything from setting up food co-operatives to community-initiated action research projects.

An example of one of these programmes was recently undertaken in the Ty Sign area of the borough. In early 2005, the Community partnership approached the Health Alliance for assistance in addressing local issues around access to healthy food choices. In order to identify both the foods and the health issues involved, a company was engaged to train and support community volunteers, along with practitioners from a diverse range of backgrounds, to undertake a 'community action appraisal'. This participatory action process was undertaken over a four-month period, and, at the time of writing, an action plan is being produced to address the issues identified. The food access issues include availability, cost, cooking skills and local transport links, and the action plan includes a wide range of initiatives to address these, including a food co-operative, a community allotment and a community café.

During 2004, Health Challenge Wales (HCW, undated) was launched as a co-ordinated effort to improve health across the whole of Wales. The priorities within HCW are already reflected in the work undertaken by the Health Alliance. The development of a raft of action plans has been a major achievement of the Health Alliance: by March 2006, action plans were in place for all the priority areas and target settings. The implementation of these plans is monitored and evaluated through a range of individually tailored programmes, and the results are widely disseminated to all partners, as well as to the communities within the borough.

Resources to fund the work of the Health Alliance are pooled between the partners and include financial contributions from the Welsh Assembly Government to support the local authority's contribution to Health Challenge Wales, the council and the local health board. Other valuable resources contributed in kind by all partners include skills, time and expertise. Although the work of the Health Alliance is borough wide, all work is targeted according to the needs of the population.

(Adapted from Welsh Local Government Association, undated)

The Caerphilly Health Alliance is an example of a top–down approach which has incorporated participatory approaches effectively so that local needs can be identified and met within the wider policy agenda. Communities and other smaller local partnerships are actively involved in the alliance processes, so bottom–up initiatives can be successfully introduced, such as the food access initiative. The key element in the success of the partnership is the strong local political support for health improvement, with the Health Alliance being chaired by the leader of the local authority. Also important are a high-level commitment by senior managers of all partner organisations and the enthusiasm of all representatives involved in the work, including the community members. The problems that might arise from this relate to power imbalance, but on the positive side, with strong strategic support, there is a greater likelihood of sufficient resources to meet the community-defined needs.

Thinking point: what are the main benefits of the alliance partnerships presented in the three case-studies?

In terms of the benefits achieved, all three examples of alliance partnerships above have been able to mobilise resources and support from statutory departments, such as housing and social services. They have all generated networks between the local community groups and the statutory bodies involved. This has allowed for open exchange through different partnership structures that have broadened the base of information and increased the range of skills, ideas and approaches. In so doing, they have widened the boundaries of responsibility for health, and, through co-operation, have achieved common goals. They are also breaking down barriers by opening up a range of facilities hitherto unused by the community.

All three local alliance partnerships appear successful and are sustainable, sometimes against considerable odds, particularly to do with funding. There is a range of reasons why alliances may not be easy to sustain, as discussed earlier. They can sometimes collapse after a few meetings, are mere 'talking shops', fail to make decisions, become inward-looking and exclusive, have vague or unrealistic goals or are insensitive to different points of view. However, the three partnerships discussed here have managed to avoid all these pitfalls.

Although community involvement is recognised as a valuable approach to promoting public health at the local level (Rifkin et al., 2000), enabling the participation of local people, as described in the case-studies above, is not an easy matter. While acknowledging the importance of community participation to public health as explored here and earlier, in Chapter 7, it is important to reflect on the realties of participation in local alliance partnership working. This is discussed in the next section.

9.4 The promise of participation and collaboration

Implicit in the notion of local alliance partnership working is that the community is fully participant. As you read in Chapter 7, this process of participation is not the same as the process of consultation, where a government agency, local authority or planning group consult with members of the community on an issue that is on their agenda. There is an important distinction between the processes involving information giving or consultation and those that require fuller participation or empowerment.

Although the rhetoric of community participation has become embedded in mainstream health discourses, policies and strategies, there is no universal agreement about what 'participation' means in practice and how it can be operationalised. As seen in earlier chapters, the term 'community' is also a multidimensional concept involving a complexity of horizontal and vertical relationships between people and organisations. For the purposes of the discussion in this chapter, 'community' will be used to describe a group of people who share an interest, a neighbourhood or a common set of circumstances (WHO, 2002). Similarly, there are important distinctions to be made between participation and consultation, many of which will be addressed in the following sections.

9.4.1 What is participation?

'Participation' as a term is used in many different ways to describe a process of taking part or being actively involved. There appears to be a wide range of understanding of what it means when participation applies to the community. Drawing on key literature, the WHO has defined community participation as: 'A process by which people are enabled to become actively and genuinely involved in defining the issues of concern to them, in making decisions about factors that affect their lives, in formulating and implementing policies, in planning, developing and delivering services and in taking action to achieve change' (WHO, 2002, p. 10).

Although this is a useful definition, it describes an ideal situation and fails to articulate the different levels at which participation takes place within local alliances, and what the underlying motivation for participation might be. Morgan (2001) outlines two distinct perspectives on community participation. The utilitarian perspective sees participation as a means to an end, the end being to accomplish the aims of the public health project more efficiently, effectively and cheaply. This fits the interpretation of participation as collaboration in which people voluntarily, or as a result of persuasion or incentive, agree to collaborate and contribute their labour and other resources in return for some expected benefit. The second way of perceiving participation is as an end in itself: participation used as an empowerment tool through which local communities take responsibility for diagnosing and working to solve their own health problems. These two broad perspectives are also open to interpretation. What does empowerment mean, for example, as it applies to participation? A radical view on this is that empowerment is an essential element of participation, and that only by stimulating conflict in partnership arrangements will the goal of more equitable distribution of power to the community be achieved, meaning that the community representatives may have to assert their positions and seize power (Morgan, 2001).

Participation can also be used synonymously with involvement, and it can apply to both individuals and communities. Williamson (2004) locates user involvement in the dramatic shift from passive recipient to active participant in service provision since the mid-1980s, from provider-led services to user-centred provision. This shift has been reflected in international and national policy initiatives. The policy analysis undertaken on user involvement and participation by Baggott (2005) presents a somewhat cynical perspective by suggesting that it can bolster professional and managerial power (Hogg and Williamson, 2001; Tritter et al., 2003) and also be used to legitimise decisions made by government. The important point to note is that access to decision making in health through consultation and participation does not automatically impact on decisions (Milewa, 2004). However, there are strong arguments that involvement and participation should be about influencing policy and service delivery in public health. The WHO demonstrate their commitment to real participation and involvement when arguing that:

> People, as part of the civil society, form the core of health systems. They use health services, contribute finances, are care givers and have a role in developing health policies and in shaping health systems ... the extent to which civil society actors are recognized and included in health policies and programmes, [is one] of the critical factors determining the course of public health today.
>
> (WHO, 2001, p. 3)

Participation within the community health movement is concerned to bring about change in the conditions of mainly disadvantaged communities, and is a significant approach in the neighbourhood regeneration, sustainable development and social exclusion agendas across the UK. By acting collectively, marginalised or disadvantaged groups can pool resources in order to influence the social context that may be damaging to their health and wellbeing. This might be achieved either by acting politically to bring about a change in policy or by taking direct action to bring about the necessary change. For example, people on a local housing estate might campaign to persuade the local council to provide a safe play area for young children or, alternatively, they may construct one themselves.

There is certainly a great deal of rhetoric attached to the notion of community participation, but how far is it achieved and what are the dilemmas posed? It is generally recognised that there are different degrees of participation. These are charted in Figure 9.1.

Control	Participant's action	Examples
High	Has control	Public health agency asks community to identify the problem and make all key decisions on goals and means. Willing to help community at each step to accomplish goals.
	Has delegated authority	Public health agency identifies and presents a problem to the community and asks community to make a series of decisions that can be embodied in a plan.
	Plans jointly	Public health agency presents tentative plan subject to change and open to change by those affected. Expects to modify plan at least slightly and perhaps more subsequently.
	Advises	Public health agency presents a plan and invites questions. Prepared to change plan only if absolutely necessary.
	Is consulted	Public health agency tries to promote a plan. Seeks to develop support to facilitate acceptance or give sufficient sanction to plan so that administrative compliance can be expected.
	Receives information	Public health agency makes plan and announces it. Community is convened for informational purposes. Compliance is expected.
Low	None	Community told nothing.

Figure 9.1   A ladder of community participation: degree of participation, participant's action and illustrative modes of achieving it (Source: adapted from WHO, 2002, p. 14, Figure 1)

The ladder metaphor has been used in many works on participation. It has proved useful in clarifying the difference between active engagement and passive information sharing, with the top rung of the ladder denoting community empowerment and the bottom rungs reflecting tokenism and community manipulation. There are, however, a number of drawbacks to the ladder metaphor, one of which is that it is easy to interpret it as hierarchical and to assume that, on all occasions, one should strive to be at the top of the ladder. Kimmerling (1999, in WHO, 2002) and Burton (2003) make a case for realism and pragmatism and the acceptance that it is not always appropriate, desirable or possible to aim for the upper rungs of the ladder in some local alliance partnership arrangements. In interpreting the different levels at which communities can be involved, the ladder has given way to a wheel metaphor (see Figure 9.2), which moves clockwise from minimal communication in the information mode to entrusted control in the empowerment mode.

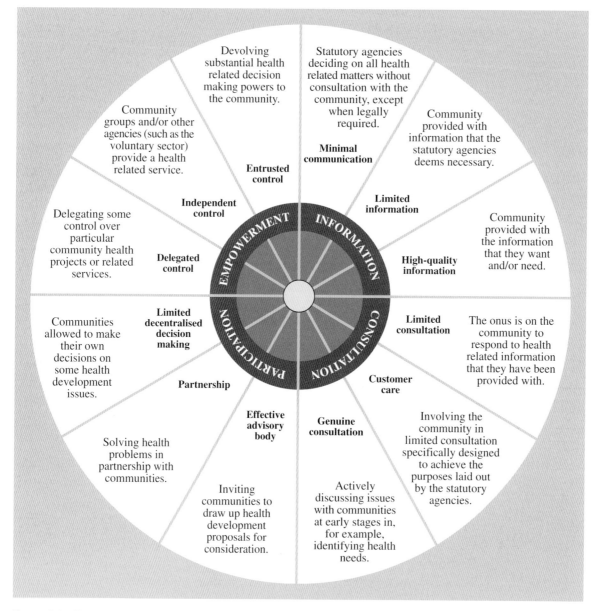

Figure 9.2   The wheel of participation (Source: adapted from WHO, 2002; Davidson, 1998)

Achieving the high degree of participation required for local partnership and the types of delegated control found in the empowerment section of the wheel might be threatening to some professionals, who may resist the implicit transference of knowledge and power. The challenge for both professionals and communities is to find a means to move up the ladder of participation or around the wheel of participation, finding new tools and techniques that promote active, balanced and genuine involvement and empowerment, rather than settling for the more passive processes of providing information and consultation (WHO, 2002).

The top of the ladder and the left-hand, top sections of the wheel of participation would describe the level of participation that would represent a more community-dominant partnership as opposed to a professionally dominated partnership. Figure 9.3 outlines the differences between professional and community dominated partnerships. When the community is dominant, this is reflected in a greater emphasis on community autonomy, inclusivity and flexibility. In any one community there are likely to be local alliance partnerships that span a spectrum of power, from professional to community dominant.

Figure 9.3   Spectrum of community-professional partnerships (Source: adapted from Krieger and Ciske, 2000, p. 2, Table 1)

Feature	Professional dominated (top–down alliances)	Negotiated partnership	Community dominated (bottom–up alliances)
Identification of health problem/need/issue	Defined by professionals	Defined jointly	Defined by community
Partnership goals	Narrow, predefined	Broad, predefined but flexible goals that can be modified	Broad, may change during process
Community definition	Population with a health problem	Combined	Existing social/identity networks
Leadership	Professional elites	Community as senior partner	Emphasis on grass-roots leadership development
Participants	Limited, exclusive, selected by professionals	Joint selection, open to additions	Open, inclusive, self-selected
Organisation	Structured and linear	Mixed	Flexible and fluid
Decision making	Agency/professional	Joint/negotiated	Community decides
Accountability	Hierarchical	Shared	Community

Thinking point: what factors might influence whether the local alliance partnership is community dominant or dominated by professionals?

The level and type of community involvement in local health alliances will be influenced by a number of factors, including the nature of the community, the motivation of professionals for engaging the community in participatory approaches, and whether the issue or problem has been identified by the community, which has then mobilised support (such as the partnership examples in Boxes 9.1 and 9.2). Resources that are available, including time, will also be a determining factor. Figure 9.4 indicates the type of questions that might be posed by professionals before initiating a participatory approach with the community.

Figure 9.4   Determining the level of community participation in local alliances: a checklist of questions (Source: adapted from WHO, 2002, p. 22)

Question	
What is the motivation for and the focus of the community participation?	Why are you engaging in community participation? Are you viewing participation as a means or an end? Do you want to hear stakeholders' views on a particular issue or on a specific planning proposal? Do you want to review service delivery? Do you want to identify community concerns and agree on an action plan for health? Different levels of participation are needed for different purposes.
Who is the community?	What is the nature of the community itself? Is your focus a specific geographical neighbourhood, a particular population group, the whole local authority population or a range of community stakeholders?
What level of participation is appropriate?	Community participation can operate at several different levels, as indicated by the ladder and wheel of participation discussed above.
How important are quantity and quality?	Are a small number of community representative stakeholders best for the participatory process, perhaps drawn through community or voluntary agencies, or would legitimacy best be achieved through participation of large numbers of the community – stakeholder rather than broadly based public participation?
How much time and other resources are available?	Community participation is resource intensive.

Another dilemma, raised earlier in this chapter, is the question of who gets to participate. Communities do not necessarily speak with one voice. Some interest groups can be dominant and serve to exclude others. Traditionally, the better educated middle-class elements in the community have the confidence and skills to ensure that their voices are heard. With the rhetoric of participation and public involvement clearly holding sway, attention must focus on obstacles to greater involvement (Burton, 2003). The non-participation of certain groups can fuel the view that their difficulties are to do with their own inadequacies. It is essential to discriminate positively to encourage those who are least likely to participate, such as poor and disadvantaged groups in society. This might involve the allocation of resources such as crèche facilities, travelling expenses, capacity building, and training and administrative help.

At its worst, participation can be little more than a window-dressing activity that gives the impression of open and democratic decision making. It is important to try to increase people's active and authentic involvement and use this to:

- enable active and positive communication from the bottom up
- determine people's experiences of services
- change or improve services or strategies as a result of what users want, to meet users' needs
- empower individuals and communities
- encourage citizenship and democracy
- achieve better health outcomes for communities.

(Adapted from Tritter, 2004)

At the heart of both the problems and the possibilities of involvement and participation lies the issue of power and control over the decision-making processes. Much of the rhetoric of community participation is concerned with empowerment. As with the terms 'participation' and 'consultation', the concept of empowerment was first touched on in earlier chapters. However, here it is examined in greater depth because of its pivotal role in local health alliance partnership working. So, what is actually meant by 'empowerment' and is it a realistic goal for community participation?

9.5 Community empowerment

At a very basic level, empowerment involves gaining power, either by being given it or by taking it. Empowerment works by raising awareness of the ways in which power is exerted, so in order to understand empowerment it is important to understand the nature of power (Laverack, 2004). Coercion as a form of control by those in power over those with no power is overt and explicit, whereas maintaining power by consent is much more subtle, involving as it can the potential for people to collude in their own subordination.

Local alliance partnerships are not usually of equals (Coulson, 2005). The effect of this can be unequal power relationships between professionals and community representatives and groups, with those holding the power having control over both the problem posing and the problem solving. In order for people to participate in the decision-making processes that affect their health, there has to be some shift in that unequal balance of power, with power being shared equitably. Laverack (2004) points to empowerment of communities as both a process and an outcome, and to the overlap between community empowerment and other concepts and processes such as community capacity building and community capital. The important point being made is that participants in alliance partnerships can gain power as a result of a change in control over the decisions that influence their lives. It is the participants themselves who achieve these outcomes by seizing or gaining power through a process of identifying problems and then implementing actions to solve them (Laverack, 2001).

In order to participate, communities need access to the political structures, organisations and institutions that affect their lives, and the creation of health alliances is part of the process. Characteristics of participation in empowering programmes have been identified by Laverack (2004) and can be adapted for use as a checklist for identifying those local health alliances that are empowering. The characteristics are:

- A strong participant base exists, involving all stakeholders, including marginalised groups, but sensitive to the cultural and social context.
- Participants are involved in defining need, solutions and actions.
- Participants are involved in decision-making mechanisms, including planning, delivery and evaluation of programmes and services, and also in policy development.
- Participation goes beyond the benefits and activities of the specific local alliance partnership and extends to broader issues.
- Mechanisms exist which allow for the free flow of information between the different stakeholders.
- Community representatives are appointed by its members

In addition to these, it must be remembered that building capacity and capability is crucial in empowering communities so that they can participate fully. This will include developing personal skills and understanding, and enabling participation through the provision of resources and practical support.

Achieving community empowerment through participation, consultation and partnership is perhaps more difficult than the advice above might suggest. In 2003, the Scottish project that developed the National Standards for Community Engagement (see Communities Scotland, 2007) provided evidence that showed that community participants frequently perceive a substantial gap between the rhetoric of community participation and empowerment and the realities in their communities. This applied equally to neighbourhood and to interest/theme-based communities. Areas that frequently elicited negative comment included:

- unrealistic timescales for community consultation

- narrowness of the scope offered for influence on policy and practice

- lack of openness in providing access to relevant information

- over-formalised participation procedures and unnecessary use of complex language and jargon

- lack of adequate investment in capacity building for agency staff and elected members to develop the skills to practise in a community-responsive manner

- lack of consistent investment in capacity building and mentoring support for community representatives and community-led initiatives

- triumphs of presentation about participation over genuinely effective practice

- political and administrative paternalism

- political cronyism

- lack of clear constitutional arrangements in partnerships that regulate the powers, roles and remits of partners

- lack of willingness to put in place procedures to manage the inherent risks involved in the pursuit of more effective solutions to community needs: for example, transfer of assets to community control, and community-led service provision.

It is hoped that the National Standards will go some way towards addressing these issues, by the production of best practice guidelines.

Conclusion

This chapter has made two fundamentally important points. The first is that developing and sustaining local health alliances through partnerships, participation and collaboration presents all those involved with a set of significant challenges. The second is that the increased emphasis on the involvement of communities and service users in policy, planning and service delivery, and in defining their own health needs, is regarded as providing a wide range of benefits. It is therefore perhaps pertinent to end by acknowledging the complexity of alliances involving community participation, and to paraphrase Morgan (2001) who describes participation as at once alluring and challenging, promising and vexing, necessary and elusive. All involved should enter into local public health alliance working with a realistic view of the challenges, vexations and intangible elements to be confronted.

Acknowledgement

Thanks go to Pamela Mckinley (Roots and Fruits), Josette Rees (Grange Park Community Partnership) and Gayle Davis (Caerphilly Health Alliance) for their support and enthusiasm for the development of the health alliances case-studies.

References

Baggott, R. (2005) 'A funny thing happened on the way to the forum? Reforming patient and public involvement in the NHS in England', *Public Administration*, vol. 83, no. 3, pp. 533–51.

Baldwin, L., Abernethy, P. and Roberts, L. (2005) 'Forming, managing and sustaining alliances for health promotion', *Health Promotion Journal of Australia*, vol. 16, no. 2, pp. 138–43.

Burton, P. (2003) *Community Involvement in Neighbourhood Regeneration: Stairway to Heaven or Road to Nowhere?* [online], http://www.bristol.ac.uk/sps/cnrpaperspdf/cnr13sum.pdf (Accessed 12 January 2007).

Communities Scotland (2007) [online], http://www.communitiesscotland.gov.uk (Accessed 12 January 2007).

Coulson, A. (2005) 'A plague on all partnerships: theory and practice in regeneration', *International Journal of Public Sector Management*, vol. 18, no. 2, pp. 151–63.

Davidson, S. (1998) 'Spinning the wheel', *Planning*, 1262, pp. 14–15.

Department for Environment, Transport and Regions (DETR) (2001) *Local Strategic Partnerships: Government Guidelines*, London, The Stationery Office.

Department of Health (DoH) (1992) *The Health of the Nation*, London, HMSO.

Department of Health (DoH) (1999) *Saving Lives: Our Healthier Nation*, London, The Stationery Office.

Department of Health (DoH) (2004a) *Choosing Health: Making Healthy Choices Easier*, London, The Stationery Office.

Department of Health (DoH) (2004b) *Making Partnerships Work for Patients, Carers and Service Users: A Strategic Agreement Between the Department of Health, the NHS and the Voluntary and Community Sector*, London, The Stationery Office.

Department of Health (DoH) (2004c) *The NHS Improvement Plan: Putting People at the Heart of Public Services*, London, The Stationery Office.

Department of Health (DoH) (2005) *Creating Healthier Communities: A Resource Pack for Local Partnerships*, London, The Stationery Office.

Department of Transport (DoT) (2003) *Evaluation of Local Strategic Partnerships: Report of a Survey of All English LSPs*, London, The Stationery Office.

East Renfrewshire Health Connect (2007) [online], http://www.eastrenfrewshire.gov.uk/healthconnect (Accessed 12 January 2007).

Entwistle, T. (2006) 'The distinctiveness of the Welsh partnership agenda', *International Journal of Public Sector Management*, vol. 19, no. 3, pp. 228–37.

Falconer, P.K. and McLaughlin, K. (2000) 'Public–private partnerships and the "New Labour" government in Britain' in Osbourne (ed.) (2000).

Health Challenge Wales (HCW) (undated) [online], http://www.new.wales.gov.uk (Accessed 18 February 2007).

HM Treasury (2004) *Voluntary and Community Sector Review 2004: Working Together, Better Together*, London, HM Treasury.

Hogg, C. and Williamson, C. (2001) 'Whose interests do lay people represent? Towards an understanding of the role of lay people as members of committees', *Health Expectations*, vol. 4, no. 1, pp. 2–9.

Huxham, C. and Vangen, S. (2000) 'What makes partnership work?' in Osbourne (ed.) (2000).

Krieger, J. and Ciske, S. (2000) 'The community as a full partner in public health initiatives', *Washington Public Health*, vol. 17, Fall, P. 2.

Laverack, G. (2001) 'An identification and interpretation of the organizational aspects of community empowerment, *Community Development Journal*, vol. 36, no. 2, pp. 40–52.

Laverack, G. (2004) *Health Promotion Practice: Power and Empowerment*, London, Sage.

Milewa, T. (2004) 'Local participatory democracy in Britain's health service: innovation or fragmentation of universal citizenship?', *Social Policy and Administration*, vol. 38, no. 3, pp. 240–52.

Morgan, L.M. (2001) 'Community participation in health: perpetual allure, persistent challenge', *Health Policy and Planning*, vol. 16, no. 3, pp. 221–30.

National Assembly for Wales (NAW) (1999) *Better Health Better Wales: Developing Local Health Alliances*, Cardiff, National Assembly for Wales.

National Assembly for Wales (NAW) (2001) *Improving Health in Wales: A Plan for the NHS with its Partners*, Cardiff, National Assembly for Wales.

National Health Service Executive (NHSE) (1999) *Patient and Public Involvement in the New NHS*, London, National Health Service Executive.

Neighbourhood Renewal Unit (2007) [online], http://www.neighbourhood.gov.uk (Accessed 12 January 2007).

NHS Scotland (2004) *Community Mobile Food Initiatives: Case Studies of Two Community Operated Mobile Food Initiatives (Report)* [online], http://www.phis.org.uk/hahp/key.asp?itemid=171 (Accessed 3 November 2005).

Office of the Deputy Prime Minster (ODPM) (2005) *Summit 2005: Delivering Sustainable Communities*, London, Office of the Deputy Prime Minster.

Osbourne, S.P. (ed.) (2000) *Public–Private Partnerships: Theory and Practice in International Perspectives*, London, Routledge.

Renwal.net (undated) *Working in Partnership* [online], http://www.renewal.net/ (Accessed 12 January 2007).

Rifkin, S.B., Lewando-Hundt, G. and Draper, A.K. (2000) *Participatory Approaches in Health Promotion and Health Planning: A Literature Review*, London, Health Development Agency.

Social Exclusion Unit (SEU) (2001) *A New Commitment to Neighbourhood Renewal: National Strategy Action Plan. A Report by the Social Exclusion Unit*, London, HMSO.

Tritter, J. (2004) '"Hands on": developing an effective approach to user involvement', Notes from Making Research Count Workshop, University of Warwick in association with Coventry University, 23 January [online], http://www2.warwick.ac.uk/fac/soc/shss/mrc/userinvolvement/tritter/notes/ (Accessed 17 May 2006).

Tritter, J., Daykin, N., Sanidas, N., Barely, V., Evans, S., McNeil, J., Palmer, N., Rimmer, J. and Turton, P. (2003) 'Divided care and the Third Way: user involvement in statutory and voluntary sector cancer services', *Sociology of Health and Illness*, vol. 25, no. 5, pp. 429–56.

Walker, R. (2002) 'Collaboration and alliances: a workforce development agenda for primary care', *Health Promotion Journal of Australia*, vol. 13, no. 1, pp. 60–4.

Welsh Local Government Association (undated) [online], http://new.wales.gov.uk/ (Accessed 1 March 2006).

Williamson, T. (2004) 'User involvement – a contemporary overview', *Mental Health Review*, vol. 9, no. 1, pp. 6–13.

World Health Organization (WHO) (1978) *Declaration of Alma Ata: International Conference on Primary Health Care*, Geneva, World Health Organization.

World Health Organization (WHO) (1986) *Ottawa Charter for Health Promotion*, Ottawa, World Health Organization.

World Health Organization (WHO) (2001) *Strategic Alliances: The Role of Civil Society in Health*, Geneva, World Health Organization.

World Health Organization (WHO) (2002) *Community Participation in Local Health and Sustainable Development: Approaches and Techniques*, European Sustainable Development and Health Series: 4, Geneva, World Health Organization.

World Health Organization (WHO) (2005) *The Bangkok Charter*, Geneva, World Health Organization.

Chapter 10

Working with communities to promote public health

Stephen Handsley and Moyra Sidell, incorporating previously published material from Pat Thornley (2002)

Introduction

Previous chapters have discussed how contemporary public health is perceived to be dedicated to a community-orientated and participatory approach, with the premise that community-based activities are essential to sound practice and research. Central to this process is the role played by the multidisciplinary public health workforce.

Given the English Government's rapid reform of the National Health Service (NHS) in 2006, it was envisaged that those working in the field would experience significant changes in the way in which they engage with communities at a local level. The English White Paper *Our Health, Our Care, Our Say: A New Direction for Community Services* (2006) outlined a twenty-first century vision in which NHS services, along with social care and primary healthcare services, were embedded in communities in which public health practitioners play a fundamental role (DoH, 2006, p. 19).

It is likely, however, that public health practitioners of the future will be found increasingly outside the institutional setting of the NHS: for example, in locally based projects. This has profound implications for the multidisciplinary public health workforce, which needs to embrace community development approaches in order to engage appropriately with the communities they serve. Whatever the setting, the role of the public health practitioner is changing rapidly.

This chapter explores some of these changes and focuses on the need for many multidisciplinary public health practitioners to adopt community development approaches to working with communities. Thus, the chapter begins by exploring the changing role of the multidisciplinary public health worker before focusing, in Sections 10.2 and 10.3, on a community development approach in order to explore the skills needed to work effectively with communities. Section 10.4 emphasises the importance of communication skills in engaging with communities in participatory ways.

Section 10.5 then brings the chapter to a close by looking at some of the ways in which community interventions and initiatives might be consolidated or sustained, and some of the difficulties and constraints of achieving this.

10.1 Making it happen: delivering multidisciplinary public health

Given that health is now thought to be 'everybody's business', the delivery of multidisciplinary public health does not fall simply to specialists in public health; rather, a much broader range of people and professionals are involved in the process and practice of public health.

10.1.1 From a specialist to a multidisciplinary public health workforce

For years, lead positions in public health have been restricted to those with a medical background. Indeed, some argue that it is almost impossible for individuals to be accredited as specialists in public health without medical training (McPherson, 2001). This fact is, as Hunter and Sengupta point out, similarly and symbolically represented through the professional bodies associated with public health: 'While the symbolic decision by the UK's Faculty of Public Health Medicine to drop "Medicine" from its title has been encouraging, its link with the Royal College of Physicians remains unchanged' (Hunter and Sengupta, 2004, p. 1). However, much work has gone into the development of a system of recognition, training and development both for specialists in public health and other public health workers from all professional backgrounds. As Wanless argues:

> Many organisations have roles in the delivery of public health and many individuals, carrying out a broad range of tasks, are part of the wider public health workforce. The Specialist public health workforce is an essential, but small, component of the public health function and to achieve greatest impact they must engage with and harness the resources of contributors across all sectors.
>
> (Wanless, 2004, p. 39)

The introduction in 2003 of the UK Voluntary Register for Public Health Specialists – a professional organisation designed to promote public confidence in specialist public health practice in the UK – has since seen specialists in public health from a variety of backgrounds, usually other than medicine, who have not in the past found an appropriate regulatory organisation, become part of their own body: a body that offers them a common core of knowledge, skills and experience. So, just who is this multidisciplinary public health workforce and what is their role?

10.1.2 The ever-changing roles and responsibilities of the community-based multidisciplinary public health worker

Given the ever-changing landscape of public health, it is important to appreciate the implication for the public health workforce. Beaglehole and Dal Poz see the public health workforce as:

> those primarily involved in protecting and promoting the health of whole or specific populations (as distinct from activities directed to the care of individuals) [Rotem et al., 1995]. The public health workforce is characterized by its diversity and its complexity and includes people from a wide range of occupational backgrounds – for example, physicians, nurses, health managers, occupational health and safety personnel, health economists, environmental health specialists, health promotion specialists and community development workers. The public health workforce is trained in a variety of institutional settings.
>
> (Beaglehole and Dal Poz, 2003, p. 3)

Thinking point: consider the types of role in which multidisciplinary public health is now practised.

Perhaps you immediately thought of public health practitioners as those who provide formal direct public health promotion (e.g. health visitors, public health doctors, public health specialists and health promotion practitioners). On the other hand, you might have thought of practitioners whose remit is not primarily health, but whose actions promote health indirectly (e.g. social services staff, or teachers); and lay people who provide informal and indirect health promotion (e.g. voluntary workers and peer groups).

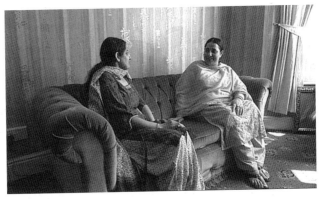

Figure 10.1   A community health development worker conducts a home visit

Although the public health practitioner's role is often difficult to summarise, in his 2001 report, *The Report of the Chief Medical Officer's Project to Strengthen the Public Health Function*, the Chief Medical Officer categorised the public health workforce into three groups:

1   public health consultants and specialists, such as those working at a strategic or senior management level

2   public health practitioners, such as those working with groups and communities as well as individuals (e.g. health visitors, environmental health officers)

3   the wider public health workforce, such as those who have a role in health improvement and reducing inequalities (e.g. teachers or social workers and the voluntary sector).

(Adapted from DoH, 2001)

A detailed categorisation of these can be found in Earle (2007).

Thus, changes in the role of community-based public health practitioners mean that these practitioners now operate in a range of settings and undertake a number of different tasks (see Figure 10.2). The statement by the Royal College of Midwives on the College's position regarding the role of the midwife in public health is testament to this change. This is given in Box 10.1.

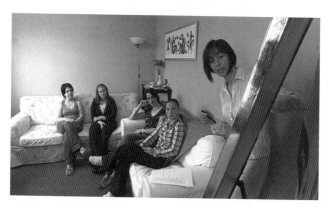

Figure 10.2   A community-based midwife offers advice on sexual health

Box 10.1 The role of the midwife in public health

Midwifery practice is rooted in public health, and for most of its history has been community-oriented. Yet the shift of management and service delivery into the acute sector has obscured midwifery's community focus and inhibited its contribution to the wider public health. It is important that midwives recognise the substantial contribution they already make to public health, working to promote the long-term wellbeing of women, their babies and their families by offering:

- Information and advice on screening and testing
- Information and advice on nutrition, exercise, and other aspects of a healthy lifestyle
- Advice on supplementation, for example with folic acid
- Support with smoking cessation
- Breastfeeding promotion and support
- Information and advice on immunisation

There is, however, considerable scope for developing the midwifery contribution to public health, through enhancing the extent of midwives' involvement in:

- Assessing the health needs of local populations through needs assessment and community profiling
- Designing, managing and evaluating maternity services with the clear aim of improving health outcomes and reducing health inequalities
- Building healthy alliances and a supportive infrastructure to provide information, resources and practical help for community development initiatives
- Engaging with local statutory and voluntary groups to work towards health-related policies and activities
- Contributing midwifery expertise and information to demographic profiling, local needs assessment, and health strategy
- Identifying groups that have particular needs, or are missing out on maternity care – such as women who are refugees, or homeless, or misusing drugs, or from minority ethnic communities – and developing services that are appropriate, acceptable and accessible to them
- Developing family-centred care, through strategies for improved parenting education, father/partner involvement, and help with domestic violence and other family problems

(Royal College of Midwives, 2001, pp. 2–3)

Thinking point: which other professional group's role has been redefined?

It is not only midwives whose role has been redefined. The UK Government's attempt to involve primary and community care services far more in addressing the social, environmental and psychological determinants of health has also seen a shift in the public health skills requirement of primary care staff. In what Sim and Mackie (2002, p. 189) refer to as 'bread and butter public health' – in short, the non-emergency, everyday public health practice that reduces health inequalities and improves health and wellbeing – the landscape for practice in multidisciplinary public health in the twenty-first century is now just as likely to be a community hall or a homeless centre as a hospital setting.

Community-based public health promotion, along with the move towards reducing health inequalities at a local level, has led many local authorities 'to create a wider "community of public health practice" – including policymakers, managers and front-line service providers within primary care, other NHS organizations, local authority services and the voluntary and community sectors' (Popay et al., 2004, p. 339). Thus, developing successful and sustainable community health promotion interventions calls for a critical understanding of the range and diversity of roles in which multidisciplinary public health is now practised. Moreover, it also requires recognition that, in many cases, in order to achieve the government's goal of improving the public's health and addressing health inequalities, the knowledge base and skills of the current public health workforce need to be broadened. For example, an audit of public health skills, carried out in 2001, found that many health visitors and school nurses experienced a lack of knowledge and key skills in areas fundamental to public health practice, including community development, partnership working, project management, team leadership, research and evaluation (HDA, 2001). Skills and competencies are the subject of the next section.

10.1.3 Achieving the vision of public health functions: skills and competencies

As touched on briefly above, while the roles and responsibilities of the twenty-first century public health practitioner are forever changing, so too are the skills required. In particular, multidisciplinary public health staff are now expected to play a key role in achieving the vision set out in the second Wanless Report (Wanless, 2004), the NHS Improvement Plan (DoH, 2004c) and the Health and Social Care Standards and Planning Framework for 2005–8 (DoH 2004b): that is, to build community capacity to understand health and help people to have control over their own health.

This same issue is flagged up in the White Paper *Choosing Health: Making Healthy Choices Easier* (DoH, 2004a), which highlights how new skills need to be developed and old-style professional boundaries broken down as a way of sharing existing skills between a wider range of public health practitioners. Such a call is, however, far from new. For instance, the need for an audit of skills within public health was mentioned as far back as 1999. In *Saving Lives: Our Healthier Nation*, the plan was to: 'make sure that the public health workforce is skilled, staffed and resourced to deal with the major task of delivering our health strategy' (DoH, 1999, paragraph 11.8). This meant ensuring that all groups of public health professionals were able to:

- manage strategic change

- act as leaders and champions of public health

- work in partnership with other agencies and individuals

- develop communities with a focus on health

- be familiar with public health concepts and use where appropriate evidence in guiding their work

- apply their professional skills and knowledge to play a part in securing the aims set out in this White Paper.

(DoH, 1999, paragraph 11.9)

Such calls for strengthening the skills base of public health practitioners were, similarly, echoed in the collaborative consultation paper *Releasing the Potential for the Public's Health*, in which it was suggested that: 'The Government should take urgent steps to build public health capacity and bring forward proposals for developing the specialist and non-specialist workforce. This should involve further attention to the development of non-medical public health career pathways' (Local Government Association et al., 2004, p. 5).

While being urged to take action, all four nations of the UK appear to agree that entry to common pathways of specialist training now exists for a diverse workforce from a wide range of backgrounds, all of whom need to achieve common recognised and validated standards of professional practice. For these reasons, the Faculty of Public Health, along with other recognised professional bodies, has created a framework based on the ten key areas of specialist practice derived in consultation with a wide variety of specialists and agreed with the four Chief Medical Officers in England, Scotland, Wales and Northern Ireland in June 2002 (Earle, 2007). These are outlined in Section 10.1.4 below.

Ensuring the implementation of public health interventions thus calls for a highly trained and skilled workforce. However, there are concerns that this has not yet been achieved. During a survey of training needs in the south-west of England, Freudenstein and Yates (2001), found evidence of a lack of key skills and training among many in the multidisciplinary public health workforce. The most recent Public Health Skills Audit (in 2001) similarly drew attention to a lack of skills needed to take a community development approach. They saw this as a challenging area, particularly for public health nurses, since it is, they argue, quite different from the individual caseload focus of their traditional roles (HDA, 2001).

How, in the twenty-first century, do these promoters and practitioners make multidisciplinary public health happen at a community level? And what skills, therefore, are required to deliver multidisciplinary public health successfully at the local level?

10.1.4 Delivering multidisciplinary public health using a community development approach

Delivering multidisciplinary public health, using a community development approach, calls for a symbiotic relationship in which professionals and lay people work together. Given that, historically, public health and health promotion have frequently operated within a top–down framework, the development of new ways of working in public health often requires fundamental changes in understandings of roles, identities and responsibilities at the level of individual workers and agencies, on the part of both community members and professionals working in the field. The ten key areas of specialist practice required of a multidisciplinary public health practitioner, mentioned in Section 10.1.3 above, can be mapped against aspects of a community development approach. The role of the public health practitioner working with communities can then be identified as shown in Figure 10.3.

Figure 10.3   Addressing public health developments (Source: adapted from HDA, 2001)

	Main areas of public health development	Contribution of a community development approach	Role of the public health practitioner
1	Surveillance and assessment of the population's health and wellbeing	Community profile	Ensure users' views form part of needs assessment
2	Protecting and promoting health and wellbeing	Many projects led by community, for example, community safety	Co-ordinate Safe Routes to School project
3	Developing quality and an evaluative culture which encourages the use of research evidence in practice and manages risk	Emphasise qualitative aspects of research	Member of steering group considering evaluating Safe Routes to School project
4	Collaborative working for health	Collaboration is part of community development principles	Ensure all stakeholders are involved
5	Developing health programmes and services and reducing inequalities	Community residents' advice as well as professionals' advice	Community safety officer

6	Policy and strategy development and implementation	Ensure community members involved	Member of steering group
7	Working with and for communities	Ensure communities drive the community project forward	Facilitator in the process, but not leader
8	Strategic leadership for health and wellbeing across all sectors	A community development approach would try to ensure that community voices are heard and are seen as equal partners at the strategic leadership level. For example, representatives of local community groups could be members of the steering group for the local health improvement programme	Community safety strategy part of health improvement programme, Health Action Zone and other partnerships
9	Research and development	Provides much valuable qualitative data: for example, narratives and vignettes (short, descriptive essays or character sketches)	Contribute to this qualitative data
10	Managing self, people and resources, and practising ethically	Values and principles of community development	Ensure they are up-to-date in their practice

This changing role of the public health practitioner is best illustrated by considering the sheer range of tasks a community health development worker might undertake during a typical week:

- identifying community issues, needs and problems
- developing new community-based programmes and resources
- evaluating and monitoring existing programmes
- enlisting the co-operation of government bodies, community organisations, and sponsors
- helping to raise public awareness on issues relevant to the community
- providing leadership and co-ordination of programmes
- acting as facilitator to promote self-help in the community
- preparing reports and policies
- networking to build contacts
- developing and agreeing strategies
- liaising with interested groups and individuals to set up new services

- mediating and negotiating with opposing parties
- recruiting and training paid and voluntary staff
- planning, attending and co-ordinating meetings and events
- overseeing the financial management of a limited budget
- fundraising
- encouraging participation in activities
- challenging inappropriate behaviour and political structures
- carrying out various administrative tasks.

(AGCAS/Graduate Prospects, 2005, p. 1)

The next two sections discuss the community development approach in more detail. Section 10.2 looks at what is involved in getting to know a community, and Section 10.3 explores what it means to engage with communities.

10.2 Working with a community development approach: planning and negotiating entry into a community

There are two main elements to planning and negotiating entry into a community, which could naturally run in parallel with each other:

1 building an initial picture and profile of the community
2 getting to know the community, both formally and informally.

10.2.1 Building an initial picture and profile of the community

As discussed in earlier chapters, assessing local need and profiling the local community is the first step towards developing a local plan. However, simply 'jumping' into the community without first considering its social, demographic and environmental make-up is likely to result in failure. Communities are not simply homogeneous, but consist of a range of social and cultural groups. People's thoughts, ideas, perceptions and needs may therefore differ.

In order to open doors, it is necessary to build up an initial picture and profile of the community. For example, part of the midwife's role discussed above is the ability to assess the particular health needs of local populations through community profiling, although it should be noted that this may not necessarily apply to the roles of all midwives. The aim of a community profile is to develop a written snapshot of the community's natural and built environment, together with the social, economic, political, cultural and religious structures of support within this. A health needs assessment can then inform local plans by looking at unmet need for services, and provide information that will allow services to be tailored to local populations.

Planning an effective strategy of entry armed with the necessary information is, therefore, an essential part of the community public health worker's role. For example, there are a number of quantitative sources – both nationally, such as the census data which gives information on a regional basis, and more locally, such as health authority and public health reports – which can help develop a picture of the community in question (see Sidell and Lloyd, 2007). Similarly, using qualitative data, such as vignettes or face-to-face interviews, provides valuable local insights into the likely impact of community-based initiatives and interventions.

Thinking point: why do you think it is important to understand the perspective of local people as well as the statistical picture?

Community profiling uses social research in a community primarily in order to listen to the voice of (often) marginalised people and then to feed that voice into an assessment of their collective needs, with a view to creating what Moran and Butler (2001, p. 60) refer to as a 'living health profile'.

A community profile draws on the following information:

- the demographic and social mix of the people – taking into account such factors as age, class, gender, ethnicity, religion and disability
- the housing available to them in the area
- access to jobs, training and income in, and accessible from, the area
- public services and facilities, schools, colleges, health centres, police services, etc., in the area and accessible nearby
- shops, entertainment, sport and culture in the area and nearby
- voluntary organisations and services, local associations and political parties
- family and community networks to which people contribute and on which they can call.

In assessing the health needs of a particular community, the following questions need to be asked:

- How healthy is the community?
- What does it need to be healthier?
- What does it need to stay healthy?
- What are the best ways to accomplish these goals?

An example of a community profile and needs assessment is given in Figure 10.4.

Figure 10.4   The revelations of a community profile and a needs assessment: key factors affecting health, social care and wellbeing in Powys (Source: adapted from Health Challenge Powys, 2005)

Context	Key factors
United Kingdom	Ageing population, more people living alone
	Decline in public transport, increasing cost of private transport
	Smoking, alcohol abuse – including among children – and drug misuse
Wales	Cardiovascular disease, cancer, diabetes and mental illness, obesity
Powys	Extreme rurality: large mountainous area, sparse population, agricultural dependency
	Small communities with diverse character and health and social care needs, no large towns or major shopping centres
	Breakdown of traditional communities and social support networks, accelerated by migration trends
	Vulnerable workforce: low incomes, seasonality, high self-employment, long hours of work
	Frail agricultural economy, highly vulnerable to market forces and external catastrophe: for example, foot and mouth disease
	Cost and potential inefficiency of service delivery to scattered small settlements
	Mainly 'rural deprivation' (housing deprivation, transport poverty, isolation, low income) with pockets of 'urban deprivation' (unemployment, benefits dependency) in some towns
	Transport poverty: lack of public transport; dependence on cars for work, shopping and healthcare; burden on household budgets; cars often old and in poor condition; road traffic accidents
	Added risks of isolation, food poverty and health inequality for residents without use of car (e.g. children; older people; people on low incomes; disabled people; those who are sick; and those who are the second adult in a one-car household)
	Rural stress a major influence on health and wellbeing
	Housing deprivation: poor condition of private housing stock, high house prices relative to incomes, high dependence on private rental, fuel poverty
	Lack of anonymity in small communities leads to health inequality and isolation for vulnerable groups and deters take-up of benefits. Combined with high self-employment, this tends to delay the seeking of both medical and financial advice

The regional profile given in Figure 10.4 revealed the following areas that required integrated joint action in the short and long term:

- geographical access and transport

- poverty and deprivation; in particular, child poverty

- restricted employment opportunities
- poor quality private sector housing, and other housing issues
- diet
- physical exercise and sport
- smoking
- substance misuse; in particular, alcohol misuse
- community development
- lifelong learning
- care and support for the most vulnerable groups
- caring for carers
- retaining and attracting young people back to the county
- sexual health; in particular, teenage pregnancy
- coronary heart disease, cancer, cerebrovascular disease, obesity, mental health and emotional wellbeing, accidents and diabetes.

An audit of local skills is also an important aspect of needs assessment and community profiling. There will be a need for appropriate personal and professional development for a wide range of people. This will include not just health professionals, but other professional groups involved in planning and delivering services (e.g. local authority officers, teachers, social workers, youth leaders and voluntary sector staff) and members of the public involved in needs assessment and in delivering community-based programmes.

Having carried out a provisional community profile and health needs assessment, it is necessary to get to know the community better.

10.2.2 Getting to know the community, both formally and informally

From the discussion in Chapter 9, it is clear that if communities are to be able to participate in the decision-making processes and achieve partnership ways of working, then public health practitioners need to work with the community and understand and value their needs and perspectives. This can take time and patience as well as a great deal of tact and diplomacy. Thus, the public health worker needs to be aware of the cultural and political sensitivities of the area. Burman et al. (2004) have, for example, shown how 'culture' can be a barrier in the delivery of domestic violence services.

'Networking' is a term frequently heard in community work. Basically, it is about making contacts, building trust, developing alliances, tapping into local knowledge and listening and learning from as wide a range of people within the community as possible. The following ideas have been suggested for building good networks:

1   Walk, don't ride. Always try to walk from A to B, and ensure that you visit areas that are unfamiliar to you.

2   Never pass up the opportunity to make or renew a contact (unless you are fairly sure that to do so at that point will damage another area of work).

3   Learn how to listen and notice.

4   In order to get you must give. People are prepared to give best when it is clear that they will get something in return.

(Twelvetrees, 1982, quoted in Thornley, 2002, p. 72)

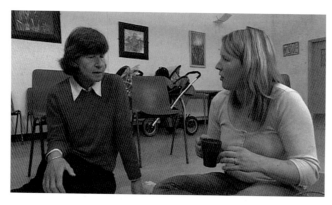

Figure 10.5   A health visitor networks with a member of the community

'Snowballing' is a useful technique in building networks. Essentially, this is about using existing contacts to suggest others who might also be contacted, who in turn are asked to suggest yet others. One of the drawbacks of this technique is that one could end up with only one real network based on the original person contacted. To avoid this, it is best to initiate more than one snowball. Community workers who are very unfamiliar with an area will need to immerse themselves in the community by frequenting local shopping centres, sitting in cafes or pubs and generally talking informally to as many people as possible.

Making both formal and informal contacts will allow the community worker the opportunity to talk and, more importantly, to listen to people who live and work in the community about what they think constitutes a 'healthy' person and community; what the particular health needs of their area are; whether they think that these are being met and, if not, what they think might be the solution to them; and whether they might want to be involved with future developments. In order to do this, the community worker can use a range of methods, such as one-to-one discussion, questionnaires, workshops, focus groups and public meetings.

The process of networking and building up community contacts can raise a number of dilemmas in terms of who can be said to represent the community's views and interests. As discussed in the previous chapter, at a practical level community leaders or representatives will be able to give a particular perspective or overall view, but it may not be representative of the whole community. The skill of the community worker is to recognise and understand this and to seek as many views as is practically possible. They also need to be aware of the community's existing organisational structures; and to clarify what local residents see as the boundary to their community, which may be different from the geographical one based on the electoral ward.

Other issues that may emerge are those related to what can be achieved and how this is to be done, particularly if any proposed local action is an 'intervention' based on a time-limited project. Local residents and/or community groups may have low expectations as to what may be achieved, particularly if they have had little or no resources in the past or, in their view, statutory agencies have 'failed to deliver'.

Thinking point: at the other end of the scale, what do you think might be some of the pitfalls of having high expectations?

'Unrealistic' expectations of what is achievable could eventually lead to demoralisation if timescales and outcomes do not match those expectations. However, low expectations are a more common problem. For various reasons (such as lack of self-confidence, the inaccessibility of an organisation, or institutional racism), local people may feel unable to raise with the appropriate agency the issues they feel strongly about.

In such situations the community worker would need to act as a conduit or communication channel to enable those voices to be heard and the issues put on the relevant agenda. They would also need to work with local people to develop their skills and confidence. This process of empowerment is crucial if local people are to be able to determine how they want to take action to get their needs met. The worker's role would be to enable them to develop appropriate ways of taking action, such as campaigning and lobbying, or developing activities to suit their needs. Local people would start to take action to set the agenda rather than having it set for them.

The role of the community worker is to build on initial research and contact with people living and working in the community, so that the needs identified can be expanded upon and solutions developed. The worker's overall role would be to support and facilitate that process, particularly in terms of existing organisational structures and the creation of new ones.

The next section addresses more specifically these aspects of engaging with a community.

10.3 Working with a community development approach: engaging with communities

Public health seeks to improve the population's health through measures aimed at large groups, and to complement clinical medicine's treatment of individuals by working to maximise the health of communities. As discussed above, effective public health practice depends on co-ordinated planning across a wide range of technical, medical and social disciplines. Those working in the field have a long-established tradition of responding to and managing the threats to community health posed by communicable and non-communicable diseases or dead bodies (Morgan, 2004). They have also developed expertise in tackling the broader determinants of health, including housing and regeneration initiatives, and work to promote the health of disadvantaged communities (Robinson et al., 2005). How, then, might one recognise, realise and respond to the potential of communities to promote public health?

10.3.1 Recognising, realising and responding to the potential of communities

There are no simple answers to what works in facilitating community engagement, but the local context is of central importance. A variety of techniques, methods and support has to be adopted to ensure optimal conditions for community engagement. However, as you have already read, much has been written on the skills and practices which seem generally effective in facilitating community engagement for health. Effective practices fall under the following main headings:

- identify local circumstances that may present barriers to effective community involvement (e.g. lack of transport infrastructure) and act on these

- acknowledge the diversity of local communities and develop both targeted and universal strategies to reach all members of the local community, including traditionally 'hard-to-reach' groups such as women, young people, people with a disability and members of minority ethnic groups

- budget and plan for community development, training and capacity building from the start, ideally involving the local residents in the planning process

- provide a variety of opportunities for training and support for local people and professionals

- use regular evaluation as a tool to identify barriers to community involvement and actions to address these

- establish effective ways of partnership working between statutory and non-statutory agencies and the local community.

Figure 10.6 is an illustration of one particular strategy used by Be Active Stay Active (BASA), a community-based mental health project in Scotland, to reach and engage with communities.

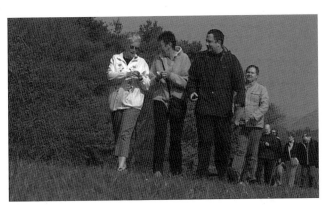

Figure 10.6   Public health practitioners are seen working with communities

The public health practitioner at a community level has a developmental role in the process of bringing together a group of people who share a common need or interest, in order to realise their hopes of taking the appropriate action to meet that need or follow that interest. Task groups or subgroups, such as a Health Action Group, can be set up to work on particular issues. Within this structure, focus groups could be organised to enable more in-depth research of the needs and solutions identified. As discussed in Chapter 8, these methods may include either a participatory action research approach or community-based participatory research, both of which favour rapid participatory appraisal techniques. This involves communities identifying and challenging their own health-related needs utilising rapid information gathering. Here, the community role is seen as critical to the development of rapid appraisal originating in the social/ community tradition. It is this feature which distinguishes this approach from the rapid epidemiological approach (which uses epidemiological and statistical methods alone for a rapid assessment) (Rifkin, 1992). Either or both of these groups could, through the composition of their membership, provide the foundations for developing a partnership between the local residents and statutory, non-statutory, voluntary and community organisations.

The setting up and development of a group to address an identified public health issue, whether it be to deal with a single issue or a variety of issues, requires the public health worker to have a range of skills to enable the group both to develop, as a cohesive force with a shared vision and common identity, and to achieve its objectives. Community development workers often seem like the glue that keeps people working together.

Realising the potential of communities calls for good organisational skills, along with the ability to manage both people and budgets. Skills in fundraising and marketing are especially useful in consolidating, sustaining and mainstreaming projects or interventions. Both community and professional members will bring different skills and experiences, together with their different commitments outside the group process. This can raise some important questions in terms of ownership and control, the development of an equitable partnership and the commitment expected from each member. This will be the case particularly for an interagency group, because its members may have differing expectations, as well as competing needs, interests and priorities. The group may also have a naturally limited lifespan because:

- it has a particular task to achieve

- it is part of a time-limited project for which the funding ceases

- there is no longer a perceived need for this particular type of group and something else might replace it.

10.3.2 Working together: prioritising needs, and agreeing and progressing solutions

Once the community worker has brought the group together, their first task will be to define its purpose, clarify and prioritise its goals, set realistic targets for action, and agree the mechanisms for monitoring and reviewing the outcomes. In the light of this, they will also need to review the group's membership in terms of the skills mix and training needs, particularly if they see the group as working towards a long-term future. This stage will form the basis for developing a framework for action which will include a timescale and timetable for meeting the agreed objectives, and a common agreement and shared understanding of the members' roles and responsibilities within this. It will also start the process of establishing effective team building and developing partnership ways of working, as well as providing opportunities for flagging up potential areas of conflict when particular dilemmas and contradictions may emerge for group members.

Central to this process will be the issue of the group achieving its objectives while building and developing the organisational structure to enable this. A prime example would be the emphasis on delivering concrete measurable outcomes as a measure of achievement.

Thinking point: what other achievements do you think should be taken into account?

Although important, quantifiable measures of concrete outcomes do not acknowledge the importance of the building of organisational structures and the empowerment of individuals and communities which this entails. It can, therefore, be difficult to translate the rhetoric (about community development and community action) into the concrete reality of achieving action and change. Thus, the community's action plan should include the development of an organisational structure to meet its particular needs and what it sees as its terms of reference. This may be done informally, agreeing the processes of recruitment/membership, decision making, communication and accountability, or more formal arrangements may be made which, as a first step, include a written constitution with agreed policies and procedures. However, the community group may also wish to seek limited company status and/or charitable status. Although this provides the group with a legal framework and also other opportunities for fundraising and income generation, it also brings additional levels of responsibility and accountability.

The process can be quite lengthy and time-consuming, demanding high levels of commitment, particularly if the group also needs to raise funds in order to support its activities. Indeed, at this point, the original purpose of the group can become subsumed under these demands, and members may become disenchanted and disillusioned as they struggle with their other various competing commitments outside the group. The community worker's skills in supporting these processes will be crucial, in terms of maintaining the impetus of the group and the commitment of its members. There is a need for perseverance, a good deal of realism and a sense of humour. The community worker will also need the ability to collect and provide information, give administrative and organisational support, and enable the group to network and liaise with other organisations so that the relevant expertise, advice and support can either be brought into or made available to the group. They may, as you read in Chapter 8, also need to resolve areas of conflict, which may be internal or external to the group. What they will certainly need is effective communication skills, which is the subject of the next section.

10.4 Communication in the engagement and consultation process

Communication is best seen as a partnership with respect for and understanding of the background, attitudes and agenda of each party. Moreover, effective communication with stakeholders generates invaluable information, insights and learning that can be used to shape services in accordance with stakeholder requirements. Poor communication, on the other hand, can often leave people feeling disillusioned and demoralised.

10.4.1 Communication skills

Communication is an everyday activity and the skills involved may seem to be quite simple. Communication skills are such a fundamental part of our everyday life that they are often taken for granted, yet there can be considerable variations in the quality of health professional communication. As communication skills are fundamental to all relationships and interactions, these are often taught in professional training courses, especially in the health field. Communications link every part, or process, of health and healthcare. In fact, for those involved in multidisciplinary public health, they are thought to sit at its core. In *Shaping the Future of Public Health: Promoting Health in the NHS*, a report aimed at public health workforce development, communication is seen as integral to the public health practitioner role: '[s]upporting people to develop health literacy and personal health skills, helping them to make informed choices. This calls for creative communication skills and partnership with appropriate, often community-based, organizations' (DoH, 2005, p. 26).

Despite such calls, according to the English White Paper *Our Health, Our Care, Our Say: A New Direction for Community Services* (DoH, 2006), only 25 per cent of NHS employees hold a basic communication qualification, a situation which, the White Paper argues, is not acceptable. As far back as 2001, the *Public Health Skills Audit* also identified communication as one of a number of public health-related skills in need of improvement (HDA, 2001).

Poor communication between health professionals and certain groups in the population is, therefore, a cause for concern. Some groups, such as older people, disabled people and those from minority ethnic backgrounds, can be disadvantaged by the poor communication skills of professional gatekeepers to health and healthcare. For example, Bryan et al. (2002) – as part of the evaluation of a one-day training package aimed at enabling care staff to communicate with older people who have a variety of communication difficulties – highlighted the need for carers to receive training to develop their own communication skills, and to enable them to communicate effectively with older people who may have a range of complex difficulties with communication. It is, therefore, important to explore the nature of communication and, in particular, to improve communication in multidisciplinary public health activities.

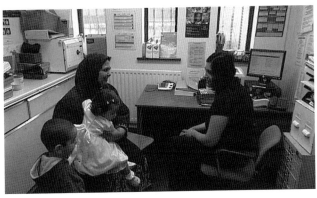

Figure 10.7 Communication skills are a major factor in delivering public health

Some may view the purpose of communicating in both public health and health promotion as conveying health messages through interventions. However, it is increasingly being acknowledged that most interactions can in some way be health enhancing, whether in a physical or a mental health context (Macleod Clark and Maben, 1998). It is the way in which communication takes place that can help to break down traditional power structures in order to foster participatory relationships where information is shared in a health-promoting way. Box 10.2 highlights some potential benefits of developing effective communication skills.

Box 10.2 Benefits of effective communication and consultation

Effective communication and consultation:

- strengthen relationships between organisations so that they understand each other's roles and responsibilities
- recognise that a two-way process means receiving as well as giving messages, listening as well as talking
- mean sharing significant changes or progress so that partner agencies are not taken by surprise
- enable the sharing of information in a language and formats that are accessible to all
- enable partners to have reasonable expectations of each other

- allow the public health professional to understand roles and boundaries in order to reduce duplication and make better use of resources

- reduce the potential for misunderstandings, disagreements and disputes

- prevent a problem from turning into a crisis

- provide a means of sharing best practice, innovative ideas and experience in specialist fields

- enable the public health professional to develop a shared vision in which everyone has clear targets towards a common goal

- enable others to contribute to the policy-making process

- value the input from participants

- lead to more realistic and robust policy that better reflects people's needs and wishes

- help in the planning, prioritising and delivery of better services

- can create a working partnership and mutual understanding with those consulted

- identify problems quickly, enabling matters to be put right early on

- help to avoid incorrect assumptions and misunderstanding at later stages

- help to keep organisations involved in and informed about policy developments, and avoid unnecessary surprises

(Adapted from Wiltshire Compact, 2005)

Although communication should be all about the exchange of ideas, there are times when this process can be extremely one-sided: for example, when the community group or the individual simply receive information from a public health professional, or when the practitioner is active and those 'receiving' the 'message' are quiet and passively listen. So it is important that any form of information giving is framed in such a way that the recipient feels valued and respected. Indeed, face-to-face communication should never be simply the one-sided conveying of information from the informed to the uninformed, but an acknowledgement of the sharing of information between equals. Good listening skills are a vital component of effective communication.

Thinking point: what other aspects of communication can make people feel valued and respected?

Non-verbal signs affect the meaning of what is being conveyed and can reveal feelings and attitudes towards others. On a positive level, non-verbal cues can demonstrate an intention to establish a good relationship with the other person, and a sensitivity to their concerns. On a negative level, however, keeping people waiting can make them feel devalued, as will being rushed, so it is important to appear to have enough time to respond to individual concerns. Eye contact is also very important. Avoidance of eye contact, for example, suggests a reluctance to become involved. Likewise, excessive gazing at the other person can be disturbing, just as much as gazing at documentation can (Inman, 1996).

From this discussion it can be seen that non-verbal and verbal communication are obviously linked, and the speed of speech, its tone, pitch and volume, along with body language, all convey feelings that contribute to whether or not people feel valued and respected.

Storytelling is another form of communication that can be used to bridge the relationship between health professionals and communities (Kim and Ball-Rokeach, 2006). For example, the rich oral traditions found in many black and minority ethnic communities can be enlisted as the principal both for transmitting important health messages and for involving the community in public health interventions. As Kim and Ball-Rokeach point out: 'When embedded in a neighborhood environment where key community storytellers encourage each other to talk about the neighborhood, individual residents are more likely to belong to their community, to have a strong sense of collective efficacy, and to participate in civic actions' (Kim and Ball-Rokeach, 2006, p. 173).

Despite the many successful communication strategies, there are sometimes barriers to effective communication.

10.4.2 Barriers to effective communication

No matter how good the communication strategy is, unfortunately barriers can and do often occur (Maguire, 2002). Effective communication with people of different cultures is especially challenging. Cultures provide people with ways of thinking, and with ways of seeing, hearing and interpreting the world. Thus, the same words can mean different things to people from different cultures, even when they talk the 'same' language. When the languages are different, and translation has to be used to communicate, the potential for misunderstandings increases.

Shashi Carter, a health development officer working for Coventry City Council's Health Development Unit, highlights some of the potential communication barriers to promoting public health:

> I'm dealing with men's health okay and within that I actually deal with refugees and asylum seekers ... I cannot categorically say that the people I deal with are from one country with the same culture, same religion, same language. So if I've got a group of women I could be dealing with somebody who is in their twenties or somebody who is sixty-five in one group ... and they could be coming from a culture who speak one or two of the Asian languages that I speak or they could be women who speak either Somalian or they speak French or Italian or Arabic ... so ... it's quite varied and I have to be able to communicate whether it's sign language, whether it's drawing pictures; whether it's just ... broken English, I have to communicate my message and try and find out what they want.
>
> (Open University, 2007)

Public health practitioners can also be viewed as a cultural, or at least a subcultural group, with its own words, language patterns and world view. It has been suggested that: 'The processing and control of knowledge by a particular group, its development of procedures for handling the lay public in those matters, and its power to manage the realities of others are all major questions which emerge from enquiry into the use of language' (Esland, 1973).

The 'power' to which Esland refers should be seen as a form of 'expert power' which is invested in the expert knowledge of the public health practitioner. This can be conveyed in the use of specialist language, which can be confusing and may sometimes be employed to exclude people or to emphasise the status of the professional. Maguire and Pitceathly (2002) advocate the careful introduction of specialised language if this is necessary, so that recipients are not confused or alienated but become well versed in understanding the terminology.

Working in collaboration with communities to promote public health, therefore, calls for recognition of the power of the professional in the communication process. Indeed, good communication and consultation will lead to better and more effective partnership working, which helps to ensure the delivery of high-quality services and improved planning that meets the needs and aspirations of local communities. Good communication is vital to the long-term sustainability of any public health intervention, although sustainability is also dependent on many other factors. These are addressed in the next section.

10.5 Consolidation and sustainability

Community public health is often project based, and much of the public health practitioner's role is therefore involved in consolidating and sustaining the project to ensure its long-term future. Consolidation refers to the period in which those involved work out their roles, territories are defined and the project either becomes stronger or weaker. Sustainability refers to the continuation and long-term viability of programmes or interventions.

There are two ways to secure the long-term future of a project: one is to secure funding to continue the project or bring it into mainstream provision, while the other is to develop a community's own resources to enable it to take over the long-term running of the project. Section 10.5.1 looks at the first of these ways; what is involved in 'letting go' and 'moving on' is then addressed in Section 10.5.2.

10.5.1 Funding and mainstreaming

Any type of project whose objective is the provision of long-term services/ activities, whether or not it complements or fills a gap in existing provision, has to be extremely creative in terms of the sustainability of these. Funding is also often a problem. For example, successful projects may collapse if funding is suddenly withdrawn at the end of a committed period, leaving the community concerned newly deprived, rather than enriched and empowered.

Given a lack of either resources or political will, in order to consolidate or sustain a health project it is often necessary to work in partnership. Despite commitments to collaborative ways of working and the promotion of public health through the empowerment of communities, it may be difficult for statutory agencies to put these into practice. One way around this is for local authorities or public health organisations to work in partnership with non-governmental organisations.

Thinking point: can you see any possible disadvantages to this?

The voluntary nature of non-governmental organisations, and the often precarious state of their funding, can mean that they also have a wide range of experience of rejection and loss. To help overcome this, an alternative approach to consolidation and sustainability is one that relies on match or co-funding for its sources of income. So, what exactly is match funding?

Match funding refers to the financial commitment put forward as a contribution to the eligible costs of a project, and can either come from private or public sources, such as central or local government or non-profit making organisations. There are two types of match funding:

1. Actual match funding

This includes hard cash and contribution of staff costs, which reflect the responsibilities of the individuals involved, and the amount of time spent on the administration of the project.

2. Match funding in kind

This refers to any service or product which is provided free of charge. It covers the donation of equipment, materials and resources. For example, where the local authority allows a community group to use a photocopier for free, providing that the match funding in kind is an eligible cost and the provider, in this case the local authority agrees to its use as match funding and can provide evidence of costs.

(Tameside Metropolitan Borough Council, 2006)

Attracting further funding, in the form of match funding, to consolidate and sustain a project often means convincing any prospective funding body that the project is worth their support in terms of time, energy and money. This may mean providing evidence in the form of, for instance, an evaluation report. Box 10.3 gives the example of St Helens Healthy Living Programme, for which match funding came from both the statutory and the voluntary sectors. This enabled the project to achieve its objective of improving the health and wellbeing of the people of St Helens. Without such a joint approach, this and similar projects might well flounder.

Box 10.3 Match funding can make a difference: St Helens Healthy Living Programme

The St Helens Healthy Living Programme is a borough-wide partnership project based within Adult Social Care and Health and managed by the Public Health Department within St Helens Primary Care Trust.

The overall aim of the programme is to make a significant ongoing contribution to the improvement of the physical and mental health, wellbeing and quality of life of people of St Helens. Based at Bold Miners Neighbourhood Centre in Parr, the project is funded until September 2007 by the New Opportunities Fund, the Neighbourhood Renewal Fund, St Helens Health Partnership and St Helens Primary Care Trust. Match funding is provided by Age Concern St Helens and St Helens Council. The project has five main cross-cutting themes:

1   **healthy living network**: promoting full and effective use of resources and information available between those organisations affiliated to the Healthy Living Network

2   **healthy active ageing:** to prevent social exclusion, to enhance health and social wellbeing of older people and to prevent deterioration in physical and mental health, to maintain independence within the community and improve quality of life

3   **increasing physical activity and wellbeing:** local people referred from local health professionals, such as GPs and cardiac nurses, are offered a structured course of physical activity and given encouragement and support to adopt a healthier lifestyle

4   **volunteering and supporting each other:** the recruitment, training and support of a network of volunteers to target people who are at risk of poor health and who, in some cases may be unlikely to use mainstream health facilities

4   **healthy eating:** developing a community food and nutrition project within schools and communities and supporting other initiatives such as Healthy Schools and the community 5 A DAY project.

(Adapted from St Helens Healthy Living Programme, 2006)

Such co-funding has been responsible for the success of Healthy Living Centres (HLCs) in the UK. Here the most common choice of partner organisation was a health organisation – perhaps unsurprisingly given the aims of the HLCs and the fact that in many cases, part of their funding or support in kind comes from this sector (see Figure 10.8). Local authorities are also a popular choice of partner, as are voluntary organisations. Given the community focus of HLCs, the other main group is community organisations – these vary, from large, well-established community-based voluntary organisations to relatively small and informal groups representing a particular sector of the community.

Figure 10.8   Type of partner by country (Source: adapted from Big Lottery Fund, 2005)

Type of partner	England (N=257)	Northern Ireland (N=19)	Scotland (N=46)	Wales (N=28)	All countries (N=350)
Health	226	16	39	25	306 (87%)
Local authority	210	11	37	24	282 (80%)
Voluntary sector	195	12	30	24	261 (74%)
Community sector	166	15	25	11	217 (62%)
Education	107	7	13	11	138 (39%)

Most HLCs have a broad mix of funding. Data shows that, overall, 193 of 330 HLCs have between three and six sources of funding, although those in Scotland, Northern Ireland and Wales have tended to have fewer partners than English HLCs (Big Lottery Fund, 2005).

While match funding from, for example, local authorities can certainly help make a difference to short-term funded projects, the onus remains on all those organisations involved in locally based health interventions to mainstream practice that is shown to be more effective than current practice. In a collaborative consultation paper, which calls for the improvement and sustainability of the public's health, the Local Government Association, the UK Public Health Association and the NHS Confederation make a number of key recommendations, one of which is that:

> the Government ensures that the barriers to mainstreaming proven effective interventions are removed – this may include commissioning research into interventions where there is a weak or insufficient evidence base to support wider roll-out. This needs to be backed up by clarification of statutory agencies' responsibilities for mainstreaming effective interventions and for monitoring progress on mainstreaming.
>
> (Local Government Association, UKPHA and
> NHS Confederation, 2004, p. 13)

However, the Health Development Agency (HDA) remains sceptical: 'After years of implementing inequalities focused initiatives, the "quick fix" mentality still means many projects are struggling to maintain funding. A long-term view to success would better facilitate mainstreaming of policy, project and practice levels' (HDA, 2005, p. 2).

What, then, can be done to ensure that effective mainstreaming decisions are made? The HDA has made a number of suggestions, some of which are strategic, others dependent on the project itself:

Strategic

- A clear understanding of the different levels of mainstreaming.

- An agreed process for mainstreaming projects.

- Named individuals (champions) to be responsible for assisting the mainstreaming process of specific projects.

- Decision-makers need to be regularly updated with progress and new evidence from projects.

- Mainstreaming decisions should be informed by project evaluations.

- The decision-making process around mainstreaming projects should begin well in advance of the funding period ending (and preferably before the original funding is allocated).

- Wide involvement of stakeholders to agree how learning from projects can be used to adapt current mainstream practice/ services.

- Organisations need to be aware of the consequences of not mainstreaming specific projects, e.g. lack of continuity, gaps in services, increased tensions between partners and communities, failure to achieve national and local targets.

- Organisations need to be willing to disinvest in current practice if new learning is shown to be more effective.

Project
- Jointly agreed aims/objectives between projects and mainstream services from the outset.

- It is important for projects to understand how their project outcomes contribute to local and national targets.

- All short-term projects need to build evaluation into their programmes to provide an evidence base about what will work, and its cost effectiveness.

- Projects need to identify learning from their work that is relevant for commissioning organisations.

- The projects need to demonstrate a positive impact on health inequalities.

- Frontline staff/communities need to have flexibility, time and money to use learning from projects to help influence strategy and service development.

(HDA, 2005, pp. 1–2)

If community health projects are to attract long-term funding, they clearly need to demonstrate their long-term value. Sound evaluation is key to this and is the subject of the next chapter. But another way to secure sustainability is to develop communities' own resources in such a way that the public health worker becomes redundant.

10.5.2 Community development or professional detachment?

Creating opportunities for community involvement and participation sits at the heart of the community development worker's role. This, as you have read, includes acting as a catalyst, energiser, facilitator and manager, and, as such, having a range of skills and the flexibility to enable them to move between these roles when the need arises. However, is there a point when this connectedness might come to an end? Does empowering communities mean having to withdraw from the role? If so, is self-sufficiency the answer? For many, in order for community development and, by definition, community action to remain a dynamic process, the community worker must be able to 'let go' and 'move on'.

Although delivering community-based multidisciplinary public health calls for a hands-on approach, the changing responses to the various needs of the community, and the consolidation of ownership and control of the project or intervention mean that it may no longer be possible or practical for the community public health practitioner to continue in their current role. Indeed, having once unlocked the potential of the community, it may be time for the community public health practitioner to 'move on'. For example, in terms of time-limited projects, exit strategies need to be devised to ensure the project's survival. The community worker(s) may, in effect, cease to be employed. Similarly, a group's organisational structure may have evolved so that it is now functioning as an independent autonomous group employing, or in the process of employing, its own staff.

However, although the discourses of development flag up the potential and possibilities of empowerment, self-determination and independence, some argue that achieving such autonomy is likely to damage projects, and that moving on would simply undo much of the valuable work that often goes into initiating and facilitating community projects (Simpson et al., 2003). In fact, for Berner and Phillips (2005), the whole community empowerment philosophy is misguided since – particularly in the case of the most disadvantaged and marginalised communities – instead of boosting self-esteem by 'letting' people take care of themselves, it simply leaves them exposed and exploited.

Much depends on the type of project and the nature of the community involved as to whether its long-term sustainability is best secured by mainstreaming or self-sufficiency. In practice, a degree of statutory support in terms of funding, as well as some form of continued support and advice from the community worker is likely to be needed. The role of the community worker, however, would need to be redefined, and the boundaries and responsibilities clearly worked out.

Conclusion

Working with communities to promote public health is a dynamic process which can provide the framework and foundations for innovatory and creative approaches. However, although community participation can be a force to influence change and, as such, presents a challenge to professional autonomy, it may be extremely difficult for communities to achieve fundamental change. Therefore, in order to maximise this potential, such enthusiasm needs to be harnessed with the skills of the twenty-first century public health workforce. These processes are fundamental to achieving improvements in the community's health status.

Bridging the gap between professionals and communities calls for ways of working which are possibly alien to their current role. Equally, the capacity-building opportunities provided by the community development worker should be accepted, acted on and valued by the community as examples of its steadfastness in tackling health inequalities and improving health. This commitment to and pursuit of a common vision maximises the resources available by effectively harnessing the skills and talents of those who live and work in the community. The synergy and reciprocal energy created by this joint vision is a far cry from the democratic deficit of previous locally based health strategies: those in which communities 'had things done to them' instead of the communities themselves instigating and influencing the agenda.

Such a change in philosophy has been helped in part by evaluation and health impact assessment techniques, which have enabled governments, local authorities, primary care trusts and other funding bodies to judge the worth, or otherwise, of projects. The next chapter looks at some of the ways in which this has been achieved.

References

Association of Graduate Careers Advisory Service (AGCAS)/Graduate Prospects (2005) *Occupational Profile: Community Development Worker* [online], http://www.prospects.ac.uk/downloads/occprofiles/profile_pdfs/B5_Community_development_worker.pdf (Accessed 18 January 2007).

Beaglehole, R. and Dal Poz, M.R. (2003) 'Public health workforce: challenges and policy issues', *Human Resources for Health*, vol. 1, no. 4 [online], http://www.human-resources-health.com/content/1/1/4 (Accessed 18 January 2007).

Berner, E. and Phillips, B. (2005) 'Left to their own devices? Community self-help between alternative development and neo-liberalism', *Community Development Journal*, vol. 40, no. 1, pp. 17–29.

Big Lottery Fund (2005) *The Evaluation of the Big Lottery Fund Healthy Living Centres*, Third Annual Report of the Bridge Consortium, London, Big Lottery Fund.

Bryan, K., Axelrod, L., Maxim, J., Bell, L. and Jordan, L. (2002) 'Working with older people with communication difficulties: an evaluation of care worker training', *Ageing and Mental Health*, vol. 6, no. 3, pp. 248–54.

Burman, E., Smailes, S.L. and Chantler, K. (2004) '"Culture" as a barrier to service provision and delivery: domestic violence services for minoritised women', *Critical Social Policy*, vol. 24, no. 3, pp. 332–57.

Department of Health (DoH) (1999) *Saving Lives: Our Healthier Nation*, London, The Stationery Office.

Department of Health (DoH) (2001) *The Report of the Chief Medical Officer's Project to Strengthen the Public Health Function*, London, The Stationery Office.

Department of Health (DoH) (2004a) *Choosing Health: Making Healthy Choices Easier*, London, The Stationery Office.

Department of Health (DoH) (2004b) *National Standards, Local Action Health and Social Care Standards and Planning Framework 2005/06–2007/08*, London, The Stationery Office.

Department of Health (DoH) (2004c) *NHS Improvement Plan 2004: Putting People at the Heart of Public Services*, London, The Stationery Office.

Department of Health (DoH) (2005*) Shaping the Future of Public Health: Promoting Health in the NHS. Project Report. The Role of Specialized Health Promotion Staff in Improving Health: Delivering 'Choosing Health' and 'Health Challenge Wales'*, London, The Stationery Office.

Department of Health (DoH) (2006) *Our Health, Our Care, Our Say: A New Direction for Community Services*, London, The Stationery Office.

Earle, S. (2007) 'Promoting public health: exploring the issues', in Earle et al. (eds) (2007).

Earle, S., Lloyd, C.E., Sidell, M. and Spurr, S. (eds) (2007) *Theory and Research in Promoting Public Health*, London, Sage/Milton Keynes, The Open University.

Esland, G. (1973) 'Language and social reality', E262 *Language and Learning*, Block 2, Milton Keynes, The Open University.

Freudenstein, U. and Yates, B. (2001) 'Public health skills in primary care in South West England – a survey of training needs, obstacles and solutions', *Public Health*, vol. 115, no. 6, pp 407–11.

Health Challenge Powys (2005) *The Powys Health, Social Care and Well-Being Strategy and Action Plan 2005–2008*, Powys, Health Challenge Wales.

Health Development Agency (HDA) (2001) *Public Health Skills Audit: Facilitator's Pack*, London, Health Development Agency.

Health Development Agency (HDA) (2005) *Briefing Paper: Tackling Health Inequalities – Learning from the East and West Midlands*, London, Health Development Agency.

Hunter, D. and Sengupta, S. (2004) Editorial, 'Building multidisciplinary public health', *Critical Public Health*, vol. 14, no. 1, pp. 1–5.

Inman, W.H. (1996) *Building the Data Warehouse* (2nd edn), New York, Wiley.

Kim, Y.C. and Ball-Rokeach, S.J. (2006) 'Civic engagement from a communication infrastructure perspective', *Communication Theory*, vol. 16, no. 2, pp. 173–97.

Local Government Association, UK Public Health Association (UKPHA) and NHS Confederation (2004) *Releasing the Potential for the Public's Health*, London, The NHS Confederation.

Macleod Clark, J. and Maben, J. (1998) 'Health promotion: perceptions of Project 2000, educated nurses', *Health Education Research*, vol. 13, no. 2, pp 185–96.

Maguire, P. and Pitceathly, C. (2002) 'Key communication skills and how to acquire them', *British Medical Journal*, vol. 325, pp. 697–700.

Maguire, T. (2002) 'Barriers to communication – how things go wrong', *The Pharmaceutical Journal*, vol. 268, pp. 246–7.

McPherson, K. (2001) 'For and against: public health does not need to be led by doctors', *British Medical Journal*, vol. 322, pp. 1593–6.

Moran, R.A. and Butler, D.S. (2001) 'Whose health profile?', *Critical Public Health*, vol. 11, no. 1, pp 59–74.

Morgan, O. (2004) 'Infectious disease risks from dead bodies following natural disasters', *Revista panamericana de salud pública*, vol. 15, no. 5, pp. 307–12.

Open University (2007) K311 *Promoting Public Health: Skills, Perspectives and Practice*, DVD, Milton Keynes, The Open University.

Popay, J., Mallinson, S., Kowarzik, U., MacKian, S., Busby, H. and Elliot, H. (2004) 'Developing public health work in local health systems', *Primary Health Care Research and Development*, vol. 5, no. 4, pp. 338–50.

Rifkin, S. (1992) 'Rapid appraisals for health; an overview', *PRA Notes*, no. 16, pp. 7–12, London, International Institute for Environment and Development.

Robinson, F., Shaw, K. and Davidson, G. (2005) 'On the side of the angels: community involvement in the governance of neighbourhood renewal', *Local Economy*, vol. 20, no. 1, pp. 13–26.

Rotem, A. et al. (1995) *The Public Health Workforce Education and Training Study: Overview of Findings*, Canberra, Australian Government Publishing Service.

Royal College of Midwives (2001) *The Midwife's Position in Public Health*, Position Paper No. 24, London, Royal College of Midwives.

Sidell, M. and Lloyd, C. (2007) 'Studying the population's health' in Earle et al. (eds) (2007).

Sim, F. and Mackie, P. (2002) Editorial, 'Bread and butter public health: when things are just important', *Public Health*, vol. 116, no. 4, pp. 189–90.

Simpson, L., Wood, L. and Daws, L. (2003) 'Community capacity building: starting with people not projects', *Community Development Journal*, vol. 38, no. 4, pp. 277–86.

St Helens Healthy Living Programme (2006) [online], http://www.sthelens.gov.uk/ (Accessed 19 June 2006).

Tameside Metropolitan Borough Council (2006) *Match Funding: What Is It? Do We Need It? How Do We Get It?* [online], http://www.tameside.gov.uk/tmbc5/matchfunding.htm (Accessed 18 January 2007).

Thornley, P. (2002) 'Working at the local level' in Jones, L., Sidell, M. and Douglas, J. (eds) *The Challenge of Promoting Health: Exploration and Action* (2nd edn), Basingstoke, Palgrave Macmillan/Milton Keynes, The Open University.

Twelvetrees, A. (1982) *Community Work*, London, Macmillan.

Wanless, D. (2004) *Securing Good Health for the Whole Population: Final Report*, London, HM Treasury.

Wiltshire Compact (2005) *Code of Practice on Communication and Consultation* [online], http:www.northwilts.gov.uk/consultation-3.pdf (Accessed 10 July 2006).

Chapter 11

Gauging the effectiveness of community-based public health projects

Stephen Handsley, Anita Noguera and Kythé Beaumont

Introduction

Given the ever-increasing push towards locating public health projects and interventions in the community, it is essential that there are ways of capturing their effectiveness. Indeed, in an era in which there is considerable pressure within the public sector to demonstrate the efficacy of all spending, there is now much emphasis on capturing what is achieved from that expenditure, along with the time and energy invested. Similarly, measuring the 'value-added' dimension, of both the public health practitioner's ability to enhance community capacity and the implementation of health interventions, is now considered fundamental to most community-based public health projects and programmes. Thus, developing frameworks for measuring either the potential or the outcome of community-based public health projects has become part of the remit of many public health practitioners. To achieve this, practitioners should possess a sound understanding of how research helps inform this process (Pearson et al., 2007).

This chapter explores some of the strategies that can be utilised to assess the effectiveness of community-based public health projects. Section 11.1 examines some of the reasons why it is important to measure the effectiveness of community action for health. Section 11.2 then considers the values underpinning evaluations of community action for health. Section 11.3 looks at the forms that such evaluations can take, the methods and methodology employed in making them, and the use made of different forms of evidence. The final section moves away from the more general ideas around evaluating community-based projects to focus on a somewhat different kind of evaluation: that of Health Impact Assessment (HIA). HIA is a way of assessing the health consequences of a policy or project that may not have health as its primary objective (HDA, 2004). In other words, rather than an evaluation of projects specifically designed to improve health, HIA is a method of evaluating any type of intervention, project or change in society that has a *potential* impact on health. Many of the principles and values underpinning HIA are the same as those underpinning the evaluation of community action more generally. Furthermore, both forms of evaluation share many methodological considerations.

11.1 Reasons for gauging the effectiveness of community-based public health projects

As you have already read in previous chapters, it is now generally accepted that the health and wellbeing of individuals, and of communities as a whole, is affected by a wide range of social and environmental issues. Proposals to make changes, of any kind, in a community could potentially greatly influence, both in the long and the short term, the health and wellbeing of those living and working in that community. For this reason, public health policy is aimed increasingly at generating a community-owned sense of health and decision making, in which the personal experiences of the target population are integral to the formulation of policy (WHO and ECHP, 1999). This is reflected in *A New Commitment to Neighbourhood Renewal: National Strategy Action Plan*, a report by the Social Exclusion Unit (SEU), which states that: 'Communities need to be listened to and the most effective interventions are those where communities are actively involved in their design and delivery, and where possible, in the driving seat' (SEU, 2001, p. 19).

Nevertheless, despite the deeply held conviction among many practitioners, community organisers, researchers and funding organisations of the intrinsic value of coalition building in multidisciplinary public health projects and programmes, there is still a strong requirement for such collaborative mechanisms to demonstrate that they are effective in changing health status. For many practitioners, this is the means by which such assessment should be carried out (Douglas et al., 2007).

According to Derek Wanless (2004, p. 15), in his report into the future cost of healthcare in England, 'there is generally little evidence about the ... effectiveness of public health'. One way of overcoming this is to employ evaluation – as Smith and Glass (1987, p. 10), state: 'Evaluation is the process of establishing value judgements based on evidence about a program or product.'

Although the terms are often used interchangeably, evaluation does not mean monitoring. Both involve measuring what has actually been achieved against what was planned (the objectives), the difference being that monitoring involves continuous measurement of progress whereas evaluation involves measurement at a given point in time. Thus, according to the Home Office Crime Reduction College:

> Evaluation is the process of assessing, at a particular point in time, whether or not a project is achieving or has achieved its objectives.
>
> Evaluation:
>
> *   provides evidence of a project's success (or failure)
> *   shows whether resources have been used cost effectively
> *   helps to avoid mistakes if the project is repeated
> *   allows improvements to be made to future work
> *   allows improvements to be made to current projects
> *   provides information for others who may want to run a similar project
> *   is an important stage in the process of accountability.
>
> Evaluation can be used to measure:
>
> *   individual projects
> *   programmes of several projects
> *   strategies.
>
> The timing of evaluation can be:
>
> *   pre-project
> *   mid-project
> *   post-project.
>
> Evaluation should form part of a project planning and management system, where evaluation measures are built in at the planning stage.
>
> (Home Office Crime Reduction College, 2002, p. 36)

11.1.1 The drive towards evaluation

The increased emphasis on evaluation derives generally, on the one hand, from the 'evidence-based' approach to policy and practice and, on the other hand, from the growing awareness of complexity in the health field (Douglas et al., 2007). Essentially, this means that we should not rely on either popular common sense or the received wisdom of the 'experts' in deciding what to do or whether or not something works. People engage in evaluation either because it is required or expected, or because they believe it is necessary and valuable.

Thinking point:　why evaluate community-based public health projects and programmes?

Hills, in a literature review of the evaluation of community-level health interventions commissioned by the Health Development Agency (HDA), identifies three key reasons for the evaluation of activities of this kind:

1　The size of these programmes has meant that they represent a major commitment of public funds, and are seen to warrant a similarly serious investment in terms of evaluation.

2　Unlike previous community-based activities, these programmes are seen as addressing major policy concerns such as social exclusion and health inequalities. Evaluations of them are therefore seen to have much greater public and political visibility, and are subject to a whole new set of pressures relating to public accountability.

3　The sheer scale of many of these community-based health interventions – for example, Health Action Zones (HAZs), Healthy Living Centres (HLCs) and Sure Start – means that they require close monitoring and evaluation in order to measure their effectiveness. This often calls for a multilayered approach which has required mechanisms for linking national and local evaluations closely together. For instance, in addition to national evaluation teams, local projects are also being encouraged to undertake their own evaluations.

(Adapted from Hills, 2004, p. 17)

Further reasons for carrying out evaluations of community-based public health projects and programmes include:

- A desire to promote the underlying philosophy of community action and prove the worth of community work in health.

- A desire to learn from experience, developing skills and understanding and informing future decision making.

- Increasing demands from funders, employers and managers of community development workers for accountability in terms of quantitative and qualitative evaluations. They need to ensure that their funding has been used wisely and as expected, and that the activity or project being evaluated is good value for money.

- A desire on the part of funders, managers and employers, as a result of pressure to meet government targets, to know the impact and outcomes of an activity. Has the activity achieved what it was meant to achieve? Have time and money been used effectively? Impact and outcome evaluations and assessments not only ask whether the activity or project achieved what it set out to do, but also identify additional or unintended consequences.

- To calculate the extent to which members of the 'target' community are interested in and affected by the way in which an activity or project actually involves and empowers them. Evaluation and assessment may ask whether and how community members' participation works.

A more long-term motive for encouraging critical evaluation of community-based public health projects is that policy makers, planners and academics could all potentially benefit from a collective body of experience that would contribute to engaging with vital questions relating to community action for health (some of which have been addressed in previous chapters in this part of the book). These include:

- Is community participation real or rhetorical?
- Can community action provoke any meaningful shift in power?
- Who initiates community action and community development projects?
- Are the projects essentially about a form of social engineering?
- Is community development more about social amelioration than radical change?
- Does the carrying out of community action and community development have more to do with enhancing the careers of health workers than with benefiting the communities concerned?

(Adapted from Baum et al., 1992, p. 14)

There is, however, often a tension between the increasing demand for evidence-based practice and the needs of local people. This is particularly relevant in relation to community-based interventions with their multiple activities addressing different aspects of health, and their community-level involvement. In fact, although evaluations may influence both policy and practice, the problem remains that, in many instances, evaluation is something that is 'done to' a community, irrespective of its needs, rather than a collaborative and equitable process undertaken with that community (Gibbon, 2002).

Fetterman (2001, p. 12) argues that, rather than using the evaluation process as a form of governance and surveillance, 'empowerment evaluation' provides opportunities for evaluators to play such diverse roles as trainers, facilitators, advocates and co-liberators. In these roles, evaluators are empowering members of the community, and other stakeholders, to carry out their own evaluations and assessments of community activities in which they are involved. Empowerment evaluation, thus, emphasises and promotes stakeholder involvement: in short, the participation of those who are affected by the project or programme.

Thinking point: can community involvement and civic engagement be evaluated?

According to an evaluation guide published by the Scottish Executive's Effective Interventions Unit (EIU) (2002), they certainly can be. The

EIU has produced a set of guidelines which looks at evaluating both community involvement and civic engagement strategies and activities, and suggests that it is possible to take a structured approach to such evaluation (community involvement and civic engagement were explained in Chapter 7; a structured approach is one that has clearly defined aims and objectives). An important distinction to be made at this stage is between the evaluation of the involvement and engagement strategy per se, and the evaluation of specific approaches or exercises that form a component part of that strategy.

This section has shown that evaluations are performed for a wide range of reasons. Nonetheless, in planning any evaluation, or assessing a completed evaluation report, it is always important to try to identify the underlying principles and values that influence the questions that are asked. You turn to these considerations in the next section.

11.2 Factors underlying the evaluation of community action for health

The discussion in the previous section explains many of the 'policy' reasons for evaluation, but these are essentially about judging the performance and economic value of an activity or project. This section considers some of the factors and principles that underpin the evaluation of community action in the broadest sense.

11.2.1 Evaluating community involvement and civic engagement strategies

Evaluation of a community engagement strategy or project is made easier if a number of factors are decided on during the strategy development stage. Ideally, a strategy will have a clarity of mission manifested in:

- a set of defined aims and objectives (what the engagement strategy expects to achieve)
- a set of defined inputs (what resources have been dedicated to community engagement)
- the process of engagement (how engagement will actually be implemented)
- a set of defined outputs (what the expected products of engagement are)
- a set of defined outcomes (what the expected effects of engagement are).

As mentioned in Section 11.1, an evaluation of a strategy will focus on whether the aims and objectives have been achieved, with a view to revising these and adjusting the strategy to be more inclusive.

A number of key principles should be taken into account in the evaluation of community engagement strategies. These are set out in a useful framework devised for the Achieving Better Community Development (ABCD) programme (see Box 11.1), which was developed as a result of a lack of systematic evaluation of community development interventions. It provides a framework for planning and learning from community development initiatives by encouraging those involved in community development to be clear about their aims, how they plan to achieve these, and how revisions can be made in light of experience.

Box 11.1 The Achieving Better Community Development (ABCD) programme

The ABCD evaluation model is based on community development principles and sets out some key considerations for evaluation, namely:

- Evaluation should be an integral part of community engagement, and should continuously inform planning and action.

- All stakeholders (including the community) should participate.

- Criteria and design should reflect the aims and objectives of all stakeholders.

- Attention should be given to evaluating the empowerment developed by communities, and the changes in the quality of community life that result.

(Adapted from EIU, 2002)

In discussing the principles that underpin evaluation, it is also important to recognise that these may be influenced by value judgements.

11.2.2 Values

The reasons for carrying out an evaluation will depend on who commissions it and their role in the activity or project in question. Funders, managers, community workers, the community itself and the different agencies involved may each have different reasons, informed by different values, expectations, interests and experiences.

Thinking point: what values might underpin the development of an evaluation of a community-based public health intervention?

Those who undertake, support, commission and use evaluations of community-based public health interventions can be generally expected to embrace the following values which, in turn, inform the chosen methodology:

- **democracy:** emphasising people's right to participate, directly or through their chosen representatives, in the formulation of policies that affect their lives; promotion of choice for individuals and communities; accessibility; working in partnership

- **equity:** working to redress the injustice that results from avoidable and unfair differences in health status between different people; equality; social inclusion

- **sustainable development:** development to meet the needs of the present without compromising future generations' ability to meet their own needs; improving the environment; promoting independence for individuals and communities

- **scientific, evidence-based practice:** ensuring that transparent, systematic and impartial processes are employed and that these are based on the best evidence available from a range of scientific disciplines and methodologies; credibility; legitimacy

- **holistic approach to health:** emphasising that health is determined by a broad range of factors from all sectors of society (known as the wider determinants of health); promotion of physical and mental wellbeing and prevention of illhealth; promotion of quality of life; promotion of social interaction.

(Adapted from Health Impact Assessment Gateway, 2006a)

Despite such a positive outlook, there are still many involved in community-based public health who view such an approach to evaluation with suspicion. For these practitioners, that a community should gain control over its affairs is not part of their agenda, and such an approach is seen simply as lacking in scientific integrity. Such opposition notwithstanding, the change of emphasis from top–down provision – based on a professionally determined health agenda – to community-based provision has meant that many public health practitioners now work according to the set of principles or values outlined above.

11.2.3 Contexts

Whenever decisions that may impact on a community's health and wellbeing are made, evaluations are invaluable tools for informing decision making at different levels and in a variety of contexts, including:

- community health profiling

- policy development and analysis

- strategy development and planning
- programme and/or project development
- commissioning or providing services
- resource allocation and capital investment
- community participation/service user involvement
- community development and planning
- preparing or assessing funding bids and obtaining sustainable funding.

(Adapted from Health Impact Assessment Gateway, 2006c)

Although evaluation as a tool might well prove invaluable, it may have to be tailored to suit the specific context. For example, the National Society for the Prevention of Cruelty to Children (NSPCC) views its evaluation service as:

> useful for organisations who want to understand whether their child protection training or training strategies:
>
> - provide value for money
>
> - develop the competence of practitioners
>
> - provide effective support for the implementation of policies and procedures
>
> - identify gaps in policies, skills and service provision
>
> - enable them to measure progress following inquiry or inspection reports.
>
> (NSPCC inform, 2006)

Economic considerations may be another factor that influences the type or level of evaluation undertaken.

11.2.4 Economic considerations

According to Byrne, in *Enabling Good Health for All*, 'Good health is not just quality of life. Good health is key to economic growth and sustainable development' (Byrne, 2004, p. 1). This fact is particularly relevant to socially and economically disadvantaged areas as it could be said to justify extra investment in all aspects of promoting public health. Population health may be considered to be an evolving capacity which results from the combined effects of social, economic and cultural factors (the so-called social determinants of health). Project, or programme, evaluation is one response to the political and economic changes that have been brought about by the impact of these social determinants of health, and which have increased the demand for accountability in the public services sector.

It is, then, essential for those responsible for improving public health, including those commissioned to carry out evaluations of community-based public health projects and programmes, to work out how the wider policy process can be developed without becoming excessively influenced by traditional public health policies and 'top–down' governmental priorities. Community-based initiatives that involve prior consultation with the members of the target community are now widely considered to be an effective way of confronting this challenge. However, in order to assess their effectiveness accurately, prior and periodic evaluations of such activities are essential, as well as adding value to the policy-making process.

Any community health promotion project or initiative that has as its objective the addressing of such issues must, therefore, be evaluated. This evaluation should address not only a project's potential impacts and outcomes (Nutbeam, 1998, 1999), but also its viability and sustainability, with a view to further promoting the wellbeing of disadvantaged communities. Since the mid-1990s, at both national and local levels, many governments have committed a substantial proportion of their budgets to promoting healthier communities and addressing widening health inequalities. However, they often fail to plan adequately for and subsequently monitor or measure the outcomes of many of these projects and their sustainability. This can result in potentially valuable, life-changing health promotion projects drawing to a premature close, primarily because their value has not been assessed and consequently recognised, at either public or policy-making level, and their long-term sustainability has consequently not been assured. This has, for example, been the case with some health projects funded by Single Regeneration Project money, which worked effectively in socially disadvantaged communities during the three years of the funding, but then closed down at the end of this time, due to mismanagement and lack of sustainable funding, leaving the affected community feeling newly 'disadvantaged' (DTLR, 2002). (The Single Regeneration Budget was set up in 1994 to provide resources to enhance the employment prospects, education and skills of local people and to tackle the needs of communities in the most deprived areas of England.)

As mentioned earlier in this section, choice of methodology is influenced by a number of different factors or values. The different forms and methods of evaluation are explored in the next section.

11.3 Forms and methods of evaluation

Addressing health inequalities in and by communities is not unlike other aspects of health policy, in so far as it is increasingly subject to severe financial constraints. The consequence is the demand, described above, for evidence-based policy, which addresses the need for all policy makers to account for and justify their expenditure. This illustrates a long-term trend in changing state–societal relations, in which results-based management and performance indicators are indispensable tools for managers and policy makers under increasing pressure to rationalise an ever-decreasing pot of social investment funding. The question that health planners and funders ultimately have to answer is therefore: what type of evidence base can be provided to convince external funding agencies of the effectiveness of the interventions being assessed?

11.3.1 Forms of evaluation

One way of thinking about the different types of evaluation is from the perspective of a temporal dimension. Some evaluations take place prior to the development and implementation of a programme. Others take place either during or near the end of a programme, as Christala Sophocleous, evaluator of the Powys Sure Start, in Wales, points out (See Box 11.2).

Box 11.2 Evaluation of Powys Sure Start

The starting point for the evaluation I think was slightly different than it might have been and that was because I was taking it on half way through the life of the project, so the projects had been up and running for a little while, or in some instances a number of years, so for me the starting point was having to develop a very quick understanding of the actual projects themselves ... so I had to do a lot of very quick learning about what they were doing and who they were doing it with. I think if evaluation had have been built in at the beginning and I'd been in at the start I think we could have tried to build the evaluation focus into projects.

(Open University, 2007)

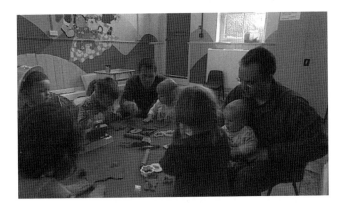

Figure 11.1   Evaluating
Powys Sure Start

Norheim (1999) illustrates how the stages of a programme's activity influence the way in which an evaluation is carried out. The key stages are summarised below.

Before

Evaluability or needs assessment is an assessment carried out prior to commencing an evaluation in order to establish whether a programme or policy can be evaluated and what might be the barriers to an effective and useful evaluation. It requires a review of the coherence and logic of a programme; clarification of data availability; and an assessment of the extent to which managers or stakeholders are likely to use evaluation findings, given their interests and the timing of any evaluation vis-à-vis future programme or policy decisions. When such activities take place prior to the development and implementation of a programme, they are primarily concerned with the systematic identification of needs or gaps in agency activities, or of client needs. A variety of methods is available, from social indicator analysis (e.g. social trends or census data) to community forums and focus groups that include community members (Sidell and Lloyd, 2007).

During

Formative evaluation: when evaluation is primarily concerned with improving a programme, it is termed 'formative'. The main purpose of formative evaluation is to identify issues and problems. Such evaluation is likely to occur during the formation or initial implementation of a programme.

After

Summative evaluation: when the primary purpose of an evaluation is to reach summary judgement of value, then the evaluation is properly termed a 'summative evaluation'. Summative evaluation may involve a decision to continue or discontinue a programme, or a decision to increase or decrease availability of resources.

11.3.2 Methods of evaluation

Methods of evaluation have changed over time. For example, the common approaches, developed during the early 1990s evaluation of community-level interventions, were largely influenced by three different traditions:

- **Experimental** and **quasi-experimental** designs
- **Participatory methods** including empowerment, stakeholder, participatory and illuminative research strategies [e.g. drawing and writing techniques]

- **Multi-method strategies** that bring together a variety of research approaches, usually incorporating considerable use of qualitative data and process indicators.

(Hills, 2004, p. 2)

According to Hills, these have proved both problematic and unpopular, at the same time failing to generate generalisable results. By contrast, more recent evaluation approaches include:

- **Theory-based** and **realistic** evaluation strategies: these challenge the lack of attention to context, programme theory and the mechanisms of change in earlier experimental and quasi-experimental approaches

- **New evaluation frameworks**: these build on earlier multi-method approaches by providing frameworks that indicate different evaluation strategies at various stages, and at different levels, in a programme or project

- New thinking about the **nature of complexity** and adoption of **socio-ecological theoretical frameworks**: these are still at an early stage of development in terms of evaluation, and have yet to be developed into fully operational evaluation strategies

- Fresh thinking in the area of **indicators and outcome measures**: provides new ways of evaluating the structural changes that arise as a result of community-based projects

- Development of **new approaches to systematic reviews** that are less dependent on experimental and quasi-experimental designs.

(Hills, 2004, p. 2)

Whatever the format of the evaluation, for many the key principles for the success of community-based evaluation include the development of trust, recognition of the importance of the knowledge and personal experiences of all stakeholders, and joint development of the evaluation agenda (Fetterman, 2001).

Thinking point: in thinking about starting to plan an evaluation, what might you need to consider?

Cockerill et al. (2000) have identified what they see as the key questions to be answered during the first stage of organising and structuring an evaluation. These, they argue, centre on the identification of stakeholders, and on the aims and objectives of the project and the extent to which there is agreement on these. They suggest that the following questions need to be discussed from the outset:

- Who are the key stakeholders, and which communities do they represent?

- What are the intended consequences or outcomes of the investigation for each stakeholder?

- What are the potential benefits of, and concerns with, the project to the individuals and institutions involved?

- Is theory development and testing an element, or a by-product, of the project, and how does this relate to other project objectives and the roles of stakeholders involved?

- Is there an action agenda, and how does this relate to other project objectives and the roles of stakeholders involved?

(Adapted from Cockerill et al., 2000)

Such an approach is designed to forge a collaborative relationship with communities: one that is in contrast to research that has historically relied exclusively on randomised controlled trial (RCT) evidence as the solution to demonstrating effectiveness (Hills and Carroll, 2004). Indeed, such recent approaches go deeper and now represent an alternative critique of the positivistic understanding of social science to the more well-known, phenomenological and constructivist critiques (Pearson et al., 2007). More 'philosophical' reflections of this type directly concern evaluators because of their implications for the way in which complex social interaction and change are theorised. In turn, such reflections influence whether public health promotion projects succeed or fail.

11.3.3 Target or process driven?

In undertaking an evaluation, practical decisions, such as whether the focus of an evaluation is to be on process or outcome, and whether the methods used are to be predominantly qualitative or quantitative, also have to be addressed (Finlay, 2007). Those who work directly in community action for health tend to favour qualitative approaches because these emphasise and explore processes, shifts in power, fulfilment of human potential, and so on. Qualitative approaches integrate the views of as many interested parties as possible, including community members, and professionals and agencies working in the community. However, the wider environment in which these workers operate tends to stress economic factors, such as value for money, and consequently requires evaluation to incorporate quantitative information and analysis relevant to these.

The current target-orientated approach to health, too, has specific, measurable aims. An example might be the measurement of the number of people attending 'Quit Smoking' groups. Where the emphasis is mainly on achieving targets, evaluation requires the identification of whether or not the targets have been met within a specific community. Process is, consequently, considered relatively unimportant. This approach might well be preferred by, for instance, a health service manager whose approach to evaluation will be predominantly centrist and bureaucratic, and who considers that evaluation is purely about demonstrating (preferably by means of rapidly assimilated tables and graphs) how well the defined targets have been met.

The process-orientated approach to health, on the other hand, gives greater value to areas of health that are less tangible in terms of numerical evidence, such as increased empowerment, better social networks and community solidarity. This approach considers that what people learn as a result of becoming involved in community action for health is no less relevant than reaching pre-set targets. Describing and analysing the process, rather than impacts and outcomes, becomes the key feature of the evaluation. As a result, the evaluation might be more acceptable to community development workers and community activists, who may take a more radical or democratic view of what evaluation should be and have as much interest in long-term benefits as short-term targets and statistical 'success'.

There has been much debate about appropriate methods, and it is generally acknowledged that there is no 'standard' way of carrying out community action for health evaluations (Douglas et al., 2001). The researcher's skill lies in selecting the right combination of methods for a *particular* policy or project. This requires balancing a method for reliably collecting essential data, and meeting other objectives of the evaluation, with the need to meet those constraints imposed by the commissioners and the context of the project under consideration. Nonetheless, methods must be chosen to complement one another and to create a holistic picture.

11.3.4 Selecting a toolkit

To date, many evaluators have developed their own 'toolkit' of methods for obtaining information. For example, an evaluation of the Inner City South Belfast Sure Start Project favoured the use of focus groups as a tool to assess what parents had gained from their involvement with the project (Field, 2003). The selection of tools and how they are applied depends on:

- the specific objectives and purpose of the evaluation
- the use to which the information is to be put
- the degree of rigour required
- the composition, skills and experience of the evaluating team

- the target audience's ethnic, cultural and religious contexts
- the resources available
- the financial and time constraints.

The evaluative approach usually adopted is based on a combination of both quantitative and qualitative methods in order to achieve the intended goal: that is, a realistic and ultimately useful report. Before embarking on any evaluation, therefore, consideration needs to be given, first, to the tools that are to be used to assess or measure the effectiveness of a programme or activity, and, second, to the likely impact of their use.

Thinking point: what might you need to take into consideration when selecting a toolkit of methods?

In selecting a toolkit, a number of key points need to be considered:

- Will the tools that you have selected address the issues of the intervention or project?
- Will the tools produce the information that you want participants to know, rather than small, irrelevant facts?
- Will the type of tool be valid? That is, will it measure what you want it to measure?
- Could the process be repeated over time? Will the data collected be consistent? That is, will the tool be reliable?
- Will the evaluation be feasible for your use? In other words, could it be relatively easily incorporated into your practice or performance, and do you have the resources to obtain and interpret the results?

If a toolkit that fits these criteria cannot be found, then one should be developed or adapted. In this case, the measure should be piloted before use.

As discussed above, in a narrow sense evaluation can involve collecting information and checking that a project has done what it set out to do, and reviewing, in the light of this, whether its objectives and approach need to be changed – in other words, the *monitoring of activities*. In the fullest sense, however, evaluation is about charting change and assessing the extent to which this is the result of project interventions or other influences – in other words, undertaking an *evaluation of outcomes*. Good practice requires not only that *what* works is explained, but also *why* it works. A good evaluation, therefore, will both monitor activities and evaluate outcomes, and the two processes will be linked: some of the information collected as part of the monitoring process will also be valid for the purposes of fuller evaluation.

11.3.5 Types of evidence

A good community action for health evaluation must ensure that different types of evidence are properly identified and analysed. However, the evidence base available to support the evaluative process may be insufficient in some areas, or difficult to locate and access. For this reason, it is important to acknowledge that researchers can make use only of the best available evidence, given the time and other resource constraints to which they are subject. Regardless of constraints, though, evidence must be collected in a methodologically rigorous manner from as many different sources as possible. That is to say, that it must be linked to the health needs and present and potential impacts and outcomes identified in the community action for health report. To this end, the input of local community members and workers is clearly essential. Many of their recommendations may be at the margins of the project or programme under consideration (i.e. they may not seem obvious). Nonetheless, they could achieve important positive impacts, both direct and indirect, in terms of addressing inequalities in health and the priority needs identified by the community itself. Such an approach to evaluation is, as Hills (2004) argues, influenced by emancipatory and participatory research traditions, which have a different epistemological base from the experimental research traditions currently favoured in the health field. As mentioned at the end of Section 11.3.2 above, these different approaches to evaluation reflect other changes that are taking place in the assumptions underlying research practice more generally.

One way to go about seeking evidence of the effectiveness of public health programmes or projects is to test the impact of a programme by using an outcomes-led approach. For Nutbeam (1998), the connection between the impact and outcomes of a policy or project and the broader health and social outcomes for the population involved in the evaluation is complex. Nutbeam provides a framework for defining the outcomes associated with health promotion activity. Within this, three broad areas of public health promotion are defined (education, social mobilisation and advocacy), which are linked in a dynamic relationship to a hierarchy of outcomes: the immediate health promotion outcomes (programme impact measures), intermediate health outcomes (modifiable determinants of health), and the desired long-term health and social outcomes (reductions in morbidity, avoidable mortality and disability, improved quality of life, functional independence, and equity) (Wimbush and Watson, 2000).

As Wimbush and Watson argue:

> Implicit in this model is the notion that changes unfold over time and that outcomes need to be differentiated on the basis of a time dimension. This model also emphasizes that public health promotion programmes often involve a diverse range of actions

aimed at different levels: for example, educational forms of action that seek change at the level of the individual; community development projects whose efforts are concerned with community empowerment and improving the quality of community life; advocacy approaches that may seek changes in environments or legislative reform. Such diversity in the range of possible actions and in the outcomes sought can make the link between public health promotion actions and eventual health outcomes complex and difficult to track. This is particularly the case where there are multiple level actions and where the time lapse between health promotion actions and outcomes is extensive.

(Wimbush and Watson, 2000, p. 36)

11.3.6 Assessing the evidence

Although based on evidence, a good community-based health evaluation goes beyond merely examining the evidence. As evidence from a variety of sources can often be mixed, contradictory or incomplete, it is important to be able to assess its significance. This involves discussion and engagement with key stakeholders at all stages of the evaluation or assessment and following the first draft of the final report. This in turn will ensure that the strengths and weaknesses identified by, and the recommendations made in, the report are grounded in a clear understanding of their different perspectives. Box 11.3 illustrates how the process works in practice.

Box 11.3 Evaluation of a new health centre pharmacy

Background – This case study describes the evaluation of a primary care intervention in the Isle of Wight, United Kingdom, arising from the decision to move a medical practice from its town location into a new health centre in a nearby village. The new centre incorporated a new community pharmacy within the practice.

Aim – To determine stakeholders' views on whether there was any perceived benefit resulting from the location of a pharmacy within the new health centre, over and above that of supply.

Method – The evaluation explored both process and outcome features by means of self-completion questionnaires with patients and semi-structured interviews with health centre staff. The first phase of the study was undertaken prior to the medical practice move into the new health centre in July, 1996, and the second phase 12 months after the move. An interim report was used to influence change by making recommendations to the health authority to provide support and resources for the new pharmacist.

Key findings – Prior to the move: three-quarters of medical practice patients surveyed expected to use the new pharmacy, and 55 per cent expected to receive a better service. The health centre staff and pharmacist were enthusiastic about the potential for service development in the pharmacy. The general practitioners (GPs) had the clearest ideas about possible additional services but there was no implementation strategy. Based on these findings, the evaluators made specific recommendations on action to be taken by the health authority. After the move: 88 per cent of patients surveyed had used the pharmacy and considered that the service was better. The perception was based on matters of convenience. Health centre staff and GPs considered that the pharmacy was providing services beyond supply and had raised awareness of prescribing issues.

Conclusion – A pharmacy located within a health centre can, given appropriate support, enhance the pharmacist's contribution to primary health care over and above supply, and provide a mechanism for developing pharmaceutical support for the prescribing function. Evaluation can help to provide insight into ways of ensuring a more satisfactory outcome following organisational change.

(Wilson et al., 2000, p. 97)

Having explored different forms and methods of evaluation in this section, the next section turns to health impact assessment (HIA) as a way of *assessing* community-based public health projects.

11.4 Using Health Impact Assessment to assess community-based public health projects

Throughout this chapter you have considered different ways of assessing the effectiveness of community-based projects designed to improve health. Health Impact Assessment (HIA) is another increasingly popular tool used to measure the *potential* impact on health of a proposed project or intervention. Specifically, HIA is used not only to help improve health and reduce health inequalities, but also, more strategically, to inform policy and programme proposals. Its primary output is a set of evidence-based recommendations geared to informing the decision-making process associated with a proposal. These recommendations aim to highlight practical ways of enhancing the positive aspects of a proposal, and of removing or minimising any negative impacts on health and inequalities (a process known as a prospective HIA) (HDA, 2004). So, what exactly is Health Impact Assessment and how does it differ from evaluation?

11.4.1 Health Impact Assessment: a different type of evaluation?

Health Impact Assessment is said to have its roots in environmental impact assessment and public health policy initiatives of the last two decades of the twentieth century (Lock, 2000; Bruce, 2002). As with an evaluation, an HIA might be used to estimate 'the effects of a specified action on the health of a defined population' (Scott-Samuel, 1998, p. 704). More specifically, HIAs can be utilised to gauge the effectiveness of many different types of community-based health projects. For example, Yazbeck et al. (2005) carried out a HIA in northern France to evaluate the health impact of boron – a naturally occurring element that is found in the form of borates in the oceans, sedimentary rocks, coal, shale, and some soils – in drinking water. By contrast, in Sweden, Finer et al. (2005) used HIA as a tool for determining how the health of different groups was affected by the proposed policy decisions taken by local policy makers. Thus, HIA is used to assess the *possible* influence on health of a *proposed* initiative.

Health Impact Assessment was established through the Gothenburg Consensus Paper (WHO and ECHP, 1999) as a process that, ideally, should be carried out as a prospective task. The Paper encouraged policy makers and funders to take into consideration any effects that their decisions might have on population health. According to the Gothenburg Consensus Paper, HIA can be defined as: 'a combination of procedures, methods and tools by which a policy, programme or project may be judged as to its potential effects on the health of a population, and the distribution of those effects within the population' (WHO and ECHP, 1999, p. 4).

Health Impact Assessment is a tool that has been developed to assess the needs, experiences and aspirations of a community designated to participate in a community health action project. It is intended to provide an opportunity for increased community participation in public policy in the target community, providing a 'bottom–up', rather than a 'top–down', approach to health improvements. HIA can also develop and/or strengthen interagency working and partnerships within the community by raising awareness not only of all the broader determinants of health, but also of the fact that all agencies working in the same community have many common interests and objectives. Similarly, HIA can potentially identify ways and means of encouraging community members to become proactive in supporting health-related initiatives, as a result of recommending that their views are instrumental in the planning and execution of these.

Thinking point: why carry out a Health Impact Assessment?

Although policies in other sectors frequently influence health, morbidity and mortality, until quite recently this fact was considered only relatively important. However, more integrated approaches to health and community development are now being adopted at national, local and regional levels. These place HIA high on the agenda of many governments and national and international organisations, such as the National Institute for Health and Clinical Excellence (NICE) in the UK, the World Bank and the World Health Organization (WHO). In research circles, too, interest in HIA has greatly increased (Scott-Samuel, 1998; Parry and Stevens, 2001; Scott-Samuel et al., 2001).

Health Impact Assessment produces a set of evidence-based recommendations in a format appropriate to decision making. In addition, the Gothenburg Consensus Paper states that it should:

- provide sustainable development
- recognise the need for different types of evidence (quantitative, qualitative, professional, expert and lay knowledge, and public opinion)
- ensure that all evidence obtained is employed in an ethical manner
- generate a sensation among the members of the community that their own experiences are what guide local policies and decision making on health matters.

In the UK, the importance of applying HIA to all public health policies has been increasingly recognised, and the government has indicated its commitment to promoting HIA in, for example, *Saving Lives: Our Healthier Nation* (DoH, 1999b) and *Tackling Health Inequalities: A Programme for Action* (DoH, 2003). Many examples of commitment to HIA at European level also exist, as the European Commission's Treaty of Amsterdam, Article 152 (European Commission, 1997) and the previously mentioned Gothenburg Consensus Paper (WHO and ECHP, 1999) indicate. In England, the Department of Health (DoH) has supported the development of HIA methodologies by establishing a cross-departmental HIA working group (DoH, 1999a).

At local level, HIA can make a valuable contribution to many areas of activity and policy, as Box 11.4 illustrates.

Box 11.4 Swansea Health Social Care and Well Being Strategy

The Swansea Health Social Care and Well Being Strategy identified the development of a local nutrition policy as a priority for preventative action. A partnership group was set up under the Swansea Children and Young People Framework to develop an initial focus on healthy eating and food health in schools, which would contribute to wider local policy development during 2006–2007. This group organised a health inequalities impact assessment consultation in the autumn of 2005.

The reason for using the impact assessment process is to improve the health of the overall population group while helping to narrow the health divide by ensuring that any intervention supports the most disadvantaged within that group. In the case of school-based nutrition and healthy eating for children and young people in Swansea, this had the potential to make a real and lasting impact on the health of that specific population. The local impact assessment and consultation – which engaged local school representatives, including headteachers, catering staff, health professionals and other key partners from organisations across Swansea – enabled a comprehensive appraisal to be made of the scale of impact that food in schools has on the health of pupils in Swansea. The perceived barriers to improving and changing practices in the school setting have been explored at local level and the opportunities for change have been summarised. The process has helped to provide clear information, to the range of stakeholders, about the relationship between good nutrition and health for children and young people in Swansea. The implications of poor eating habits, cultural influences, lack of knowledge and skills, and unsatisfactory food provision in schools have become clear.

(Adapted from WHIASU, 2006)

In view of the fact that one of the underpinning principles of HIA is to focus on health inequalities and socio-economic disadvantage, it is not surprising that many, but not *all*, HIAs in England are related to regeneration initiatives and projects designed to address social exclusion. Notable exceptions are a HIA commissioned to assess the health impacts of the development of a second runway at Manchester International Airport (Will et al., 1994), and a HIA, commissioned by Brent Council, of the new National Stadium at Wembley (Barnes et al., 2004).

According to the former NHS Health Development Agency (HDA, 2004) – now integrated with the National Institute for Health and Clinical Excellence (NICE) – HIA is also a valuable tool for local strategic partnership work in areas as diverse as:

- neighbourhood renewal
- community strategies
- tackling inequalities and social exclusion
- equity audits

- regeneration initiatives, such as Single Regeneration Budgets
- enhancing the social, economic or environmental wellbeing of communities
- fulfilling local government policies and requirements, such as those to promote health.

That the use of HIA is now a requirement under professional competencies for public health specialists is hardly surprising given that it is recommended in many national policy, programme and guidance documents, such as, for example:

- *New Deal for Transport* (DETR, 1998)
- *New Deal for Communities* (Neighbourhood Renewal Unit, 2002)
- *Coronary Heart Disease, National Service Framework* (DoH, 2000)
- *Modernising Government* (Cabinet Office, 1999)
- *Health and Neighbourhood Renewal* (DoH and Neighbourhood Renewal Unit, 2002)
- *Tackling Health Inequalities: A Programme for Action* (DoH, 2003).

Although HIA has become popular in political circles, at international, national and local levels, it is, as discussed earlier, underpinned by a number of key principles.

11.4.2 How to implement HIA: process, stages and choices

The starting point in any HIA should be analysis. A major problem, particularly in quantitative research, is that much of the data collected is not used at all. Thus, when designing and conducting research, and in order to be prudent in the use of resources, it is essential to consider for what purposes the data is being collected. Part of the tools selection process, therefore, should be to look at the data a particular tool will produce and to think about how this will be processed and analysed.

The HIA process has five main stages: these can be sequential, but may sometimes be iterative, and they can be adjusted to meet local needs. They ensure a coherent and systematic approach to HIA. The stages are:

Screening: to establish quickly whether a particular policy, programme or project is relevant to health. This may involve the use of check-lists or other tools, such as a Venn diagram (a diagram of overlapping circles, illustrating the links and the common elements between them) to determine whether there is indeed a relationship between health and the proposed project. It will also flag up whether there is a need for a more detailed assessment.

Scoping: to identify the relevant health issues and public concerns that need to be addressed during the appraisal. Scoping generates questions, maps out possible connections, and sets the boundaries and terms of reference for appraisal.

Appraisal: to identify and, when possible, quantify the potential impacts of policies or programmes on health and wellbeing in the context of available evidence and the knowledge, experience and opinions of stakeholders. It can be a *rapid* or an *in-depth* appraisal, depending on the level of detail and quantification needed to inform the policy decision, and may include mitigation and health-promoting measures.

Reporting: communicating with stakeholders about the expected impacts on health and about how the policy, programme or other development could be modified to minimise negative and maximise positive impacts.

Monitoring and evaluation: of compliance with recommendations and of expected health impacts following the implementation of the policy or programme. This allows the existing evidence base to be expanded.

(Adapted from Handsley and Noguera, 2005)

Essentially, what differentiates a HIA from evaluation is that HIAs are normally applied *prospectively* (before policy, programme or project implementation), although they may also be made during and at the conclusion of a project. Indeed, there are demonstrable benefits from HIA evaluations carried out *concurrently* – during the implementation of a project or policy – in terms of informing the ongoing development of the existing work and future funding arrangements; or *retrospectively* – once a project has concluded – to inform future policies, programmes and projects by identifying, not just outcomes, but also lessons to be learned and models of good practice.

11.4.3 Methodology

Although the basic process of carrying out a HIA is as described in Section 11.3 for evaluations, what is specific to HIA is that it is designed to estimate the effects of a specified action on the health of a defined population. It has much in common with the relatively long-established environmental impact assessment (EIA), as mentioned above, and although a preferred methodology for HIA has yet to be established, current thinking (see, for example, Health Impact Assessment Gateway, 2007) suggests that it should be based on a process that takes into consideration:

• both qualitative and quantitative data

• the potential effects and impact on the target population of the proposed policy, programme or project

• the opinions, experience and expectations of the members of the affected community, taking local factors into account

- making practical recommendations to aid decision makers in reaching fully informed decisions and maximising positive impacts and minimising negative ones

- the need for information and recommendations that can be used to continually shape the project or programme in question, providing evidence of both strengths to be developed and weaknesses to be addressed.

Thinking point: what sort of socio-economic determinants of health or social regeneration policies could HIAs be applied to?

The principles mentioned above can be employed in assessing the impact on health of socio-economic determinants of health and social regeneration policies, such as:

- modification of the physical environment for people who have physical and/or sensory impairments: including better facilities, such as playgrounds and parks, and better services, such as litter collection

- lifestyle changes: encouraging healthier lifestyles in the community, such as 'Quit Smoking' groups

- improved leisure facilities: for example, access to fitness centres and youth clubs

- enhanced training and employment prospects: for example, literacy classes and parenting skills

- reduced crime/improved policing: for example, community patrols, encouraging Neighbourhood Watch

- fostering empowerment and people's control over their own lives: for example, public consultations, home helps for older people and disabled people, carers' support groups

- improved access to public services: for example, signposting, better transport

- enhanced relationships between local residents and public sector agencies: for example, better information sharing, consultations.

Having taken these considerations into account, HIA can also be integrated with other forms of impact assessment, such as:

- **Integrated Impact Assessment (IIA)**   This is a good practice tool designed to help assess the impact of a policy and is useful to anyone involved in a policy development exercise. It is intended to provide both a mechanism for screening and a format for presenting the results of more detailed impact assessment of a policy.

- **Strategic Environmental Assessment (SEA)**   This is the process of appraisal by which environmental protection and sustainable development are considered and factored into national and local decisions regarding government (and other) plans and programmes.

- **Environmental Impact Assessment (EIA)**   This term describes a procedure that must be followed for certain types of project before they can be given 'development consent'. The procedure is a means of drawing together, in a systematic way, an assessment of a project's likely significant environmental effects. This helps to ensure that the importance of the predicted effects, and the scope for reducing them, are properly understood by the public and the relevant competent authority before it makes its decision.

- **Social Impact Assessment (SIA)**   This is a subfield of the social sciences that is developing a knowledge base to provide a systematic appraisal in advance of the impacts on the day-to-day quality of life of people and communities whose environment is likely to be affected by a proposed project, plan or policy change. Social impacts (also effects and consequences) refer to changes to communities and to the daily lives of individuals due to a proposed action that alters the day-to-day way in which people live, work, play, relate to one another, organise to meet their needs and generally cope as members of society.

(Adapted from Health Impact Assessment Gateway, 2006a)

However, when impact assessments such as those mentioned above are necessary, it should also be asked:

> whether a separate HIA would be useful, or whether it should be integrated with the other assessments. For example, there is a health element in environmental impact assessments, and in some situations it may be worth considering enhancing the health and equity element of environmental assessment, rather than undertaking a separate HIA. Many IIA and SIA tools and methods would fulfil the definition of HIA, and this is not surprising when comparing the wider determinants of health approach used in HIA with the broad approaches used in integrated and social assessments.

(Health Impact Assessment Gateway, 2006b)

Whether 'integrated' with another impact assessment or not, although (as in the case of Manchester International Airport and the Wembley Stadium) a HIA will be only one part of the evidence necessary to the sustainability of the policy or project assessed, it will highlight the health impacts inherent in this, as well as future uses of the learning and experience acquired. Nonetheless, all these recommendations will be worthless if they are not strongly evidence-based and this evidence obtained from a variety of sources, principle among these being the community in which the project is to take place.

Thinking point: are there any disadvantages to undertaking a HIA?

It should be stressed that HIA is not a magic formula; nor does it replace decision making. It is not a form of comparative risk assessment, nor is it, in itself, community development. Although the importance of HIA has been widely acknowledged throughout the world, it has also been criticised for:

- being just another bureaucratic process which slows down decision-making

- trying to make pseudo-scientific measurements of the immeasurable

- making the health effects of a project dominate decision making, stopping progress in other areas

- adding excessive costs to planning and policy making.

(Adapted from Mindell et al., 2004)

Nevertheless, it does provide policy makers and practitioners with valuable information to inform and influence decision making. Although a HIA could theoretically be undertaken without the active involvement of policy makers, funders and community members, as this chapter has shown, it is only likely to be truly effective if these are actively involved from the earliest stages. However, many factors influence decision making, and HIA is just one of these. There are also other ways to ensure that health and equity are considered when a proposal is developed and implemented. Given current interest in HIA, it is important to be realistic about what it can achieve, and to ensure that it is employed in those situations in which it can most effectively contribute to the decision-making process and to addressing health inequalities.

Conclusion

Considerable resources are spent implementing community-based health programmes that are discontinued soon after initial funding. Measuring and assessing the impact of such programmes is now considered to be key in determining their effectiveness and influencing their longevity and sustainability. Both evaluation and HIA are useful tools in achieving this. Evaluation, as this chapter has demonstrated, helps to provide evidence of a project's success (or failure) and shows whether resources have been used cost-effectively. HIA aims to identify the potential changes in health determinants that might result from a new policy or project – for example, an employment or transport policy – and the effects these changes might have on the health of a population.

Given the short-term horizon of governments and funding agencies – and due to a crisis mode of operation, short budget cycles and internal political pressures – this has meant that projects and programmes constantly have to justify their existence and prove their worth. As for other health professionals, evaluation and HIA have become vital tools in the public health practitioner's toolbox in helping to accomplish this.

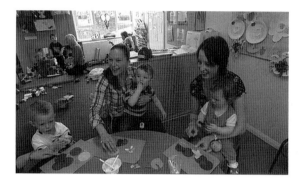 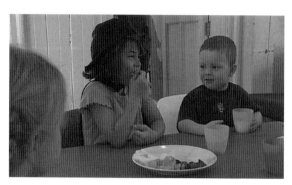

Figure 11.2   Sure Start: a community-based public health project

References

Barnes, R., Nelson, P. and Stanton, J. (2004) *Delivering a New Wembley: Health Impact Assessment*, London, Brent NHS Teaching Primary Care Trust.

Baum, F., Fry, D. and Lennie, I. (eds) (1992) *Community Health: Policy and Practice in Australia*, Leichardt, NSW, Pluto.

Bruce, N. (2002) 'Health impact assessment: a Liverpool perspective', *Urban Voice*, vol. 1, no. 3, pp. 2–5.

Byrne, D. (2004) *Enabling Good Health for All*, Geneva, World Health Organization.

Cabinet Office (1999) *Modernising Government*, London, The Stationery Office.

Cockerill, R., Myers, T. and Allman, D. (2000) 'Planning for community based evaluation', *American Journal of Evaluation*, vol. 21, no. 3, pp. 351–7.

Department for the Environment, Transport and the Regions (DETR) (1998) *New Deal for Transport*, London, The Stationery Office.

Department for Transport, Local Government and the Regions (DTLR) (2002) *Neighbourhood Regeneration: Lessons and Evaluation Evidence from Ten Single Regeneration Budget Cases*, Urban Research Summary No. 1, London, Department for Transport, Local Government and the Regions/The Stationery Office.

Department of Health (DoH) (1999a) *Health Impact Assessment: Report of a Methodological Seminar*, London, The Stationery Office.

Department of Health (DoH) (1999b) *Saving Lives: Our Healthier Nation*, London, The Stationery Office.

Department of Health (DoH) (2000) *Coronary Heart Disease: National Service Framework*, London, The Stationery Office.

Department of Health (DoH) (2003) *Tackling Health Inequalities: A Programme for Action*, London, The Stationery Office.

Department of Health (DoH) and Neighbourhood Renewal Unit (2002) *Health and Neighbourhood Renewal*, London, The Stationery Office.

Douglas, J., Sidell, M., Lloyd. C., Earle, S. (2007) 'Evaluating public health interventions' in Earle et al. (eds) (2007).

Douglas, M., Conway, L., Gorman, D., Gavin, S. and Hanlon, P. (2001) 'Developing principles for health impact assessment', *Journal of Public Health Medicine*, vol. 23, no. 2, pp. 148–54.

Earle, S., Lloyd, C.E., Sidell, M. and Spurr, S. (eds) (2007) *Theory and Research in Promoting Public Health*, London, Sage/Milton Keynes, The Open University.

Effective Intervention Unit (EIU) (2002) *Evaluation Guide 10: Evaluating Community Engagement*, Edinburgh, Scottish Executive.

European Commission (1997) *Treaty of Amsterdam*, Article 152, Brussels, European Commission.

Fetterman, D. (2001) *Foundations of Empowerment Evaluation*, Thousand Oaks, CA, Sage.

Field, J. (2003) *Evaluating Community Projects*, Leicester, National Institute of Adult Continuing Education.

Finer, D., Tillgren, P., Berensson, K., Guldbrand, K. and Haglund, B.J.A. (2005) 'Implementation of a Health Impact Assessment (HIA) tool in a regional health organization in Sweden – a feasibility study', *Health Promotion International*, vol. 20, no. 3, pp. 277–84.

Finlay, L. (2007) 'Qualitative research towards public health' in Earle et al. (eds) (2007).

Gibbon, M. (2002) 'Doing a doctorate using a participatory action research framework in the context of community health', *Qualitative Health Research*, vol. 12, no. 4, pp. 546–58.

Handsley, S. and Noguera, A. (2005) *"With a Glad Heart": Phoenix Health Inequalities Project, Health Impact Assessment*, London, Independent Consultants in Community Research.

Health Development Agency (HDA) 2004) *Clarifying Health Impact Assessment, Integrated Impact Assessment and Health Needs Assessment*, London, Health Development Agency.

Health Impact Assessment Gateway (2006a) *HIA Glossary* [online], http://www.hiagateway.org.uk/page.aspx?o=HIAGlossary (Accessed 15 February 2007).

Health Impact Assessment Gateway (2006b) *Underpinning Principles of Health Impact Assessment* [online], http://www.hiagateway.org.uk/page.aspx?o=Underpinningprinciples (Accessed 26 February 2007).

Health Impact Assessment Gateway (2006c) *Why Should I Bother?* [online], http://www.hiagateway.org.uk/page.aspx?o=WhyshouldIbother (Accessed 7 November 2006).

Health Impact Assessment Gateway (2007) [online],http://www.hiagateway.org.uk (Accessed 25 January 2007).

Hills, D. (2004) *Evaluation of Community-Level Interventions for Health Improvement: A Review of Experience in the UK*, London, Health Development Agency.

Hills, M. and Carroll, S. (2004) 'Health promotion evaluation, realist synthesis and participation', *Ciência e saude coletiva*, vol. 9, no. 3, pp. 536–9.

Home Office Crime Reduction College (2002) *Passport to Evaluation*, York, Home Office Crime Reduction College.

Lock, K. (2000) 'Health Impact Assessment', *British Medical Journal*, vol. 320, pp. 1395–8.

Mindell, J., Boaz, A., Joffe, M., Curtis, S. and Birley, M. (2004) 'Enhancing the evidence base for health impact assessment', *Journal of Epidemiology and Community Health*, vol. 58, no. 7, pp. 546–51.

Neighbourhood Renewal Unit (2002) NDC Reflections: A Study in Community Engagement [online], http://www.neighbourhood.gov.uk/publications.asp (Accessed 15 February 2007).

Norheim, L. (1999) *Community Development for Health: A Resource Guide for Health Workers*, Lancaster, Lancaster University Public Health and Health Professional Development Unit.

NSPCC inform (2006) *Evaluation and Audit Service: An Immediate or Tailored Evaluation and Audit Service to Report on Impact and Effectiveness of Learning and Development Programmes* [online], http://www.nspcc.org.uk/inform/trainingandconsultancy/training/evaluationandauditservice/evaluation_asp_ifega23725.html (Accessed 7 November 2006).

Nutbeam, D. (1998) 'Evaluating health promotion – Progress, problems and solutions', *Health Promotion International*, vol. 13, no. 1, pp. 27–44.

Nutbeam, D. (1999) 'The challenge to provide "evidence" in health promotion', *Health Promotion International*, vol. 14, no. 2, pp. 99–101.

Open University (2007) K311 *Promoting Public Health: Skills, Perspectives and Practice*, DVD, Milton Keynes, The Open University.

Parry, J. and Stevens, A. (2001) 'Prospective health impact assessment: pitfalls, problems and possible ways forward', *British Medical Journal*, vol. 323, pp. 1177–82.

Pearson, C., Thomas, J. and Lloyd, C. (2007) 'Researching health' in Earle et al. (eds) (2007).

Scott-Samuel, A. (1998) 'Health Impact Assessment – theory into practice', *Journal of Epidemiology and Community Health*, vol. 52, no. 11, pp. 704–5.

Scott-Samuel, A., Birley, M. and Ardern, K. (2001) *The Merseyside Guidelines for Health Impact Assessment* (2nd edn), Liverpool, University of Liverpool, International Health Impact Assessment Consortium (IMPACT).

Sidell, M. and Lloyd, C. (2007) 'Studying the population's health' in Earle et al. (eds) (2007).

Smith, M.L. and Glass, G.V. (1987) *Research and Evaluation in Education and the Social Sciences*, Englewood Cliffs, NJ, Prentice-Hall.

Social Exclusion Unit (SEU) (2001) *A New Commitment to Neighbourhood Renewal: National Strategy Action Plan*, London, Cabinet Office/HMSO.

Wanless, D. (2004) *Securing Good Health for the Whole Population: Final Report*, London, HM Treasury.

Welsh Health Impact Assessment Support Unit (WHIASU) (2006) *Food in Schools: The Impact on the Health of Children and Young People in Swansea*, Swansea, Welsh Health Impact Assessment Support Unit.

Will, S., Ardern, K., Spencely, M. and Watkins, S. (1994) *A Prospective Health Impact Assessment of the Proposed Development of a Second Runway at Manchester International Airport*, Manchester and Stockport Health Commissions (report submitted to the public inquiry).

Wilson, K.A., Jesson, J.K. and Staunton, N. (2000) 'Evaluation of a new health centre pharmacy: a case study', *International Journal of Pharmaceutical Practice*, vol. 8, pp. 97–102.

Wimbush, R. and Watson, E. (2000) 'An evaluation framework for health promotion: theory, quality and effectiveness', *Evaluation*, vol. 6, no. 3, pp. 301–21.

World Health Organization (WHO) and European Centre for Health Policy (ECHP) (1999) *Health Impact Assessment*, Gothenburg Consensus Paper, Brussels, World Health Organization Regional Office for Europe and European Centre for Health Policy.

Yazbeck, C., Kloppmann, W., Cottier, R., Sahuquillo, J., Debotte, G. and Huel, G. (2005) 'Health impact evaluation of boron in drinking water: a geographical risk assessment in Northern France', *Environmental Geochemistry and Health*, vol. 27, no. 5/6, pp. 419–27.

Chapter 12

Promoting mental health and social inclusion

Stephen Handsley

Introduction

Throughout Part II of this book, the focus has been on community-orientated approaches to promoting public health. In this final chapter, you are asked to consider the effectiveness of this approach with respect to mental health and mental health promotion. Mental health problems are not uncommon among all sections of the general population (Layard, 2006; Age Concern and Mental Health Foundation, 2006). Although they are thought by many to be a taboo subject (McCulloch and Boxer, 1997), in fact, the rise in mental health problems with the concomitant increase in public and professional concern has seen the issue of public mental health placed firmly on the public health agenda (DoH, 2004a).

So what is being done to address this situation? What measures are government departments, health authorities, primary care trusts and other statutory sector agencies taking to improve and promote mental health? What is the role of the voluntary sector in helping to promote mental health? Although in many cases policy makers have at last begun to grasp the seriousness and exclusionary nature of mental illhealth, this is not always reflected in current legislation.

This chapter begins by examining what is meant by mental health and mental health promotion before summarising some of the risks and protective factors for mental health problems. Section 12.2 then puts mental health promotion in context by discussing how the respective public health promotion practices and policies of each of the four nations of the UK grapple with the issue of mental health, and the strategies that are in place to foster a climate that facilitates positive mental health and emotional wellbeing. Turning to mental health promotion at the community level, Section 12.3 looks at the way in which local communities and providers of services can engage effectively with each other to define their needs and plan and provide services with respect to mental health. The final section draws together this part of the book by looking towards the future for multidisciplinary public health and mental health promotion at a community level.

Before unpacking the topic in any great depth, however, it is important to explain the rationale, not only for including mental health promotion in this book, but also for situating it in this second part of the book, the focus of which is promoting public health at a community level. Many of the themes at the heart of community strategies are relevant to mental health promotion: for example, improving community governance, tackling social exclusion, and building community capacity and social capital. Some authorities are establishing staff training in community development, providing an important opportunity for shared learning between mental health promotion and local government. In addition, Standard One of the National Service Framework (NSF) for Mental Health (DoH, 1999) identifies communities as a target setting for mental health promotion. For these reasons, then, this is the perfect place for the discussion to appear.

12.1 What is mental health and mental health promotion?

As with general health (Earle, 2007), mental health can be approached and defined in many ways. Most essential in grasping the concept of 'mental health' is that it should be seen as a broad issue, rather than as relating only to mental disorders or being a matter just for psychiatrists and psychologists. According to a 2004 report published by European Communities and STAKES (the Finnish National Research and Development Centre for Welfare and Health), there is, in fact, no health without mental health and, further, mental health ought to be seen as an indivisible part of public health generally.

What exactly is mental health, then, and what is its importance? Moreover, what is meant by the term 'mental health promotion'? And how does mental health differ from mental illness?

12.1.1 What is mental health and why is it important?

In addressing these questions, it should be noted first of all that there is a lack of clarity and some confusion surrounding the meaning and significance of different terminology associated with mental health, which can, as Friedli (2004) has pointed out, hinder communication and lead to misunderstanding. For example, as Read and Wallcraft (1995) have argued, the phrase 'service user' is particularly problematic, especially for those under an element of the Mental Health Act. The difficulties in defining the concept of service user involvement have been well documented (Anthony and Crawford, 2000). For instance, user involvement is seen by some as merging and blurring 'with "negotiated care", "collaborative care", "patient participation" and "person-centred care"' (Anthony and Crawford, 2000, p. 426).

Mental health is important for a number of reasons. Not only does it help facilitate the successful performance of mental functions, but it also affects people's capacity to manage, to communicate and to form and sustain relationships. Mental health is essentially about how people think and feel about themselves and others, and how they interpret the world around them. It affects the capacity to cope with change and major life transitions, such as having a baby, getting married, divorce and bereavement, as well as impacting on physical health and wellbeing.

Thinking point: how would you define mental health?

Definitions of mental health are, it seems, difficult to pin down. According to the Mental Health Foundation, good mental health is not just the absence of mental health problems. Individuals with good mental health:

- develop emotionally, creatively, intellectually and spiritually
- initiate, develop and sustain mutually satisfying personal relationships
- face problems, resolve them and learn from them
- are confident and assertive
- are aware of others and empathise with them
- use and enjoy solitude
- play, have fun and laugh, both at themselves and at the world.

(Adapted from Mental Health Foundation, 2005)

Drawing on the report from European Communities and STAKES (2004) mentioned above, mental health, as an indivisible component of general health, reflects the equilibrium between the individual and his or her environment. It is influenced by:

- individual biological and psychological factors
- social interactions
- societal structures and resources
- cultural values.

(European Communities and STAKES, 2004, p. 5)

In this context, mental health can be seen as both a process and a product, comprising predisposing factors (e.g. childhood experiences), actual precipitating factors (e.g. stressful life events) and supporting factors (e.g. social networks), as well as various consequences and outcomes (e.g. creativity or health behaviour). Mental health has two dimensions:

1   Positive mental health can be conceptualised as a value in itself (feeling well); or as a capacity to perceive, comprehend and interpret our surroundings, to adapt to them and to change them if necessary; and the capacity to think and to communicate with each other.

2   Negative mental health (or mental illhealth) is concerned with mental disorders, symptoms and problems.

Although such definitions appear to confirm and clarify the meaning of mental health, the terminology associated with the concept has changed drastically since the mid-1980s. For example, whereas mental illness was commonly perceived as some sort of biological disorder, many now argue that it is simply socially constructed (Flick, 1998). For these scholars, such terms as 'mental illness' or 'mental health problems' are constructed as a form of social control, largely orchestrated by psychiatrists and other health professionals as a form of dominance and surveillance of those who do not quite conform to the existing norms of society.

For others, establishing a basic, universally applicable concept of mental health is impossible (Kamal and Loewenthal, 2002; Secker, 2005). For them, no objective definitions and standards are possible since behaviour that is regarded as healthy or normal in one culture may be regarded as neurotic or aberrant in another. A cross-cultural example is suicide. In many countries, such as the USA and the UK, a person who commits suicide or attempts to do so, or even thinks about it seriously, is considered to be mentally ill. In contrast, neither Hinduism nor Buddhism have any intrinsic objections to suicide, and in some forms of Buddhism self-incineration is believed to confer special merit (Kamal and Loewenthal, 2002). All criteria, these scholars conclude, are a matter of 'cultural bias'.

According to Secker (2005), approaches to mental health have traditionally adopted a reductionist perspective. This conceptualises mental health in terms of 'component parts': a psychological approach consisting of lists of cognitive and behavioural skills, or developmental attributes, which clearly sits uneasily with the emphasis of a twenty-first century public health agenda that focuses on holistic understandings of health. As Secker notes, in this model the implied focus for improving mental health remains the individual, at the expense of work at structural as well as at community levels.

In contrast, despite the general, largely negative, perception that mental illhealth is closely associated with psychology and mental disorders, it is equally the case that the many determinants of mental illhealth are linked more to physical, social and cultural factors.

Thinking point: should we really be concerned over the type of terminology used when discussing mental health?

Perhaps you feel that, whether or not it is right to employ such terms as 'mental health' or 'mental illness', mental illhealth does indeed constitute some sort of biological disorder. On the other hand, perhaps you perceive mental health as a concept grounded in cultural traits or particularities? Given that people who suffer from mental health problems are often marginalised and, at times, even demonised – usually as a result of ignorance or misinformation. As you read about the experience, in Box 12.1, of a former service user, you may recognise the importance attached both to the way in which 'mental health' is defined and the impact this might have on those 'real people' who may suffer with mental health problems. Box 12.1 illustrates the work of Be Active Stay Active (BASA), a community-based mental health project in Scotland, which has used activity and exercise as a way of promoting positive mental health.

Box 12.1 BASA activities for promoting positive mental health: walking

Forbes Winter, a former service user from Alloa in Scotland, talks about the way in which BASA has helped to change his life:

> I was an outpatient at Alloa Community Hospital and joined BASA to help me to get out and about. BASA organises a range of activities and I attended a keep fit class at first. However this was too strenuous, so we began walking instead. I have been walking with BASA since May 2003. That was a good summer and it meant we were out walking in lovely weather – although the group walks in rain, hail or snow. I became a walk leader the following May. I have noticed my fitness improve and I can walk more quickly now. I recently had an operation, so have been unable to walk with the group. I miss the company but am looking forward to going back. Walking regularly increased my fitness so that I was able to manage longer walks with my family when we holidayed in Shetland last summer. I enjoy the company – the group mixes really well and we always go for a coffee or something to eat after the walks. It's great to visit new and interesting places on the walks and I often take my camera along. I have been surprised to visit places that I had never been to in Alloa, and I've lived here 35 years. If you have a problem, BASA co-ordinators are always happy to help. As a walk leader, I find this particularly reassuring and it can be therapeutic to talk over problems. The walks do lead to other things, such as a football group or going to the allotments. We've also introduced a creative walk, where someone might bring along a sketch book, and I've started taking my camera a lot now. For me, the walks have also stimulated an interest in local history. I'd like to see more people attending our walking group and to have social events. However, even if only one or two people attend, the most important thing is that they enjoy attending the group.

(Open University, 2007)

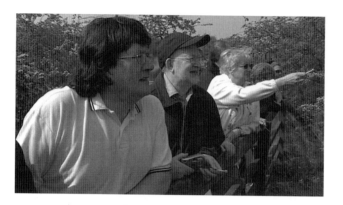

Figure 12.1   Walking with the BASA project

Thus, the misuse and abuse of such terms as mental health and mental illness may well create a culture that further stigmatises and marginalises those with mental health problems, which in turn prevents them from taking part in such community-based activities as keep fit classes or healthy walks.

You will read more about BASA later in the chapter.

12.1.2 The public face of mental health

The stigma usually associated with mental health often marginalises those who are most in need of help and support. And yet, no one can safely assume that one day, they too might not experience such problems. Given this, how confident can people be of receiving the necessary care and treatment? Do such negative connotations create barriers to promoting mental health? Many argue that they do; indeed, although since the mid-1990s positive attitudes to mental health have increased greatly, there has been a decline in tolerance for people with serious mental health problems. For example, many of the media representations of mental health service users during a similar period appear to emphasise violence, dangerousness and criminality (Cutcliffe and Hannigan, 2001). Mental health groups have long complained that media coverage of issues such as care in the community has played on public fears at the cost of sensible debate. Box 12.2 illustrates the type of feelings expressed towards those experiencing mental distress.

Box 12.2 Feelings towards those experiencing mental distress

A survey at the start of the Royal College of Psychiatrists' five-year campaign to reduce the stigma of mental illness showed just how prevalent are such stereotypical images of mental distress as those mentioned above. In the survey, 1,737 adults were asked about seven common mental health problems: severe depression, panic attacks, schizophrenia, dementia, eating disorders, alcoholism and drug addiction. In the survey, people with schizophrenia, alcoholism and drug addiction were seen as unpredictable and dangerous, although this opinion was less common in people over the age of 65. There was a widespread view that people with any of these conditions are hard to talk to. The respondents generally saw people with mental health problems as being difficult to communicate and empathise with. There was also little sympathy for problems that were seen to be self-inflicted, such as addiction problems and eating disorders.

(Adapted from Royal College of Psychiatrists, 2003)

Box 12.3 Examples of newspaper headlines portraying mental health issues

Maniac killed twin sisters
(Front page headline, *London Evening Standard*, 18 April 2005)

Knife maniac freed to kill. Mental patient ran amok in the park
(Front page headline, *Daily Mail*, 26 February 2005)

Violent, mad. So Docs set him free. New 'Community Care' scandal
(*The Sun*, 26 February 2005)

(Adapted from Thornicroft, 2006)

What, then, can be done to overcome the types of negative image of mental health illustrated above? One way is to be much more proactive in promoting the positive dimensions of mental health. Indeed, it has been argued that a framework for public mental health promotion should be designed to address the wider determinants of mental health, reducing the enduring inequalities in the distribution of mental distress and improving the mental health of the population as a whole (Friedli, 2004).

12.1.3 Mental health promotion

Having considered the meaning of mental health, what, then, is mental health promotion? And does it differ from the more general public health strategies discussed earlier in this book? According to Friedli, mental health promotion is: 'both any action to enhance the mental well-being of individuals, families, organisations and communities, and a set of principles which recognise that how people feel is not an abstract and elusive concept, but a significant influence on health' (Friedli, 2000, p. 15).

For Friedli and others, mental health promotion is the process of enhancing the capacity of individuals and communities to take control over their lives and improve their mental health. Such a philosophy echoes that discussed in earlier chapters in which communities were seen as a key driver in the process of empowerment. It can contribute to improved health and wellbeing by preventing mental health problems, improving physical health, strengthening communities, improving information and reducing work-related illhealth. Mental health promotion can be seen as working at two levels. On one level, it seeks to improve the quality of life of those with a mental health problem and to intervene early to offer appropriate treatment. On another, wider level, mental health promotion, as mentioned above, aims to improve the mental wellbeing of the whole population. If it is acknowledged that there is a two-way relationship between mental wellbeing and general wellbeing, then seeking to enhance positive mental wellbeing will improve the general health and quality of life of a community. How might this look in practice?

Returning to the BASA project mentioned in Section 12.1.1 in relation to walking as an activity to facilitate the process of mental health promotion, Box 12.4 and Figure 12.2 below illustrate how gardening has similarly been used.

Box 12.4 BASA activities for promoting active mental health: gardening

One of the BASA volunteers, himself a service user, speaks of the value of gardening in the promotion of positive mental health:

> My name is Lindsay McNab ... I've actually been involved in horticulture for about twenty-five years ... I've been to West of Scotland College and I've done two diplomas and so I quite enjoy doing this type of work ... I've also been a lecturer as well for eleven years up at Clackmannan College and Falkirk College ... Oh, I get a lot of satisfaction from trying to help people to understand how the environment works and also about the plant material ... it gives them a lot of self confidence and belief in themselves, especially from a mental health point of view, but also empowers them to be able to do things and also it helps them to socialise and it's good for me as well, to be able to pass over my skills to other people ...

(Open University, 2007)

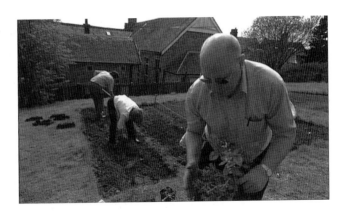

Figure 12.2 Gardening with the BASA project

On a practical level, then, this is one example of what can be done to prevent mental health problems, and to promote good mental health. Of others, among the simplest and most effective measures for individuals are regular exercise (an example of which you read about in Box 12.1) and a healthy diet. Indeed, a recently published report by the Mental Health Foundation (2006) has demonstrated a clear link between diet and mental health. *Feeding Minds: The Impact of Food on Mental Health* found growing evidence that a poor diet plays an important contributory role in specific mental health problems, including attention deficit hyperactivity disorder (ADHD), depression, schizophrenia and Alzheimer's disease. Recognising the link between mental health and physical health, the Department of Health (DoH) publication *Choosing Health: Supporting the Physical Health Needs of People with Severe Mental Illness* (DoH, 2006a) appears to have remedied the mistakes made in the original White Paper *Choosing Health: Making Healthy Choices Easier* (DoH, 2004a) in accepting that: 'People with diagnoses of severe and enduring mental illnesses (SMI) such as schizophrenia and bipolar disorder are at increased risk for a range of physical illnesses and conditions, including coronary heart disease, diabetes, infections, respiratory disease and greater levels of obesity' (DoH, 2006a, p. 3).

Although such interventions as those offered by the BASA project are to be welcomed, for a variety of reasons not everyone is able to access this type of service. For instance, by its very nature, mental illhealth often means that those who would most benefit from such interventions, slip through the net. Indeed, for many, mental health problems can become the catalyst for social exclusion, stigmatisation and marginalisation, leading to long-term unemployment, homelessness, poor physical health and lasting social isolation. This is illustrated in Box 12.5.

Box 12.5 Social exclusion: the causes

The Social Exclusion Unit has identified five main reasons why mental health problems too often lead to and reinforce social exclusion:

- **Stigma and discrimination** against people with mental health problems is pervasive throughout society. Despite a number of campaigns, there has been no significant change in attitude [Taylor Nielson Sofres, 2003]. Fewer than four in ten employers say they would recruit someone with a mental health problem [Manning and White, 1995]. Many people fear disclosing their condition, even to family and friends.

- Professionals across sectors too often have **low expectations** of what people with mental health problems can achieve. There is limited recognition in the NHS that returning to work and overcoming social isolation is associated with better health outcomes. Employment is not seen as a key objective for people with mental health problems by many health and social care professionals.

- There is a **lack of clear responsibility** for promoting vocational and social outcomes for adults with mental health problems. Services do not always work effectively together to meet individual needs and maximise the impact of available resources.

- People can **lack ongoing support to enable them to work.** £140 million a year is invested by health and social care in vocational and day services for people with mental health problems [Financial Mapping Returns, 2003]. But not all of these promote social inclusion as effectively as they could, and links with Jobcentre Plus can be weak. People on benefits often do not believe they will end up financially better off if they try to move into work. Many people lose jobs that they might have kept had they received better support.

- People face **barriers to engaging in the community.** They can struggle to access the basic services they need, in particular decent housing and transport. Education, arts, sports and leisure providers often are not aware how their services could benefit people with mental health problems and how they could make their services more accessible for this group. Many people do not want to participate in activities alone, but feel there is no one they can ask to go with them. People can also face exclusion by law from some community roles such as jury service.

(ODPM, 2004b, p. 4)

Mental health promotion, therefore, needs to be part of an ambitious strategy for public health, one that fosters an environment in which people are encouraged to seek help early. The components of such a strategy should include prevention (preventing symptoms of mental health problems and disorders) as well as promotion (promoting good mental health). As noted above, this strategy seeks to provide a framework for positive action at both levels, working with existing mental health problems and strengthening the wellbeing of communities.

12.1.4 The evidence for mental health promotion

Despite the successes of mental health promotion, some of which were illustrated above, does it really work? The DoH publication *Making It Happen: A Guide to Delivering Mental Health Promotion* (DoH, 2001) identifies several factors that are thought to have an impact on mental wellbeing. It argues that many of the factors that influence mental health lie outside the remit of health and social care: for example, housing and homelessness, employment and family relationships. It makes a distinction between factors associated with poor mental health (referred to as 'risk factors') and preventative factors (i.e. those that tend to increase good mental health or reduce the likelihood of mental illness). Preventative factors include economic security, good physical health, positive school achievement, a supportive relationship or social network, and opportunities for personal achievement. Conversely, associated (risk) factors include poverty, unemployment, poor housing, bereavement, a family history of psychiatric disorder, caring for someone with an illness/disability, misuse of drugs or alcohol, and family breakdown. How, then, might this approach to mental health work? What should a model of mental health promotion look like?

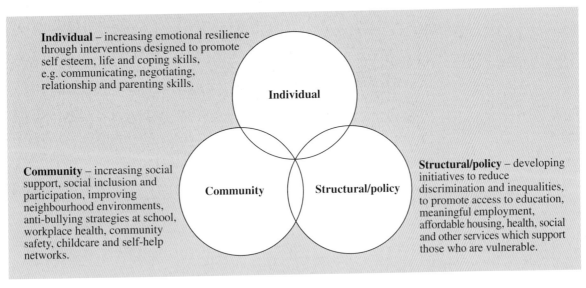

Figure 12.3   A model of mental health promotion

The model shown in Figure 12.3 illustrates not only the holistic nature of mental health promotion, but also how partnership working is key to achieving this. This model represents the way in which successful mental health promotion cannot be achieved in isolation. Rather, it is achieved by the adoption of an approach that recognises the overlap between the individual, the community and structural/policy issues.

According to the National Electronic Library for Health (NeLH), in collaboration with mentality:

> [t]he principles of effective mental health promotion interventions have been described as those which include the following approaches:
>
> • the intervention aims to influence a combination of several risk or protective factors
>
> • it involves the social network of the target group
>
> • it intervenes at a range of different times rather than once only
>
> • it involves a combination of intervention methods.
>
> (Bosma and Hosman, 1990)
>
> Key principles of effective practice include programmes that aim to:
>
> • reduce anxiety
>
> • enhance control
>
> • facilitate participation
>
> • promote social inclusion.
>
> (Department of Health, 2001)
>
> Principles that are considered to underpin effective interventions include:
>
> • non-stigmatising provision – often open access
>
> • needs-led programmes – based on mapping, current provision and priorities
>
> • effective methods of consultation with local communities and ownership
>
> • engagement with users – in the broadest sense – can be the whole community

- delivery in partnership – pan sector approach to provision
- utilising appropriate approaches – e.g. peer led (age specific), culturally relevant

(Sainsbury Centre for Mental Health and Mentality, 2004)

(NeLH in collaboration with Mentality, 2004)

A mental health promotion strategy can, therefore, be effective by seeking to strengthen preventative factors and minimising risk factors within its target population. Clearly, this involves changes to public policy far outside the remit of mental health services, and illustrates the importance of linking mental health promotion principles to wider community strategies.

In exploring mental health and mental heath promotion, you will, by now, have begun to get a feel for the way in which these are perceived and presented at a public level. The next section takes up the theme of public policy and examines some of the many polices that influence the way in which mental health is represented and perceived.

12.2 Putting mental health promotion in context: policy and perspectives

Since the end of 2000 in particular, there has been a plethora of policies – international, national, regional and local – which claim to be committed to working towards the vision of promoting positive mental health. These include, for example, *The NHS Plan* (DoH, 2000), *Action on Mental Health* (ODPM, 2004a), *Choosing Mental Health* (Mental Health Foundation, 2005), as well as strategies from the four nations of the UK. Each of these policy documents has called for a more proactive approach to mental health and mental health promotion. In fact, raising awareness of mental health has, since the 1990s, become a major theme of all four nations' public health policies.

In what might be perceived as a 'radical' move on the part of the then English Labour Government, and in response to the report by the Social Exclusion Unit entitled *Mental Health and Social Exclusion* (ODPM, 2004b), a guide intended to 'promote direct payments within mental health services as a means of facilitating greater social participation' (ODPM, 2004b, p. 4) was published (DoH, 2006b). Direct payments are payments made to individuals who have been assessed as needing social care services, to enable them to make their own arrangements to meet their needs. According to the Department of Health, the purpose of such payments is: 'to give recipients control over their own life by providing an alternative to social care services provided by a local council. This will help increase opportunities for independence, social inclusion and enhanced self-esteem' (DoH, 2006b, p. 1).

Given that social exclusion and unemployment are major indicators of mental health, the direct payments scheme was introduced by the Labour Government as way of addressing this. However, in a further report entitled *Direct Payments and Mental Health: New Directions* (Newbiggin and Lowe, 2005), it was suggested that, despite the slow but steady growth in the implementation of direct payments, the number of people with mental health needs who have taken up direct payments has remained low, particularly in comparison with other groups.

Thinking point: how serious is the drive to promote mental health and wellbeing?

Perhaps you believe that governments are doing enough to promote mental health? Or, you may wonder what lies behind the rhetoric? For example, is the direct payments scheme, as discussed above, a way forward in helping to overcome the type of social exclusion experienced by people who suffer mental health problems? As part of its drive to improve mental health and wellbeing in Scotland, the Scottish Executive has come up with a framework for public mental health with respect to different levels of influence and action. This is set out in Figure 12.4, which shows a 'map' of key protective and risk factors for mental health and wellbeing.

Figure 12.4   Key protective and risk factors for mental health and wellbeing (Source: Scottish Public Mental Health Alliance, 2002, p. 9, Table 1.1)

Level of influence and action	Protective factors	Risk factors
Individual	Meaningful role in society Self-esteem and confidence Resilience Adequate income, warm home, wholesome food, regular exercise	Living in poverty Inadequate social support Low self-esteem and poor interpersonal and social skills
Family	Planned parenthood Loving, supportive relationships Adequate income	Living in poverty Teenage parents Abusive/neglectful parenting Parental substance misuse
Work	Respectful and trusting work environment Clear expectations of role and accountability Balance between effort and reward perceived to be fair	Lack of autonomy Lack of security Low pay Discrimination

Community	High levels of interaction and good social support High levels of participation in community activity Influence over decisions that affect community Physically pleasant surroundings	Poor housing High crime rates Poor transport Poor local services Lack of trust between people
Society	Inclusive and participative Tolerant and caring Equitable	Exclusive and intolerant (e.g. racism, ageism, sexism, homophobia, sectarianism) Inequitable

Making the Mental Health National Service Framework a reality depends on expertise, resources and partnerships across all sectors and disciplines (DoH, 1999). The importance of partnerships to public health was noted in Chapter 9, but what can partnerships achieve in terms of locally based mental health projects? In Box 12.6, Pat Gilmartin, an occupational therapist working with BASA, discusses the benefits of such alliances for members of BASA.

Box 12.6 Partnership working in mental health

'So, one of the first partnerships that we recognised first of all was the partnership between the members – you know the service users – and also the allied health professions. We felt that this was one of the most important elements of the project and that we needed to get it right first of all. We then felt that there was a range of other partnerships that we could certainly speak with and one of those has been the Paths to Health Project which is based here in Clackmannanshire. It's a Scottish Executive initiative to get people walking. It is this whole kind of connection with walking and well being, and what that's allowed us to do, that has been a real boost for BASA. What's made this project different is that, through this partnership with Paths to Health, this has enabled us to really invest in the members and their well being. For example, several of our members have now trained to become walk leaders and that's benefited greatly to a point where they're actually facilitating their own walks by themselves.'

(Open University, 2007)

Such locally based alliances are a key factor in addressing many of the problems associated with mental health. However, as you will see from the next section, making mental health promotion happen at a local level can sometimes be problematic simply because policy makers and people at the 'sharp' end of society do not always look at issues in the same way.

12.3 Mental health promotion: making it happen at a local level

Throughout Part II of this book, you have read about the benefits and potential of promoting public health at a local level. In the same vein, you might ask what mental health promotion might achieve at a local level. For example, you have already read about the potential of mental health promotion to create a collective, communal and secure environment.

12.3.1 Communities and mental health

In the same way in which communities are now seen as a vital component of public health policy and practice, strong communities are seen as vital in facilitating the type of social support, inclusion and participation that helps to protect mental wellbeing (DoH, 2004a). Indeed, it is at a local level that the national and international policies mentioned earlier are both realised and operationalised. What form might this process take?

Some of the successful outcomes of using a positive mental health approach, facilitated by a community-orientated perspective, might be to:

- improve physical health and wellbeing
- prevent or reduce the risk of some mental health problems, notably behavioural disorders, depression and anxiety, and substance misuse
- assist recovery from mental health problems
- improve mental health services and the quality of life for people experiencing mental health problems
- strengthen the capacity of communities to support social inclusion, tolerance and participation, and reduce vulnerability to socio-economic stressors
- increase the mental health literacy of individuals, organisations and communities
- improve health at work, increasing productivity and reducing sickness absence.

12.3.2 Engaging communities with particular mental health needs

Engaging communities with particular mental health needs can – in much the same way as that of physical health needs – prove especially problematic. Indeed, there is a recognition that some groups face particular barriers to having their mental health and social needs addressed.

Thinking point: can you think of any particular groups that might face such barriers?

- **Black and minority ethnic groups** may feel alienated from mainstream (predominantly white) mental health services, and so tend to present late to mental health services. They may be wrongly diagnosed, based on cultural misassumptions, and in seeking work may encounter discrimination on grounds of both health status and ethnicity.

- **Young men** with mental health problems are at high risk of dropping out of education or work and of becoming involved with crime, and they are a particularly high risk group for suicide.

- **Parents** with mental health problems – particularly lone parents – have very low employment rates and may not receive sufficient family support, and their children may develop emotional problems.

- **Adults with complex needs**, arsing from, for example, substance misuse or homelessness in addition to their mental health problems, often struggle to have their needs met by statutory services.

- **Older people** with mental health problems are also at high risk because social isolation is one of the key risk factors in mental health and wellbeing.

(Adapted from ODPM, 2004b, p. 4)

Rethink, a leading national mental health membership charity, has highlighted how, in some cultures, professionals place a low priority on mental illness, with the result that treatment is poor and there is little motivation to seek help (Rethink, 2006). In addition, in providing mental health services for older people at least two generations may need to be included. For all groups, mainstream goals – such as acquiring and maintaining a home or securing ongoing employment – are likely to be severely compromised by the compounding effects of homelessness, social exclusion and poor mental health.

Thinking point: how might these barriers be overcome, and what might be the implication for mental health promotion?

In dealing with a range of 'client groups' of service users, it is important to recognise that they are made up of people who may have nothing in common except the labels professionals use for them. People do not define themselves by the categories they are put into. Rather, they are individuals with their own needs and expectations. There are ways of engaging with people that are better, or worse, suited to particular individuals and their particular circumstances, but the same broad principles of good practice apply to all. The National Occupational Standards (NOS) and National Workforce Competences (NWC) for mental health have set the following performance criteria for engaging with communities with mental health issues:

You need to:

1. encourage **people** to identify and find out about appropriate **networks**

2. obtain and provide relevant information to enable people to determine the involvement they wish to have with relevant networks

3. identify and create opportunities for people to participate in networks in which they have expressed an interest

4. identify and minimise any barriers to accessing appropriate networks

5. provide **support and assistance** as required to enable people to participate in relevant networks

6. seek appropriate advice to protect people's welfare, where involvement with a network appears to be having negative effects on their behaviour or condition

7. take action in accordance with the advice you are given to ensure a positive outcome for the people you are supporting.

(National Occupational Standards, 2005, p. 5)

For every public health project or intervention that successfully overcomes barriers, there are others that require more formal codes of practice to ensure that people are not excluded on the basis of, for instance, age, gender, ethnicity, religion or disability. For example, a report from the Joseph Rowntree Foundation (2002) found that, where mainstream advocacy services existed, they were inaccessible by and often inappropriate to the specific needs of black service users and carers. In response to such oversights, many local authorities and agencies have drawn up codes of practice for those engaging with hard-to-reach communities. For example, in England the Walsall Compact has come up with a policy statement that provides a framework for tackling inequality and discrimination against black and minority ethnic (BME) groups (see Box 12.7).

Box 12.7 Code of practice for engaging with community groups

This policy statement will provide a framework for partnership working that will help provide community cohesion and ensure adherence to the principles of equality.

We will ensure that:

- support is provided for an effective BME infrastructure
- the diversity of interests and opinions within the BME community are recognised, respected and valued
- Walsall BME communities are actively involved and fully engaged in the development of local plans and strategies
- recognition is given to the provisions of all race relations legislation.

Walsall Compact Partners agree to:

- recognise the importance of faith groups
- recognise the diversity within the BME groups
- ensure that consultation processes include all within the BME communities
- ensure that our policies and processes are impartial and free from prejudice
- promote innovative ways of working.

(Walsall Borough Strategic Partnership, 2005, p. 27)

In laying down such public messages, local authorities are helping to build bridges towards the integration of mental health promotion and public health. The next section explores this further.

12.4 Building bridges: integrating mental health promotion and public health

As discussed in earlier chapters, community-orientated approaches to promoting public health have, since the mid-1990s, proved successful, especially in addressing health inequalities and tackling social exclusion. How might this same approach be adopted by professionals and practitioners working in the field of mental health? And, if it were to be adopted, would it represent an example of the integration of mental health promotion and public health?

12.4.1 Developing a common strategy, or a missed opportunity?

Although the development of a community mental health ideology has seen community mental health teams (CMHTs) 'reach out' to those with mental health problems, it is questionable whether this community-based approach has helped to promote public mental health. For example, according to the

Mental Health Policy Implementation Guide: Community Mental Health Teams (DoH, 2002), CMHTs have an important, integral role to play in supporting service users and families in community settings. However, it could be argued that this role does not include the promotion of mental health as part of its remit, instead preferring to 'treat' the causes of mental illhealth. Similarly, as Friedli and McCulloch (2005) point out, although local government's mainstream services, such as education and social services, play a major role in promoting public health, including mental health at a community level, there is much more that could be done to develop an integrated framework that focuses on a holistic model of health and wellbeing. Friedli and McCulloch note the following additional 'powers and responsibilities' that local authorities have:

- the general duty for local authorities to promote population well-being

- flexibility for local authorities to develop local targets and work in partnership to respond to local need through the development of local area agreement pilot projects

- more support for local authorities to improve parks and public spaces and 'whole town' approaches to walking, cycling and public transport

- the national 'Healthy Schools Programme' focusing on food in schools, school travel, physical education and sport in schools

- expanding the number of school nurses working with each primary care trust (PCT) and its local schools.

(Friedli and McCulloch, 2005, p. 39)

Some positive efforts are being made to mainstream emotional wellbeing into the school setting. For example, the National Health Schools Standards have shown how school-based mental health promotion interventions are effective in improving and maintaining emotional health and wellbeing (HDA, 2004). Nonetheless, despite being widely welcomed for its principles in encouraging the public to make healthier and more informed choices with regard to their general health, in the English White Paper *Choosing Health* (DoH, 2004a), mental health is largely neglected (Friedli and McCulloch, 2005, p. 39).

Thinking point: how far is mental health promotion integrated into the wider public health debate?

Perhaps, from what you have read, the promise of mental health promotion taking its place in the wider public health framework appears to be part of government rhetoric rather than reality? Although this may be the case, there are examples of some local authorities successfully adopting a more integrated approach. For instance, in the Scottish city of Aberdeen, the city council, working with the NHS, further education and a wide range of partners from the voluntary sector, has been part of a public health project which utilises a community development approach to meet the needs of people in Aberdeen who experience economic disadvantage and mental health difficulties (Aberdeen City Alliance, 2005). This project focuses in particular on parents and children, young people, travellers, minority ethnic communities, people who are homeless, and people with mental health problems and their carers. It includes an Affordable Food Initiative and food co-operatives, an arts programme and the development of a credit union. Such an approach – which attracted over 10,000 participants in its first year – has enabled local communities to identify the priorities that would make a difference to their lives. It has made it possible to listen to practitioners 'on the ground' who have a real awareness of the needs of their target group. Given that material deprivation is consistently associated with a higher prevalence of mental health problems (Rogers and Pilgrim, 2003), this shows the value of taking a more integrated and holistic approach.

The report by the Department of Health, *Choosing Health: Supporting the Physical Health Needs of People with Severe Mental Illness* (DoH, 2006a), appears to concede that, in order to address the rise in mental health problems, it is first important to tackle the wider determinants of health. This means taking a more proactive, integrated approach to promoting public health: one that involves a national contract on mental health (i.e. a national strategy for and guidance on the development of mental health services), which takes account of social and economic interventions, environmental interventions, personal behaviour, service interventions, and spheres in which mental health is discussed in terms of its relevance to public health.

12.4.2 Community development and mental health promotion

Throughout this part of the book, you have read much about the role of community development in multidisciplinary public health. Community development (CD) plays an equally important role in mental health and mental health promotion. Indeed, in accordance with Department of Health guidelines, it was envisaged that 500 community development workers (CDWs) would be employed by the end of 2006 to work specifically with people from black and minority ethnic communities who experience mental health problems (DoH, 2004b). A key role would be to facilitate community participation and ownership for people from black and minority ethnic groups. So, why should CD present opportunities for promoting mental health?

For some, a community development approach to mental health – one that draws on the expertise of local people and facilitates the statutory sector in sharing and devolving power – can help to bring about radical changes (Seebohm et al., 2005). Many of these proposed changes have been laid out in at least two Department of Health reports on mental health: *Community Development Workers for Black and Minority Ethnic Communities* (DoH, 2004b) and *Delivering Race Equality* (DoH, 2005). In each case, CD was seen as a key element in the government's action plan to tackle discrimination and inequality in mental health services. According to Hitch, cited by Seebohm et al., community development can be an empowering process, leading to:

- Development of new skills and competencies.
- Increased feelings of control in daily life.
- Informed choices from a range of options and access to information.
- Recognition of self-worth and self-esteem.
- Meaningful participation in decision making.
- Effecting change within institutions and social groups.
- Ability to self advocate.
- A process of growth and change.

(Hitch, quoted in Seebohm et al., 2005, p. 87)

So, how effective is CD in helping to tackle mental health problems and promoting positive mental health? Box 12.8 describes a project that has successfully utilised a CD approach.

Box 12.8 The Sharing Voices Initiative

The Sharing Voices Initiative (SVI), funded by Bradford City primary care trust, has adopted a community development approach to mental health and seeks to engage local people from black and minority ethnic communities to develop innovative ways of engagement and new forms of support that are based on their own agendas and priorities. SVI has a project co-ordinator, and two community development workers, and, more recently, has received additional funding for a development worker to focus on developing the capacity of local people with mental health issues from black and minority ethnic communities to access and engage in employment, training and meaningful daytime activities. The project plays a major role in opening up possibilities for addressing the needs of diverse communities and their mental health needs. It addresses the different ways in which mental health is understood cross-culturally, using a model of social psychiatry. The community development workers work with the city mental health services, and the local communities, facilitating dialogue. Through this dialogue, the communities articulate their own understanding of mental health and distress. There are two main elements to the community development workers' work. First, the process of communication between the communities and the service means that mental health professionals have a better understanding of the diverse explanatory frameworks relating to emotional distress within the communities. Second, the community development workers participate in training mental health professionals.

(Adapted from Seebohm et al., 2005)

Gina Alexander, a volunteer development officer with the Volunteer Centre in Clackmannanshire, supports the notion that CD is the most effective approach to promoting mental health. As a supporter of a CD approach, she has worked closely with members of BASA. As she points out:

> The community development approach is about people within the community who want to get involved in planning services that affect the community that they live in. It's not about the so-called professionals winging in and saying, you know, we're going to solve all your problems; we're going to put these things in place and we're going to make your community a great place to live. That's not what it's about. That's not what a community development approach is about. It's about working alongside people that live in the community, whether they're people from a mental health background and you're talking about mental health community or people with learning disabilities or whatever. It's about getting alongside people and working with them to enable them and facilitate them to bring the services that they need into their particular area, so that, you know that they kind of feel part of it all and they feel like they've got some ownership. It's not about solving all their problems. It's about helping them to solve their own problems and issues.

(Open University, 2007)

Having discussed how mental health promotion and public health are interlinked, the final section of this chapter draws together your understanding of the primary importance of communities in promoting public health at a local level. It asks you to reflect on what you have read about community engagement, consultation and participation throughout Part II of this book, and begins to consider the future for multidisciplinary public health at a community level.

12.5 The future for multidisciplinary public health at a community level: surveillance and scrutiny or collaboration and consultation?

In exploring the potential of communities to promote public health, earlier chapters have shown a move away from a model that is almost exclusively bound up with surveillance and scrutiny to one that embraces collaboration and consultation. However, critics have argued that many locally based government initiatives, such as Sure Start, Health Action Zones and Healthy Living Centres, rather than decreasing inequalities in health, have merely increased health surveillance in communities (McLeod and Bywaters, 2000). In terms of mental health, evidence shows that many employers are using surveillance techniques to compile evidence against employees who are absent from work with stress-related illnesses (Amicus, 2005). In some cases, this has led to employees being dismissed or suspended.

What, then, does the future hold for multidisciplinary public health at a community level? Is there a move towards a more democratic model, or do communities require a more intrusive input provided by experts?

According to the Chief Medical Officer of 2001, good surveillance is the cornerstone of a system to control infectious diseases in the population (DoH, 2001). The notion of health surveillance and the politics of health are discussed elsewhere (see Earle, 2007), but critics believe that, despite government strategies aimed at empowering individuals and communities, such an approach is a political ruse (McLeod and Bywaters, 2000). Rather than empowering communities and increasing community involvement and self-determination, such inclusive initiatives, they argue, are often simply a form of community management and manipulation which increase social and political control. For example, although schemes such as Sure Start, and the many projects included in Health Action Zones, have sought to increase the communication between professionals and individuals in an attempt to reduce social exclusion, for many such interventions have been guilty of simply increasing inequalities in power by extending the forms of professional surveillance (McLeod and Bywaters, 2000). Fitzpatrick, an inner city GP, writes: 'Under the banner of health inequalities New Labour has turned health promotion into a sophisticated instrument for the regulation, not only of individual behaviour, but that of whole communities' (Fitzpatrick, 2001, p. 95).

However, effective protection of public health often requires direction from the information provided by disease surveillance: for example, in the cases of AIDS and variant Creutzfeldt-Jakob disease, surveillance data led to action that protected health (Verity and Nicoll, 2002). Thus, health surveillance relies entirely on prompt and accurate reporting of the occurrence of disease by doctors and other health professionals. So, what is meant by public health surveillance?

According to Choi et al., public health surveillance can be defined as: 'the ongoing collection, analysis, and interpretation of health data essential to public health practice, closely integrated with timely dissemination of information for intervention' (Choi et al, 2002, p. 402). For Choi et al., such scrutiny is analogous to a twenty-four hour surveillance camera (data collection) under the watchful eyes of guards (data analysis and interpretation) who have telephone access (information dissemination) to the police and firefighters (intervention).

Of the ten competences required for the practice of public health, one explicitly refers to '[the] surveillance and assessment of the population's health and well-being' (Scottish Executive, 2004), thus illustrating the role of public health practitioners in regulating individual behaviour. It is claimed that NHS Direct, the nurse-led telephone helpline introduced in 1998 in England and Wales, has in the past used its data for community surveillance, the purpose of which is to detect a local or national increase in symptoms reported by callers (Baker et al., 2003).

Such attempts by health practitioners to enforce their values on local people are, it could be argued, borne of Foucault's notion of 'panopticism' (Foucault, 1977, p. 195). Here, the transformative potential of surveillance is revealed as an unsuspecting population simply internalises the all-pervasive message that to be 'healthy' is to be a good citizen. Such subjective self-regulation does not, however, occur by accident. Rather, it is fostered and facilitated by a complex web of conscious management and stealth-like manipulation, thereby ensuring that subjects are bound into the language of expertise (Coveney, 1998). As Wood notes: 'Panopticism, the social trajectory represented by the figure of the Panopticon, the drive to self-monitoring through the belief that one is under constant scrutiny, thus becomes both a driving force and a key symbol of the modernist project' (Wood, 2003, p. 234).

Thinking point: think about these claims in relation to recent government initiatives to promote public health.

Although it could be argued that present government policy readily acknowledges and recognises the effects of poverty, inequality and social exclusion on the health of disadvantaged individuals and communities, current public health and health promotion initiatives appear to bring more people under the 'gaze' of the government and professional. This is something which, as Coker (1999) points out, creates a tension between the protection of individual civil liberties and the protection of public health. Using tuberculosis as an example, Coker suggests that, because of the size and urgency of the threat and the fact that vulnerable populations are most affected by the disease, some control programmes often include coercion.

Moreover, more people are being regarded as 'at risk', either because of their lifestyles and behaviours, or because of their social characteristics: that is, they are seen to belong to a socially excluded group. It is individuals and communities like these that community health interventions, such as Healthy Living Centres and even welfare benefit take-up schemes, are seeking to put into contact with professionals and agents of the state, in a way that a greater part of their lives comes under the scrutiny and surveillance of health and other professionals. Thus, in reality, initiatives such as Healthy Living Centres may in fact institutionalise social divisions further, and any redistribution of power may be in appearance only. This is clearly illustrated by Bandesha and Litva (2005) who, during a qualitative study into perceptions of community participation and health gain in a community project for the South Asian population, found evidence that suggests that there are important differences in perceptions of participation and its associated health gain between professionals and the lay population.

On the other hand, collaboration and consultation continue to function as key drivers in tackling health inequalities. Since the 1990s, health policy has concentrated on the *treatment* of illhealth, whereas much recent government policy aims to shift this emphasis by focusing on *prevention*, in order to tackle health-related factors within our social, economic, physical and cultural environment. This fundamental shift in policy making and delivery is enjoying the support of strong local communities which have benefited from being able to make healthy choices. For example, Robinson and Elliot (2000), during a qualitative study into heart health promotion, found that (echoing Seebohm et al., 2005) by adopting a community development approach – one that facilitates a participatory and collaborative environment – people were more inclined to heed the advice of professionals. This was illustrated by a local resident:

> We have a community that is mobilized, we have a lot of organizations with volunteers, that are manned. We also have an awful lot of partner organizations that have been brought into heart health that were here 6 years ago, but they weren't talking about heart health. We have come some distance here ... there is an energy that is ready to be applied ...
>
> (Quoted in Robinson and Elliott, 2000, p. 227)

In what appears to be the future of multidisciplinary public health at a local level, as discussed earlier, governments have apparently willingly and enthusiastically taken up the baton of participation, consultation and collaboration. As you read in earlier chapters, a key feature of the English public health White Paper, *Choosing Health*, is the commitment to fostering and expanding a range of community health improvement services that includes specialist practitioners who are able to work with communities in order to strengthen community action for health and tackle inequalities (DoH, 2004a, Chapter 6, para 21).

Reinforcing their apparent commitment to communities, in 2006 Ruth Kelly, the English Government's Secretary of State for Communities and Local Government, introduced a White Paper, *Strong and Prosperous Communities* (DCLG, 2006), which, it was claimed, would give local people and local communities more influence and power to improve their lives, while delivering better public services, primarily through the devolution of power from central government to local authorities and local people.

Such a commitment is also to be found in the other three nations of the UK. For example, a major theme of a 2004 review of the public health function in Northern Ireland, to strengthen its ability to meet the challenges of the twenty-first century, is the continuing contribution of the community in developing effective approaches that target health needs (DHSSPS, 2004). Also in 2004, a review of the public health function in Scotland called for practitioners to be mindful of the importance of community involvement to the success of public health interventions (Scottish Executive, 2004). In Wales, since the mid-1990s there has been a shift towards proposals that place the citizen at the centre of the drive to promote health and tackle health inequalities. This involves communities in the collective development of policies for health and wellbeing, and makes the process of health policy making inclusive. Accountability to communities is thus integrated into the delivery of services (NAW, 2001, p. 7).

Conclusion

Part II of this book started out by asking you to consider the potential for promoting public health at a local level. In reaching the end, it is clear that engaging communities in this process is the key to its success. For example, like public health, mental health promotion strategies and polices are now geared towards the more proactive route of prevention, rather than treatment, of illhealth. To achieve this, interventions are focusing on the provision of local knowledge and the expertise of local people. Social contact and support, such as home visiting programmes, self-help groups and involvement in social and physical activity, have all provided evidence of reducing moderate levels of depression and anxiety and thus improving people's mental health. Communities therefore provide the cornerstone for such interactions and serve as a bridge between public health practitioners and professional and lay people.

References

Aberdeen City Alliance (2005) *Joint Health Improvement Plan: Aberdeen City 2005–08*, Aberdeen, The Aberdeen City Alliance.

Age Concern and Mental Health Foundation (2006) *Promoting Mental Health and Well-Being in Later Life*, London, Age Concern and Mental Health Foundation.

Amicus (2005) *Amicus Guide to Privacy at Work*, London, Amicus.

Anthony, P. and Crawford, P. (2000) 'Service user involvement in care planning: the mental health nurse's perspective', *Journal of Psychiatric and Mental Health Nursing*, vol. 7, no. 5, pp. 425–34.

Baker, M., Smith, G.E., Cooper, D., Verlander, N.Q., Chinemana, F., Cotterill, S., Hollyoak, V. and Griffiths, R. (2003) 'Early warning and NHS Direct: a role in community surveillance?', *Journal of Public Health Medicine*, vol. 25, no. 4, pp. 362–8.

Bandesha, G. and Litva, A. (2005) 'Perceptions of community participation and health gain in a community project for the South Asian population: a qualitative study', *Journal of Public Health*, vol. 27, no. 3, pp. 241–5.

Bosma, M.W.M. and Hosman, C.M.H. (1990) *Preventie op Waarde Geschat*, Nijmegen, Beta.

Choi, B.C.K., Pak, A.W.P. and Ottoson, J.M. (2002) 'Understanding the basic concepts of public health surveillance', *Journal of Epidemiological and Community Health*, vol. 56, no. 6, p. 402.

Coker, R. (1999) 'Public health, civil liberties, and tuberculosis', *British Medical Journal*, vol. 318, pp. 1434–5.

Coveney, J. (1998) 'The government and ethics of health promotion: the importance of Michel Foucault', *Health Education Research*, vol. 13, no. 3, pp. 459–68.

Cutcliffe, J.R. and Hannigan, B. (2001) 'Mass media, "monsters" and mental health clients: the need for increased lobbying', *Journal of Psychiatric and Mental Health Nursing*, vol. 8, no. 4, pp. 315–21.

Department for Communities and Local Government (DCLG) (2006) *Strong and Prosperous Communities*, London, The Stationery Office.

Department of Health (DoH) (1999) *National Service Framework for Mental Health: Modern Standards and Service Models*, London, The Stationery Office.

Department of Health (DoH) (2000) *The NHS Plan: A Plan for Investment, a Plan for Reform*, London, The Stationery Office.

Department of Health (DoH) (2001) *Making It Happen: A Guide to Delivering Mental Health Promotion*, London, The Stationery Office.

Department of Health (DoH) (2002) *Mental Health Policy Implementation Guide: Community Mental Health Teams*, London, The Stationery Office.

Department of Health (DoH) (2004a) *Choosing Health: Making Healthy Choices Easier*, London, The Stationery Office.

Department of Health (DoH) (2004b) *Community Development Workers for Black and Minority Ethnic Communities*, London, The Stationery Office.

Department of Health (DoH) (2005) *Delivering Race Equality: A Framework for Action*, London, The Stationery Office.

Department of Health (DoH) (2006a) *Choosing Health: Supporting the Physical Health Needs of People with Severe Mental Illness*, London, The Stationery Office.

Department of Health (DoH) (2006b) *Direct Payments for People with Mental Health Problems: A Guide to Action*, London, The Stationery Office.

Department of Health, Social Services and Public Safety in Northern Ireland (DHSSPS) (2004) *The Review of the Public Health Function in Northern Ireland*, Belfast, Department of Health, Social Services and Public Safety.

Earle, S. (2007) 'Promoting public health: exploring the issues' in Earle, S., Lloyd, C.E., Sidell, M. and Spurr, S. (eds) *Theory and Research in Promoting Public Health*, London, Sage/Milton Keynes, The Open University.

European Communities and STAKES (2004) *Action for Mental Health: Activities Co-funded from European Community Public Health Programmes 1997–2004*, Luxemburg, European Communities and STAKES.

Financial Mapping Returns (2003) Collated by Mental Health Strategies, unpublished.

Fitzpatrick, M. (2001) *The Tyranny of Health: Doctors and the Regulation of Lifestyle*, London, Routledge.

Flick, U. (1998) 'The social construction of individual and public health: contributions of social representations theory to a social science of health', *Social Science Information*, vol. 37, no. 4, pp. 639–62.

Foucault, M. (1977) *Discipline and Punish*, London, Allen Lane.

Friedli, L. (2000) 'Mental health promotion: rethinking the evidence base', *Mental Health Review*, vol. 5, no. 3, pp. 15–18.

Friedli, L. (2004) 'Editorial', *Journal of Mental Health Promotion*, vol. 3, no. 1, pp. 2–6.

Friedli, L. and McCulloch, A. (2005) 'Choosing mental health: a response to the government', *Journal of Public Mental Health*, vol. 4, no. 1, pp. 35–44.

Health Development Agency (HDA) (2004) *National Healthy Schools Programme: A Briefing for Directors of Public Health*, London, Health Development Agency.

Joseph Rowntree Foundation (2002) *Mental Health Advocacy for Black and Minority Ethnic Users and Carers* [online], http://www.jrf.org.uk/ (Accessed 17 June 2006).

Kamal, Z. and Loewenthal, K.M. (2002) 'Suicide beliefs and behaviour among young Muslims and Hindus in the UK', *Mental Health, Religion and Culture*, vol. 5, no. 2, pp. 11–118.

Layard, R. (2006) Mental Health: Britain's Biggest Social Problem? [online], http://ceplse.ac.uk/layard/ (Accessed 12 May 2006).

Manning, C. and White, P.D. (1995) 'Attitudes of employers to the mentally ill', *Psychiatric Bulletin*, vol. 19, pp. 541–3.

McCulloch, G.F. and Boxer, J. (1997) *Mental Health Promotion: Policy, Practice and Partnerships*, London, Baillière Tindall.

McLeod, E. and Bywaters, P. (2000) *Social Work, Health and Equality*, London, Routledge.

Mental Health Foundation (2005) *Choosing Mental Health: A Policy Agenda for Mental Health and Public Health*, London, Mental Health Foundation.

Mental Health Foundation (2006) *Feeding Minds: The Impact of Food on Mental Health*, London, Mental Health Foundation.

National Assembly for Wales (NAW) (2001) *Improving Health in Wales: A Plan for the NHS with its Partners*, Cardiff, National Assembly for Wales.

National Electronic Library for Health (NeLH) in collaboration with mentality (2004) *Models of Mental Health Promotion* [online], http://www.dev.nelh.nhs.uk/nsf/ mentalhealth/whatworks/intro (Accessed 7 November 2006).

National Occupational Standards (2005) [online], http://www.skillsforhealth.org.uk/ frameworks.php (Accessed 9 July 2006).

Newbiggin, K. and Lowe, J. (2005) *Direct Payments and Mental Health: New Directions*, York, Joseph Rowntree Foundation.

NHS Health Scotland (2004) *Mental Health Improvement: Evidence and Practice*, Edinburgh, Health Scotland.

Office of the Deputy Prime Minister (ODPM) (2004a) *Action on Mental Health: A Guide to Promoting Social Inclusion*, London, Office of the Deputy Prime Minister.

Office of the Deputy Prime Minister (ODPM) (2004b) *Mental Health and Social Exclusion*, London, Office of the Deputy Prime Minister.

Open University (2007) K311 *Promoting Public Health: Skills, Perspectives and Practice*, DVD, Milton Keynes, The Open University.

Read, J. and Wallcraft, J. (1995) *Guidelines in Equal Opportunities and Mental Health*, London, MIND Publications.

Rethink (2006) *Black and Minority Ethnic (BME) Communities and Severe Mental Illness: Factsheet* [online], http://www.mentalhealthshop.org/products/rethink_publications/ black_minority.html (Accessed 21 February 2007).

Robinson, K.L. and Elliot, S.J. (2000) 'The practice of community development approaches in heart health promotion', *Health Education Research*, vol. 15, no. 2, pp. 219–31.

Rogers, A. and Pilgrim, D. (2003) *Mental Health and Inequality*, Basingstoke, Palgrave Macmillan.

Royal College of Psychiatrists (2003) *Stigmatisation of People with Mental Illness* [online], http://www.rcpsych.ac.uk/PDF/report_9803.pdf (Accessed 17 June 2006).

Sainsbury Centre for Mental Health and Mentality (2004) *Briefing on Standard One of the National Service Framework for Mental Health: Mental Health Promotion*, London, Sainsbury Centre for Mental Health.

Scottish Executive (2004) *Health in Scotland 2004*, Edinburgh, Scottish Executive.

Scottish Public Mental Health Alliance (2002) *With Health in Mind: Improving Mental Health and Wellbeing in Scotland*, Edinburgh, Scottish Development Centre for Mental Health.

Secker, J. (2005) 'Mental health promotion theory: review and application', *Journal of Public Mental Health*, vol. 4, no. 1, pp. 10–13.

Seebohm, P., Henderson, P., Munn-Giddings, C., Thomas, P. and Yasmeen, S. (2005) *Together We Will Change: Community Development, Mental Health and Diversity*, London, Sainsbury Centre for Mental Health.

Taylor Nielson Sofres (2003) *Attitudes to Mental Illness 2003: Report*, London, Department of Health/Office for National Statistics.

Thornicroft, G. (2006) *Newspaper Portrayals of Mental Illness* [online], http://www.mentalhealthcare.org.uk/content/?id=194 (Accessed 21 February 2007).

Verity, C. and Nicoll, A. (2002) 'Consent, confidentiality and the threat to public health surveillance', *British Medical Journal*, vol. 324, pp. 1210–30.

Walsall Borough Strategic Partnership (2005) *Walsall Local Compact: Working Together, Better Together* [online], http://www.wbsp.org.uk/acompact20052.pdf (Accessed 23 January 2007).

Wood, D. (2003) Editorial, 'Foucault and panopticism revisited', *Surveillance and Society*, vol. 1, no. 3, pp. 234–9.

Acknowledgements

Text

Page 239: Part of a poem from Gatwick House, supported by Hull DOC.

Tables

Figure 1.4: The World Health Report, (2006), 'Working Lifespan Strategies', Overview, World Health Organisation; Figure 6.1: McKay S., (2004), 'Poverty or Preference: What do "Consensual Deprivation Indicators" Really Mean?', Institute for Fiscal Studies 2004; Figure 6.2: 'Households Below Average Income' published by the DWP and HM Treasury; Figure 6.3: 'Households Below Average Income' published by the DWP and HM Treasury; Figure 9.3: Krieger, J. and Ciske, S. (2000), 'The community as a full partner in public health initiatives', Washington Public Health, Fall 2000, University of Washington; Figure 12.4: The Scottish Public Health Alliance (2002), 'With Health in Mind: Improving Mental Health and Wellbeing in Scotland'. Copyright © 2002 Scottish Development Centre for Mental Health, reproduced with permission.

Figures

Figure 1.1: Dean H., (2006), 'Principal International Governmental Organisations', Social Policy, Polity Press; Figure 2.5: Tones B.K., (1990), 'The Power to Choose Health Education and the New Public Health', Health Education Unit, Leeds Metropolitan University; Figure 2.6: Macdonald G.and Bunton R., (1993), 'Health Promotion: Disciplines and Diversity', Routledge; Figure 3.3: Townsend J., Roderick P., Cooper J., (1994), 'Cigarette Smoking by Socioeconomic Group, Sex and Age: Effects of Price Income and Health Publicity'; Figure 3.4: © STARSTOCK/Photoshot; Figure 3.4: © Schwartz Andy/Corbis Sygma – © Corbis Sygma – © Ronald Siemoneit/Corbis Sygma; Figure 3.6: © Adbusters/Advertising Archives; Figure 3.6: © Ad Busters/Advertising Archives; Figure 3.7: Edwards R., (2004), 'The Problem of Tobacco Smoking', British Medical Journal; Figure 3.8: MacKay J., and Eriksen M., (2002) 'Past and Future', The Tobacco Atlas, Geneva World Health Organisation; Figure 3.9: Copyright © Titosh. Reproduced by permission; Figure 3.10: Orchid: Copyright © blickwinkel/Alamy – Ashtray: Copyright © plainpicture GmbH & Co; Figure 5.1: 'An Innovative Public–Private Partnership', The GAVI Alliance; Figure 5.3: Bauer G., Davies J.K., and Pelikan J., (2006), 'Health Promotion International', The EUHPID Consortium; Figure 6.4: Source: World Development Indicators World Bank 2000; Figure 6.5: UNICEF, 'Child Poverty in Rich Countries

2005', Innocent Report Card No.6, UNICEF Innocent Research Centre Florence, © The United Nations Childrens Fund 2005; Figure 6.6: 'Tackling Health Inequalities: Status Report on the Programme for Action', Crown copyright material is reproduced under Class Licence Number C01W0000065 with the permission of the Controller of HMSO and the Queen's Printer for Scotland; Figure 6.7: UNICEF, 'Child Poverty in Rich Countries 2005', Innocent Report Card No.6, UNICEF Innocent Research Centre Florence, © The United Nations Childrens Fund 2005; Figure 6.8: Shaw M., Davey Smith G., Dorling D., (2005), 'Health Inequalities and New Labour: How the Promises Compare with Real Progress', British Medical Journal; Figure 7.2: Emmel N., and Conn C., (2004), 'Identifying the Goal and Objectives of Community Involvement, Towards Community Involvement: Strategies for Health and Social Care Providers', Nuffield Institute for Heal University of Leeds; Figure 9.1: WHO (2002), 'Community participation in local health and sustainable development'. Copyright © 2002. World Health Organization; Fig 9.2: WHO (2002), 'Community participation in local health and sustainable development'. Copyright © 2002. World Health Organization.

Illustrations

Page 14: Copyright © Studio Bendib; Page 50: David Hoffman Photo Library/Alamy Page 179: © Stephen Pond/News Team International/epa/ Corbis; Page 229: The Community Health Shop; Pages 36-38, 40, 51, 358 and 361: Taken from OU specially shot material on K311 DVD.

Index